护理学专业双语教材

供 护 理 学 类 专 业 用

中 医 护 理 学

Nursing Science of Traditional Chinese Medicine

主　　审　刘建平　Je Kan Alder-Collins

主　　编　郝玉芳　马良宵

副 主 编　王　琦　李晓丽　马雪玲

编译委员会（以姓氏笔画为序）

　　　　　马良宵（北京中医药大学）

　　　　　马雪玲（北京中医药大学）

　　　　　王　琦（北京中医药大学）

　　　　　乔　雪（北京中医药大学）

　　　　　刘建平（北京中医药大学）

　　　　　苏春香（北京中医药大学）

　　　　　李晓莉（北京中医药大学）

　　　　　杨晓玮（北京中医药大学）

　　　　　陈　岩（北京中医药大学）

　　　　　周　芬（北京中医药大学）

　　　　　郝玉芳（北京中医药大学）

Je Kan Alder-Collins（Fukuoka Prefectural University，Japan）

人民卫生出版社

图书在版编目（CIP）数据

中医护理学：双语版 / 郝玉芳，马良宵主编. —北京：人民
卫生出版社，2014
ISBN 978-7-117-20088-2

Ⅰ.①中… Ⅱ.①郝…②马… Ⅲ.①中医学－护理学－
双语教学－医学院校－教材 Ⅳ.①R248

中国版本图书馆 CIP 数据核字（2014）第 305607 号

| 人卫社官网 | www.pmph.com | 出版物查询，在线购书 |
| 人卫医学网 | www.ipmph.com | 医学考试辅导，医学数据库服务，医学教育资源，大众健康资讯 |

中医护理学

主　　编：郝玉芳　马良宵
出版发行：人民卫生出版社（中继线 010-59780011）
地　　址：北京市朝阳区潘家园南里 19 号
邮　　编：100021
E - mail：pmph @ pmph.com
购书热线：010-59787592　010-59787584　010-65264830
印　　刷：北京人卫印刷厂
经　　销：新华书店
开　　本：787×1092　1/16　印张：22　插页：4
字　　数：549 千字
版　　次：2015 年 2 月第 1 版　2015 年 2 月第 1 版第 1 次印刷
标准书号：ISBN 978-7-117-20088-2/R·20089
定　　价：55.00 元
打击盗版举报电话：010-59787491　E-mail：WQ @ pmph.com
（凡属印装质量问题请与本社市场营销中心联系退换）

Nursing Science of Traditional Chinese Medicine

Reviewer   Liu Jianping   Je Kan Alder-Collins
Complier-in-chief   Hao Yufang   Ma Liangxiao
Vice Complier-in-chief   Wang Qi   Li Xiaoli   Ma Xueling

Compiling and Translating Committee

Ma Liangxiao （School of Acupuncture-Moxibustion and Tuina，Beijing University of Chinese Medicine）

Ma Xueling （School of Nursing，Beijing University of Chinese Medicine）

Wang Qi （School of Nursing，Beijing University of Chinese Medicine）

Qiao Xue （School of Nursing，Beijing University of Chinese Medicine）

Liu Jianping （Institution of Evidence-based Medicine，Beijing University of Chinese Medicine）

Su Chunxiang （School of Nursing，Beijing University of Chinese Medicine）

Li Xiaoli （Humanities school，Beijing University of Chinese Medicine）

Yang Xiaowei （School of Nursing，Beijing University of Chinese Medicine）

Chen Yan （School of Nursing，Beijing University of Chinese Medicine）

Zhou Fen （School of Nursing，Beijing University of Chinese Medicine）

HaoYufang （School of Nursing，Beijing University of Chinese Medicine）

Je Kan Alder-Collins （Fukuoka Prefectural University，Japan）

People's Medical Publishing House

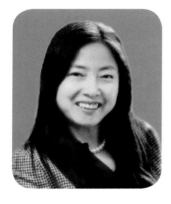

郝玉芳，护理学博士，教授，博士生导师，现任北京中医药大学护理学院院长。先后毕业于北京医科大学、北京中医药大学和上海第二军医大。分别在美国罗彻斯特大学、北京大学做访问学者 1 年。国家中医药管理局中医护理重点学科和北京市护理学一级学科重点学科带头人。教育部护理教学指导委员会委员；全国中医药高等医学教育学会护理教育研究会理事长；国家留学基金管理委员会评审专家；全国高等医学教育学会护理教育分会常务理事；CMIA 护理信息学专业委员会常务理事；中国老年学学会老年保健康复专业委员会常务委员；中国心理学会护理专业委员会委员；北京中医医院急诊及 ICU 质量评价与控制中心专家委员会委员；北京市社区服务评审专家；国内多本杂志和国外一本 SCI 杂志审稿人；国家中医药管理局中医师资格认证中心命审题专家；人民卫生出版社和中国中医药出版社教材评审专家。北京市高等学校优秀青年骨干教师；主编的教材获 2011 年北京市精品教材；获校级教学成果一、二等奖；国家中医药管理局课题三等奖。主持和参与各级课题 50 余项。公开发表学术论文 90 余篇。参加了全国 13 本统编教材的编写，其中主编 4 本，副主编 4 本。曾在加拿大 McGill、美国 Rochester、日本福冈、日本富山和韩国庆熙大学护理学院做讲座。

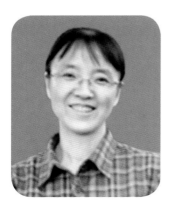

马良宵，女，北京中医药大学针灸推拿学院副教授，副主任医师，医学博士，针灸推拿专业硕士研究生导师。中国针灸学会腧穴分会副秘书长，北京针灸学会针灸技术专业委员会常务秘书，美国医学针灸学会官方杂志 Medical Acupuncture 编委。以第一作者发表学术论文 20 余篇，其中 SCI 收录 2 篇。主持校级课题 4 项，参加国家级课题 8 项，省部级课题 5 项（其中国际合作课题 4 项）。获北京市及中华中医药学会科学技术奖三等奖各 1 项、校级科学技术奖 2 项。参编教材 5 部（3 部为中英对照教材、1 部为英文教材），其中主译 1 部，副主译 1 部，编委 3 部。参编著作 8 部（其中 2 部为国外出版发行的英文版著作），副主编 2 部，编委 2 部，编写人员 4 部。

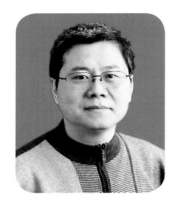

刘建平，男，医学博士，教育部长江学者奖励计划特聘教授，博士生导师。现任北京中医药大学循证医学中心主任；挪威特洛姆瑟大学国家补充与替代医学研究中心兼职教授，澳大利亚皇家墨尔本理工大学客座教授；世界卫生组织西太区传统医学顾问，国际 Cochrane 协作网肝胆疾病组编辑，美国马里兰大学医学院整合医学中心专家委员会顾问，澳大利亚皇家墨尔本理工大学卫生科学院博士学位论文评审专家，国际补充替代医学研究会（ISCAMR）董事会成员，国际中医药学会（ISCM）会员；中国中西医结合学会循证医学专业委员会副主任委员；世界中医学会联合会中医临床疗效评价专业委员会副会长；教育部科学技术委员会委员、教育部科学技术奖励评审委员、教育部高等学校公共卫生与全科医学教学指导委员会预防医学专业教学指导分委员会委员、国家留学基金评审专家、教育部长江学者通讯评审专家、国家人力资源和社会保障部国家基本医疗保险审评专家。主持国家级及国际合作项目／课题 20 余项。担任国内外 30 余种期刊编委和审稿人。主编出版专著 6 部，国内外发表论文 340 余篇，发表 SCI 论文 40 余篇。

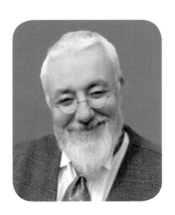

Je Kan Adler-Collins，男，英国人，教育学博士，英国注册护士，现任日本 Fukuoka Prefectural University 副教授，博士生导师。英国国际护理评述（*International Nursing Review*）杂志的副主编。生活理论行动研究专家和国际合作研究专家。多个国际合作项目的研究带头人或合作者，主要合作国家有中国、日本、英国、泰国和韩国。发表了近 20 篇学术论文或著作，担任 13 种杂志的评审专家。

前　言

中医学和护理学均是医学科学领域中重要的分支学科，在维护人类健康的医疗实践中起到了重要作用。中医学以其独特的理论体系和显著的临床效果，在国际上越来越受到人们的重视。而有中医特色的护理学科也随之受到关注。随着医学模式的转变，护理学有了更深刻的内涵和更广阔的外延。护理从"以疾病为中心"向"以人的健康为中心"转变，从附属于医疗的技术性职业转变为独立的为人类健康服务的专业。护理服务对象是整体的人，应关注人生理、心理和社会多方面的需要。护理服务于人类生命的全过程，即从出生到死亡，包括疾病的护理、康复锻炼、健康指导以及临终关怀等。护理工作的范围从个体扩展至家庭、社区，促进全民健康是护理的最终目标。

护理理念和护理服务范畴的转变，对护理专业人员提出了更大的挑战。而有中医特色的护理学凭借其独特的理论和实用的护理技术，在护理领域中将发挥更大的作用，也更具优势。中医护理学科的中医特色主要体现在慢性病管理中融入中医养生康复理念与方法和发挥中医护理技术的"简、便、廉、验、效"的优势。我国目前慢性病如高血压、糖尿病、冠心病、中风等患病率高。慢性病大多可防可控，中医的整体观和治未病的理论与方法，尤其是中医养生康复在慢病管理中发挥着重要作用，如中医健身气功、推拿按摩、中医食疗等养生方法可提高慢性病患病人群及慢性病高危人群的生活质量，改善病情。护理学科中将中医养生康复方法融入慢性病管理中，不但丰富了护理工作方法，充实了护理健康教育内容，也有力地降低了医疗成本，丰富了中医护理的内涵。中医护理的另一特色在于丰富的治疗手段和通俗易懂、简便易行的中医护理操作技术。近几年，随着国家中医药振兴计划的实施，中医护理知识和技术在预防保健、术后康复和慢性疾病护理中发挥出的优势也愈来愈显著，中医护理的特色不仅与护理预防疾病、促进健康的目标高度一致，而且更贴近生活，也更易被人们接受，人民群众对中医药卫生保健服务的需求也越来越高。

近几年，有中医特色的护理专业人才，在国内外的需求呈上升趋势。许多国外护理同仁希望学习中医护理相关理论和技术。此外，在全球护理人员短缺的现状下，国内众多护理院校纷纷开设护理涉外专业方向，而护理人才的国际化，对传统医学的需求也将越来越大。为了适应国内外对中医护理人才和中医护理国际交流与合作的需要，加快中医护理国际化进程，培养出具有对外交流能力的有中国特色的高水平护理人才。在出版社的支持和指导下，我们组织专家编写《中医护理学》双语教材。较上一版《中医护理学基础》双语教材，本教材更注重中医文化的传承，增加了中医哲学思想基础、中医文化的演变、中国传统饮食文化等内容，各章节突出实用性和可操作性，更利于国际交流。

本教材编写组成员包括护理学、中医学、针灸推拿学、循证医学、医学英语专家以及国外护理专家，各章内容经过多位专家多次审定，保证了其科学性、新颖性、系统性和实用性。

　　中医护理学包括中医护理学的基本理论、基本知识和基本技能。具体内容涵盖中医与中国传统文化、中医护理学发展简史、中医基础理论概述、经络腧穴概述、中医护理的基本特点和原则、一般护理、中医用药护理及传统的护理技术操作、中医自我调护、常见病证的中医调护。

　　本教材适用于中医及西医护理院校护理研究生、本科生作为必修或选修课程，尤其适用于涉外方向的护理本科生作为必修课程；也适用于各类对中国传统医学感兴趣的留学生；也可作为各种短期培训班教材。

　　编写中医护理双语教材，是一项艰巨的工作，编写组付出了很大的努力。尽管如此，由于经验不足和编者水平有限，仍会存在一定问题，希望大家提出宝贵意见，我们会进一步修订改进。

郝玉芳　马良宵
2014 年 12 月

Preface

Traditional Chinese medicine (TCM) and nursing, are two important disciplines within the framework of medical science and have played a key role in the medical practice of maintaining human health. TCM has a unique theoretical system and is clinically effective. Over the past decades TCM and nursing science which has the characteristics of TCM, have been attracting ever increasing attention globally. With the change of medical modes, nursing science is now of much deeper connotation and wider extension. Nursing is transcending from disease-based professional model attached to medical treatment to human health-based model and an independent specialty of healthcare. Nursing philosophy refers to man as a whole integrity, including his physiology, psychology and social needs. Nursing contents refer to the complete process of human life from birth to death, including nursing care of diseases, exercises for rehabilitation, health guidance and palliative care. Nursing practices evolve to embrace the needs of individuals, to families and communities, promoting health for all.

The constant change and evolution of nursing concepts and practices bring with them great challenges for nursing staff. Nursing science with its characteristics of TCM is well positioned toy contribute more with its unique theories and practical manipulations. The integration of the philosophy and methodology of the preservation of health and natural convalescence within chronic disease management along with its skills of symptom differentiation and diagnosis featured in TCM are its major strengths as a nursing discipline. Additionally, TCM nursing skills have traits of being "simple, convenient, cheap, efficacious and effective", combined with TCM concepts of "holism" and "treating disease before it arises" play an important role in chronic disease management which is an advantage of TCM nursing. At present, the morbidity of chronic diseases such as hypertension, diabetes, coronary heart disease and stroke are becoming prevalent in China. However, most of these chronic diseases are preventable and controllable. Incorporating the knowledge of TCM health preservation and natural convalescence is very helpful for specific chronic disease management. In this way, the condition and quality of life for citizens at high risk can be identified, improved by early interventions and planning thus contributing to the reduction in long term medical costs. TCM can enrich health education skills and practice of the content of nursing profession. The other feature of TCM nursing discipline is its use of plain and simple skills. In the last few years, with the implementation of the national TCM stimulus plan, all of the TCM hospitals in China have been strongly developing TCM nursing skills. The result is that the advantage of TCM nursing has been fully realized in preventive care, postoperative rehabilitation and chronic disease nursing. In this process, not only has client satisfaction increased, the nurse's sense of achievement has also been boosted.

The demands for nursing professionals of TCM both home and abroad have been in the ascendant over the recent years. Nursing and other health care professional abroad also expect to know about the theories and skills of Chinese nursing. In the face of international shortage of nursing resources, Chinese domestic schools of nursing have worked to offer foreign oriented nursing specialty in TCM nursing with the belief that internationalization of nursing professionals will lead to further development of traditional medicine. In direct response to needs of the market for nursing professionals and demands of international exchange and cooperation of Chinese nursing, acceleration of the processes of internationalization of Chinese nursing needs to occur with the nurturing of high-level TCM nursing professionals in promoting international communication, this Chinese-English bilingual textbook of *Nursing Science of Traditional Chinese Medicine* has been compiled under the support and guidance of the People's Medical Publishing House. This textbook pays more attention to TCM culture inheritance and adds several related chapters, such as TCM and the ancient Chinese philosophy, the evolution of TCM culture, Chinese tradition diet culture, etc. The contents of each chapter high light its practicality and operability, and are more suitable for international communication.

The compiling and translating committee of this textbook includes experts from fields of nursing, Chinese medicine, acupuncture and tuina, evidence-based medicine, medical English and nurse specialists abroad. The contents of each chapter are examined and revised repeatedly by numerous experts so as to make sure the scientific, original, systematic and practical nature of this textbook.

This textbook includes the basic theories and knowledge and techniques of Chinese nursing. The contents include TCM and traditional Chinese culture, developing history of Chinese nursing, introduction of fundamental theories of TCM, introduction of channels and acupoints, basic characteristics and principles of TCM nursing, general nursing, nursing care with TCM, traditional nursing skills, self-regulation nursing care, and nursing care of common diseases.

The textbook is designed for nursing graduate or undergraduate students in colleges and universities of both Western and Chinese medicine, especially for students of foreign oriented nursing major. It is suitable for overseas students who are interested in TCM nursing, and also recommended to students of various kinds of short-term training programs.

It is very hard work to compile a Chinese-English bilingual textbook of Chinese nursing for all editors, translators and publishers. We apologize if there are any errors in the book due to our limitation of compiling experiences and knowledge. Any suggestions are welcome for further edition.

Hao Yufang   Ma Liangxiao

Dec. 2014

目 录

总 论

各　论

Content

总　论

第一章
中医与中医护理学概述

第一节　中医与中国传统文化

中医学博大精深，广涉旁通，明代张介宾《类经·序》言其"上极天文，下穷地纪，中悉人事，大而阴阳变化，小而草木昆虫、音律象数之肇端，脏腑经络之曲折"，无所不包容涵盖，可谓是中国传统文化的一个缩影。中医学在中国传统文化的基础上形成了独特的理论体系，中医学理论中所包含着的中国传统文化元素，直接反映着中医学的主导思维方式，中医对世界的贡献不仅是一种独特的医疗体系，而且是中国传统文化的一个重要组成部分。

中国传统文化涵盖了中国古代哲学思想、医药理论、天文地理、神话传说、历史事件、音乐艺术、风俗民情等诸多方面。而以阴阳五行为代表的哲学思想，以道家、道教理论为基础的养生学，以易学为旗帜的天文学和地理学，以儒学思想为指导的医学伦理学，以及各种传统学术相互融合而构成的其他理论，则构成了中医学坚实的理论基础和文化背景。只有了解并熟悉中国传统文化，才能领会中医学的历史沿革、哲学基础、思维模式、价值观念等文化内涵，在此基础上才能熟练地运用中医药技术。

一、中医文化源流及发展简史

在中华五千年文明史上，中医药这颗璀璨明珠，对中华民族的医疗保健、繁衍生息有着不可磨灭的历史功勋。关于医学的起源，至今没有定论，大致有本能说、劳动说、大脑结构进化说、巫术说、圣人说等。而关于中医的起源，"医源于圣人说"和"医源于巫说"是目前学术界的基本认识。

（一）医源于圣人说

从医药的起源来说，古人把它推向了遥远的上古时代的神话。相传伏羲、神农、黄帝是中华民族文化、医药的开创者。

1. 伏羲——中华民族的人文始祖　《帝王世纪》记载："伏羲划卦，所以六气、六腑、五脏、五行、阴阳、四时、水火升降得以有象，百病之理得以有类，乃尝百药，制九针，以拯夭枉"。伏羲创造了中华民族的古老文化，他根据天地间阴阳变化之理，创制八卦，即以八种形状简明却寓意深刻的符号来概括、描述天地之间的事物。相传他也开创了中华医药，为民族的繁衍生息做出了重要贡献，伏羲被称为是中华民族人文始祖。

----- 知识链接 1-1 ---

伏羲八卦图

相传伏羲人首蛇身，伏羲氏对事物有着敏锐的观察力，对土地有着深厚的感情。同时他又拥有着超人的智能,伏羲氏将他观察到的一切,用一种数学符号描述了下来这就是八卦。上古时期,孟津东部有一条图河与黄河相接,龙马负图出于此河,伏羲氏依龙马之图画出了乾、兑、离、震、巽、坎、艮、坤为内容的卦图,后人称为"伏羲八卦图"(图1-1)。

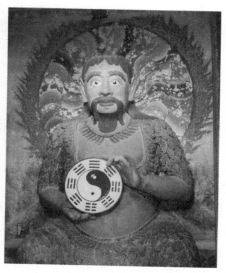

图1-1　伏羲八卦
Fig. 1-1　Fu Xi's eight diagrams

伏羲氏仰观象于天,俯察法于地,用阴阳八卦来解释天地万物的演化规律和人伦秩序。伏羲氏取火种、正婚姻、教渔猎,结束了人们茹毛饮血的历史。

2. 神农——农耕、礼乐、医学的创立者　神农氏是传说中的上古帝王,因为神农氏的部落居住在南方,"五行说"认为南方主火德,所以被称为炎帝。炎帝神农代表着人类认识的扩大与发展,人类开始更广泛地利用自然。神农氏是继伏羲、女娲之后的天下共主,传说他发明了农耕、礼乐,而且是医学的创立者,《通外纪》中记载:"民有疾病,未知药石,炎帝始味草木之滋,尝一日遇七十毒,神而化之,遂作方书,以疗民疾,而医道立矣"。

------ 知识链接 1-2 ------

神农尝百草

有关神农氏的故事,流传最广的就是神农尝百草,神话传说中神农氏是牛头人身,民间还传说神农氏生来就长了一副透明的"水晶肚",五脏六腑清晰可见,吃下什么东西,从外面都能看得清清楚楚。

远古时期,人们还不懂农耕,以采食野生瓜果,生吃动物蚌蛤为生,经常有人误食有毒的食物而中毒、死亡。炎帝神农氏为"宣药疗疾",救天伤人命,使百姓益寿延年,他跋山涉水,行遍三湘大地,尝遍百草,了解百草之平毒寒温之药性,为民找寻治病解毒良药,"神农尝百草,一日遇七十毒",他几乎嚼尝过所有植物(图1-2)。神农在尝百草的过程中,识别了百草,发现了具有攻毒祛病、养生保健作用的中药。由此令民有所就,不复为疾病,故先民封他为"药神"。

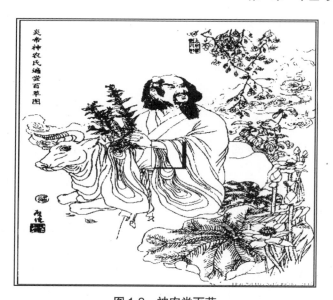

图 1-2　神农尝百草
Fig. 1-2　Shen Nong tasted hundreds of herbs

3. 黄帝——创医药之始祖　黄帝为上古传说中远古时代华夏民族的共主，五帝之首，相传其姓公孙，出生于轩辕之丘，故名号轩辕氏。中国史书记载，他在炎帝之后，统一了中国各部落。

相传黄帝为中华民族文化的创始者，举凡兵器、舟车、算术、音律、文字、养蚕、弓箭、衣服、医药等，皆创于黄帝时代。现有中医学经典著作《黄帝内经》、《黄帝八十一难经》等，均系托名而作。相传黄帝曾与其臣岐伯、伯高、少俞等谈论医道（图 1-3），故后世习称中医为"岐黄之术"。中医历来尊黄帝为创医药之始祖。"神农所创之医，为医之经验；黄帝所创之医，为医之原理"，表明医学开始由经验医学阶段走向系统的理性医学阶段。

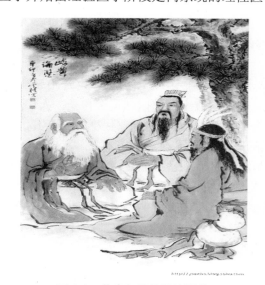

图 1-3　黄帝与岐伯谈论医道
Fig. 1-3　Huang Di and Qi Bo's talk on medicine

（二）医源于巫说

1. 巫文化　巫文化是人类最早的文化形态之一，是人类文化史上极漫长而重要的阶段。有学者认为巫是制度化之母、宗教之母、科学之母，是远古时代最重要、最全能的百科全书式的人物。

由于远古时代人类认识能力低下，对大自然的一切感到神秘莫测，尤其对疾病、死亡等现象无法理解，在怀有莫大的恐惧的同时又会加以揣测和臆想，认为是超自然的力量在左右着世界万物，由此出现了鬼神的概念。随着鬼神概念的出现，人类历史上最早的文化形态之一——"巫史文化"也就开始了。

巫术反映了人类渴望征服自然的愿望，人类对于不可知的事物的认识是一个由禁忌到崇拜，再到驱赶禁制的循序渐进的过程。虽然这一过程中的几个阶段可能交叉重叠，但基本上是符合人类认识、思维的发展规律，同时是与当时的生产力、科学技术发展水平相适应的。

2. 祝由术与中医学　巫术在中医几千年的发展历史过程中一直是存在的，其中最典型的便是祝由术。自马王堆出土的汉代帛书，到宋元明时期的大量医学著作，祝由作为一科与各种医疗技术并列。

对祝由术的内容进行仔细分析，可以发现，祝由术中确实存在不少具有科学价值的内涵，实际上祝由可以认为是心理疗法（暗示）、气功疗法、传统体育疗法的先驱。运用现代的理论解释祝由，可以说这种方法是利用患者的信仰和崇拜对象或恐惧对象，用语言和行为诱导患者进入特定的心理状态（或催眠状态），以达到治疗目的的一种医术。心理疗法主要取决于患者的主观意识状态，祝由术依赖患者信赖、畏惧鬼神的心理定势，通过暗示、慰藉等原理改善患者的精神状态，从而间接地调整患者的机体功能。调整呼吸，按摩脏腑，调和气血是气功疗法的重要组成部分，在祝由术中可以找到气功呼吸术式的源头。气功最古老的呼吸术式之一"六字诀"（吹、呼、呵、嘘、唏、呬）就是祝由术的内容。而中国最具特色的传统体育疗法导引法、武术等均继承了祝由术中的形体动作。马王堆出土的帛书祝由方中多次提及的"禹步"相传是上古酋长大禹所走的步子，这是一种按程式运动的步伐，与现代华尔兹舞步非常接近。在祝由师带领下，患者走动舞蹈，实际上是进行了体育锻炼，能够达到疏经通络的效果，从而减轻或缓解病痛，可见祝由疗法亦具有体育疗法的成分。

随着时代的发展，学术的不断进步，医学与巫术也开始逐渐分离。尤其到了春秋战国时期，学术界百家争鸣，宗教的地位不再像以前那么神圣。人们逐渐开始认识到，医学比巫术更科学、更实用，也更有根据，于是医学终于取代巫术，成为医疗卫生的主导。

（三）中医理论体系的形成与发展

虽然古人将医药的起源推向了遥远的神话，然而医药实则来自上古先民的实践。中医学的理论体系源于实践，是建立在长期临床实践基础上的一门科学。

1. 中医理论体系发展简史　早在远古时代，我们的祖先在艰难的生存环境中，就已经掌握了一些能够缓解病痛的方法：人们发现食用某些食物后能够减轻和消除某种病痛，用烧热的沙石熨烫或用尖锐的石器戳刺身体某些部位也能够缓解病痛，这些经验逐渐被积累下来，这就是中医的萌芽。

中医理论是建立在对实践经验总结的基础上，同时又受到它所处时代文化的影响，并随着实践经验的不断积累而逐渐发展起来。当人类进入文明社会之后，尤其是到了春秋战国时期，我国的医药就开始走向理论化，逐步完善，由经验医学向系统的理性医学转化。

春秋战国时期《黄帝内经》的问世，标志着中医学理论体系的初步形成。经过两汉四百年的实践，医圣张仲景所著《伤寒杂病论》确立了辨证论治的基本原则，《神农本草经》奠定了中药学的基础。经过两晋到五代七百年的医疗实践，中医理论体系不断深化发展，西晋医家皇甫谧撰成中国现存最早的一部针灸专书《针灸甲乙经》，巢元方等人集体编写的《诸病源候论》则是中国现存最早的病因证候学专著，唐代医家孙思邈集毕生之精力，著成《备急千金要方》、《千金翼方》，对临床各科、针灸、食疗、预防、养生等均有论述。宋代王惟一设计铸造的针灸铜人则是中国医学教育事业的创举。至金元时代，出现了以刘完素、张从正、李东垣、朱震亨"金元四大家"为代表的学术争鸣。后经明清五百年的实践，明代医药学家李时珍历时27年之久著成《本草纲目》，清代叶桂的《温热论》、薛雪的《湿热条辨》、吴瑭的《温病条辨》及王士雄的《温热经纬》标志着温病学说的崛起，王清任的《医林改错》发展了瘀血致病理论。医学各科的成就，使中医理论逐步走向完善和成熟。

其中《黄帝内经》与《伤寒杂病论》对中医理论体系的形成与发展具有极其深远的影响。《黄帝内经》，包括《素问》和《灵枢》两部分，是几千年来我国中医学术的指南。《黄帝内经》以"天人相应"的整体观为指导思想，以阴阳五行学说为逻辑工具，以脏腑经络学说为核心内容，建立了一个抽象度极高、涵盖极广、解释功能和推理功能极强的理论体系。《黄帝内经》最伟大的成就是将哲学思想引入经验医学。它的成书标志着我国古老的医学体系由单纯积累经验的经验医学阶段，发展到系统的理性医学阶段。《伤寒杂病论》成书于东汉末年，战争频发，瘟疫肆虐，中原地区发生瘟疫大流行十次有余，尸横遍野。医圣张仲景家族在不到十年的时间内死去三分之二的人，仲景伤痛之余，勤奋研习医术，著成《伤寒杂病论》，完成了《内经》理论与临床实践的衔接，使中医体系理法方药融会贯通，集四诊、八纲、辨因、论治、处方、用药、针灸、外治于一体，形成了中医诊治疾病的基本思想体系，即辨证论治体系。《伤寒杂病论》标志着中医体系的形成，被誉为"众方之宗，群方之祖"。

2. 中医学的成就和影响 在中医学发展史上，涌现过许多杰出的医家和浩瀚的医学典籍，有过许多令人瞩目的成就。春秋时期，名医扁鹊采用砭石、针灸、按摩、药物、熨帖等方法，在内外、妇、儿、五官等科的治疗中，取得较为理想的疗效。东晋时期，医家已论述了天花、霍乱等传染病，如葛洪详细且准确地描述了恙虫的生活形态、传染途径、临床特征、预防措施及预后等，比国外同类研究早1600多年。明代开始出现的人痘接种术，有效地控制了天花的流行，并成为现代免疫学的开端。

------ **知识链接1-3** --

尼克松访华掀起"美国针灸热"

在当今一些科学比较发达的国家里，也产生了学习、研究和应用中医药的"中医热"。20世纪70年代美国总统尼克松访华期间，在周总理的陪同下，观看了在针刺麻醉下进行的甲状腺切除手术。同年由30余人组成的尼克松访华团，也观看了由北京医科大学第三附属医院辛育龄教授主刀、在针刺麻醉下施行"右肺上叶切除术"的全过程，代表团返回美国后对"针刺麻醉"之神奇的宣传，再次引起美国民众的兴趣，小小银针的针灸技术一下轰动了美国，震惊了世界，西方有识之士像发现新大陆一项，纷至沓来，学习、研究、探求中国传统医学宝藏。

金针拨障术

中医眼科很早就采用金针拨障术治疗白内障。唐代王焘《外台秘要》中就已非常详尽地描述了金蓖术治疗白内障的方法（金蓖，由金属制成，类似箭镞的手术刀），经过历代眼科医家的临床实践，该疗法得到进一步的发展。

20 世纪 50 年代以后，中国眼科专家对金针拨障术进行了大量临床研究，成功地为患者施行金针拨障术，一些国内外重要人物都曾因接受这种疗法而重见光明。1972 年，柬埔寨首相宾努亲王患白内障，在北京 301 医院，由著名眼科专家唐由之施行针拨白内障套出术而成功治愈。1975 年 8 月，以唐由之为首的医疗组，再次采用该疗法医治毛泽东主席的白内障。

二、中医与中国古代哲学

中医药文化，就其思想体系而言，中国古代哲学占有极其重要的地位。中医与中国古代哲学的关系，主要体现在中国古代哲学中探索宇宙本源的"元气论"，认识生命本质的"阴阳学说"以及探索生命结构及其关系的"五行学说"。

在中医学的形成和发展的过程中，古代医家将当时的哲学思想和哲学概念融入到中医学中，并且与丰富的医学知识和诊疗经验相结合，形成了中医学独特的理论体系，并长期指导着临床实践，如将阴阳、五行、气等概念和理论，逐步成为中医学阐释问题的逻辑工具。另一方面，由于哲学是建立在具体学科之上的，在对气形神的关系、天人关系以及阴阳五行学说等与人体生命活动相关的哲学命题的深入探讨中，中医学又反过来丰富和发展了古代哲学，如五行学中的生克乘侮，就在中医典籍中得到充分讨论。

（一）"元气论"与"天人合一"的整体观

1. 元气论的产生　"元气"是中国古代的哲学概念，指产生和构成天地万物的原始物质。《说文解字》中，元，通"原"，"始也"，指天地万物之本原。气的概念源于"云气说"，《说文解字》："气，云气也。"云气是气的本始意义，引申之，凡与云气相类似的现象都可归结为气。古人对气的认识，从自然之气、呼吸之气而逐渐发展，认为气是构成世界万物生成的基本物质。认为世界上一切有形的物质，皆由无形之气变化而来，并认为气的运动变化是自然界一切事物发展变化的内在动力。这一思想萌生于先秦，成熟于战国及秦汉，晋代以后不断充实，对中国传统文化和古代科技有着深刻影响。

2. 元气论的内涵

（1）气是宇宙万物之本原：气是构成整个宇宙的最基本的物质，也是精神的来源，这是元气论的基本观点。《素问·五常政大论》曰："气始而生化，气散而有形，气布而蕃育，气终而象变，其致一也。"由于气的存在及其运动变化，才出现了天地，化生了宇宙万物，天地万物及人类皆为气所生。在中国古代哲学中，宇宙又称天地、天下、太虚、寰宇、乾坤、宇空等。《内经》称宇宙为太虚，在广阔无垠的宇宙虚空中，充满着无穷无尽具有生化能力的元气。

（2）气是不断运动变化的物质，气的运动变化过程是事物发展演变的过程：气分为"有形之气"和"无形之气"。所谓有形之气，指气的一种聚合状态，表现为人们能够清晰观察到的各种具有形态和结构的物体；无形之气，是指广布于宇宙空间及万物之中，无处不在、无时不在，不断运动变化的精微物质，虽然人们肉眼不能直接观察到，但却能够通过对有形之物的发展变化来认识和把握的。有形之气和无形之气随时都处在相互转化的过程之中，在有形和无形之气的不断运动变化中，才出现了万物生长转化和生命的诞生与消亡。由于气的运动，才产生了天地间的万物及各种自然现象。

元气论认为事物的发展变化过程即为"气化"的过程。自然界万物在形态、功能及表现方式上所出现的各种变化，都是气化的结果。所谓"气生形""形化气"是有形之气与无形之气的相互转化过程。而形与形、气与气以及有形之物自身内部的发展变化等，均为气化的过程和结果。人的健康与疾病状态的相互转化，亦是气化的过程与结果。因此，气化被认为是宇宙万物发展变化的内在机制。

（3）气是天、地与万物的中介：气既是构成宇宙万物的基本物质，又是宇宙万物相互作用与联系的中介。由于这一中介的存在和作用，宇宙天地万物才能形成一个整体。这个整体由弥漫于天地之间的无形之气（元气）将整个宇宙联系在一起（包括人与自然的联系）。同时这种无形之气弥散于事物内部，这就使事物之间存在着普遍的相互联系与感应。气的这种作用，构成了事物间的普遍联系及其相互影响转化的渠道与中介。

3. 元气论对中医学的影响

（1）元气论对中医学"天人合一"整体观的影响：元气论认为气是人类生命的本原，气是构成人体的基本物质，作为宇宙万物之一，人也是由天地之气聚合而生，因为人是宇宙间最高级的生物，所以认为构成人的气是宇宙的"精气"。气是构成人体生命形态和维持生命活动的基本物质。气不仅构筑了人体有形的组织器官，还弥散于整个机体，游移于各组织器官之间，从而使人体各组织之间构成了一个统一的整体。气在这一整体间的游移贯通，使人体的局部与整体、内在结构与外在功能之间形成了密切相关性，因此医家可以运用"以表知里"、"司外揣内"等方法观察、诊断疾病的性质和病位，进而确定治疗与调整的方案。

人作为自然界的万物之一，与自然界万物之间也要以气为中介进行物质交换，人体也是自然界物质整体的组成部分，人与自然的统一性，也因此表现出来。在此基础上，天人合一、天人相应以及形神统一的整体观念不断发展，并对中医学顺应季节的养生观、司外揣内的辩证方法、因人制宜的治疗思想，起到指导性的作用和影响。

1）"天人合一"整体观的内涵："天人合一"是中国古典哲学的根本观念之一，也是中国哲学异于西方的最显著的特征，在中国思想史上，"天人合一"是一个基本的信念。季羡林先生对其解释为：天，就是大自然；人，就是人类；合，就是互相理解，结成友谊。东方先哲告诫我们，人类只是天地万物中的一个部分，人与自然是息息相通的一体。如对"春生、夏长、秋收、冬藏"的规律性认识，要求养生治病要考虑到季节、气候、地理等因素对人的影响。此外，人在胚胎形成之时，由于受孕时气候、季节、时辰、运气以及父母素质等因素影响，会使胎儿所禀赋的先天因素各不相同，出生后就成为各种不同体质的人，这就是《内经》的体质学说，治疗时要"因人制宜"。

不仅如此，中医学还认为，人的身体就是一个小宇宙，人天同构是《内经》天人合一观的最直观的表达，认为人的身体结构体现了天地的结构。天有阴阳，人有脏腑；天有四季，人有四肢；天有五行，人有五脏；地有江河，人有经络。《素问·金匮真言论》及《素问·阴阳应象大论》等篇中的五行归类，正是源于事物内在的运动方式、状态或现象的同一性。将在天的方位、季节、气候、星宿，在地的品类、五谷、五畜、五音、五色、五味、五臭，在人的五脏、五声、五志，病变、病位等进行五行归类，这样就可以通过类别之间"象"的普遍联系，来识别同类运动方式的共同特征及其相互作用规律。

----- 知识链接 1-5 -----

中医学中人体的昼夜节律、月节律、四季节律

人的生命活动周期受到地球及日月星辰的运动周期的影响。人的生理和病理周期存在昼、夜、日、月、四季节律，乃至年节律。

昼夜节律：又称日节律，其周期为24小时或接近24小时。中医学中所说的日节律包括人体阴阳之气消长日节律、人体营卫之气运行节律、人体五脏之时辰节律、人体色脉日节律变化等。人体阴阳之气消长日节律又称为人体之气生、长、收、藏日节律，是人体生命活动的最基本形式。

月节律：月节律是人体对月球朔望运动的一种反应，人体气血的盛衰也与月的盈虚有关。以女子月经而言，一月一行为月信，如海水有潮汐之象，潮汐与月的盈虚有关。人体气血盛衰呈现月节律，月经与月相同步，具有按月而来的周期节律性，并认为月经节律与月相的盈亏和海潮有一定的关系。

四季节律：是人体对四季寒暑变化的一种节律性反应。中医的脉象随四季变化而呈现出不同的特点，春天以弦脉为主，夏天以洪脉为主，秋天脉象毛浮，冬天脉象沉实，此即四季脉象节律。

---

2)"天人合一"观与养生：中医学认为养生最重要的原则就是顺应自然，人与自然和谐相处。四时阴阳的消长变化是促使万物表现出"生、长、化、收、藏"的生态过程的根本原因，万物都不能违背这一规律，人的生活起居、精神情绪及养生活动也应与此相适应。《黄帝内经》许多篇章中都有顺时调摄养生的介绍。

(2)元气论在中医诊断及治疗疾病中的应用：元气论影响着中医学对生命活动现象的认识过程。精、气、神概念体系的建立，用来说明人体的生理和病理现象，解释了人的生命现象的活动过程。由先天之精气、后天水谷之气、自然之清气等共同作用于人体脏腑而产生的元气、宗气、营气、卫气、脏腑经络之气等，与血、津液、精等生命物质结合，分布贯行于全身，推动和激发人体各组织器官的功能活动，维持人体正常的生理状态。

中医学认为，人体的各种生命活动，都是在气的运行、推动下进行的。气的功能正常，人就处于健全的状态；气有余、不足或异常，人就处于病理状态。人体的正气与致病的邪气相搏，就会导致疾病的产生。《素问·举痛论》"百病生于气也，怒则气上，喜则气缓，悲则气消，恐则气下，寒则气收，炅则气泄，惊则气乱，劳则气耗，思则气结。"因此，中医学在临床诊断上，非常注重气的失调状态及病位所在，在治疗上，也离不开行气、补气、降气、调气等，直至气的状态相对平衡。

（二）阴阳学说

1. 易道与阴阳的概念　阴阳最初的概念很朴素，源于象形文字，是指日光的向背，向日者为阳，背日者为阴，之后逐渐延伸为一切事物或现象本身所存在的相互对立的两个方面。

阴阳理论来自于古代的星象学和天文学。汉代，阴阳观念已经渗透到包括哲学、自然科学及社会政治理论的几乎所有领域，特别是对于中国古代天文学、气象学、算学、化学、医学等自然学科的形成与发展产生了极为深刻的影响。如《周易·系辞》则对阴阳学说从哲学高度进行了概括，指出"一阴一阳之谓道"，即认为阴阳是天地万物运动和发展变化的根源和基本规律，阴阳之间存在对立制约、消长转化、互根互用、交感相错等关系。此后阴阳被

上升为一对独立的哲学概念,被广泛地应用于认识和改造世界的过程中。公元前8世纪的伯阳父就曾用阴阳来解释地震,把地震的原因归结为大地内部阴阳两种对立的物质运动的不协调。

2. 阴阳学说在中医学中的应用　阴阳学说在中医学中用于说明人体的组织结构。中医认为人体内部各组织系统间充满了阴阳对立互根的关系,将人体组织结构划分为既相互独立同时又相互依存的若干部分,从而使人体脏腑经络及形体组织结构,具备了各自的阴阳属性,进而可以依据其上下、内外、表里、前后各部分之间的联系,用阴阳的对立统一观点来加以认识和分析。

人体的生理活动及各组织的生理功能,均有其独特的阴阳属性,并互相联系,互相为用,共同维持和协调着人体的生命活动过程。人体的生命活动,是阴阳调和的动态平衡过程,这种平衡一旦失调,就会导致机体的异常状态,阴阳失调是人体疾病的基本病机之一。中医学运用阴阳学说来分析病因的阴阳属性,认识疾病病理变化的基本规律,并用于疾病的诊断及治疗。

------ **知识链接 1-6** --

八卦

八卦是中华古文明最具重要意义的发明之一,是阐明阴阳的多层次性及其普遍意义的学说,"易道以阴阳"。从《说文解字》对阴阳的注释,我们发现阴阳最初是指暗与光,而光暗交替则形成时序,时序又与方位相联系,因此八卦的本源与时序和方位的变化规律密切相关。

八卦表示事物自身变化的阴阳系统。用"—"代表阳,用"——"代表阴,用三个这样的符号,组成八种形式,叫做"八卦"。每一卦形代表一定的事物。乾代表天,坤代表地,坎代表水,离代表火,震代表雷,艮代表山,巽代表风,兑代表泽。八卦所对应的五行:金-乾、兑;木-震、巽;土-坤、艮;水-坎;火-离,见图1-4。八卦互相搭配又得到六十四卦,用来象征各种自然现象和人事现象,见表1-1。

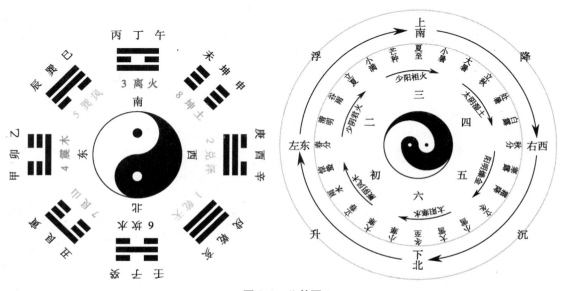

图 1-4　八卦图

表 1-1　八卦象征事物

卦名	自然	肢体	动物	方位	季节	阴阳	五行	五脏
乾	天	首	马	西北	秋冬间	阳	金	大肠
兑	泽	口	羊	西	秋	阴	金	肺
离	火	目	雉	南	夏	阴	火	小肠/心
震	雷	足	龙	东	春	阳	木	肝
巽	风	股	鸡	东南	春夏间	阴	木	胆
坎	水	耳	猪	北	冬	阳	水	肾/膀胱
艮	山	手	狗	东北	冬春间	阳	土	胃
坤	地	腹	牛	西南	夏秋间	阴	土	脾

（三）五行学说

五行的概念起源于殷商时代的五方概念。甲骨文记载，殷人把商朝的领域称为"中商"，并与于"东土""南土""西土""北土"并列，用五方总括整个空间方位。继五方说之后，出现了"五材说"，它把一切有形物质最终归纳为木、火、土、金、水这五大类。随后，又从木、火、土、金、水等五种具体物质中抽取其特性，用各自的特性与其他物体进行类比，具有类似特征的事物均化为同类。这样，五行理论就上升成为哲学概念，并采用取象比类和推演方法，将自然界中的各种事物和现象分归为五类，并以五行之间的关系来解释各种事物和现象发生发展和变化的规律。

五行学说在中医学中用于说明五脏的生理功能和特点，以及五脏之间的相互联系。中医学将五行之间的相互作用：相生与相克、制化与胜复，相乘与相侮以及母子相及的关系用以解释五脏病变的相互影响，认识疾病的传变，解释疾病与自然环境的相互关系以及指导疾病的诊断和治疗。

------ **知识链接 1-7** --

西方四液平衡学说

约在公元前 460—371 年，古希腊诞生了一位伟大的医学家希波克拉底，创立了人体的四液平衡学说，在西方被称为医学之父。四液平衡学说是在恩培多克勒的四元素学说的基础上发展而来的。恩培多克勒认为组成世界的四种基本元素是：空气、水、火和土。这四种元素与体内血液、黏液、黄胆汁和黑胆汁相对应。希波克拉底运用这四种体液在人体内的平衡和变动，来说明人体的生理病理现象。认为如果四种体液处于平衡状态，那么人体就处于健康状态，如果四种体液的失调是暂时的，则有恢复平衡的趋势。

三、中医与中国古代科技、宗教、军事、地理

《黄帝内经》嘱后世学医者，必须"上知天文，下知地理，中知人事"，说明中医学与自然科学、人文社会科学存在着密切的联系。中医学的巨著《黄帝内经》涉及天文、地理、数学、宗教、军事等学科在内的多学科知识及技术。

（一）中医学与中国古代天文学

医学与天文学的关系非常密切。天文学与人类历史一样悠久，"古者伏羲氏之王天下也，

仰则观象于天，俯则观法与地，观鸟兽之文与地之宜，进取诸身，远取诸物，于是始作八卦，以通神明之德，以类万物之情。"

1. 中国古代天文学成就　中国是世界上天文学起步最早、发展最快的国家之一，在世界天文史上有着重要的地位。中国古代天文学萌芽于原始社会。公元前 24 世纪的帝尧时代，就设立了专门从事"观象授时"的天文官，有史料记载的天文观察历史也十分悠久。

（1）天文仪器：在创制天文仪器方面，中国科学家也作出过杰出的贡献。2000 多年前制成了测量天体位置的仪器——浑仪。以后历代先后创制和改进了 10 多种天文仪器，如简仪、高表、仰仪。

（2）古代历法：古人通过观察日月星辰的位置及其变化，掌握天体运动的规律性来确定四季、编制历法，为生产和生活服务。其中节气的推算是古代历法中的主要内容。节气是通过气候变化与农业生产的关系编制出来的历法，是宝贵的科学遗产。公元前 104 年正式把二十四节气定于历法，明确了二十四节的天文位置。除了节气外，古代历法还包括每月日数的分配、月和闰月的安排，日月食发生时刻和可见情况的计算和预报，五大行星位置的推算和预报等。

二十四节气：春雨惊春清谷天，夏满芒夏暑相连，秋处露秋寒霜降，冬雪雪冬小大寒。

二十四节气与星座的关系见图 1-5。

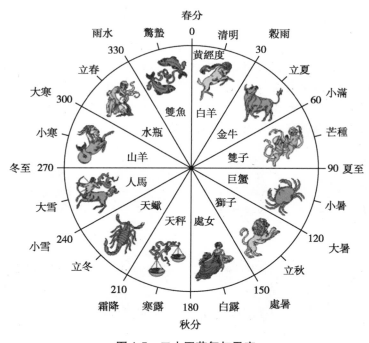

图 1-5　二十四节气与星座

（3）"干支说"：天干地支，是一个顺序符号系统，古人用天干来表述太阳对地球的引力影响周期，用木、火、土、金、水五运来表示其阶段性特征；用十二地支来表述月亮对地球接受太阳光辐射的影响周期，用三阴三阳六气表示其阶段性特征。

"干"、"支"犹如一棵千古的大树，支撑起我们对宇宙及万事万物变化法则的把握。同时，这种对宇宙及万事万物变化法则的把握又是简单明确的：由六轮天干与五轮地支构成一个六十的循环周期，（阳）天干与（阳）地支组合，（阴）天干与（阴）地支组合，然后按照阳组合与阴组合，依次交替组成六十个纪年的组合，构成的这套表示时间、空间的象数表达方式，于是便有了从第一组"甲子"到第六十位"癸亥"的循环轮转。

十个天干：（阳）甲、（阴）乙、（阳）丙、（阴）丁、（阳）戊、（阴）己、（阳）庚、（阴）辛、（阳）壬、（阴）癸。

十二地支：（阳）子、（阴）丑、（阳）寅、（阴）卯、（阳）辰、（阴）巳、（阳）午、（阴）未、（阳）申、（阴）酉、（阳）戌、（阴）亥。

天干 + 地支 = 五个阳天干配六个阳地支（5×6）+ 五个阴天干配六个阴地支（5×6）="六十甲子"纪年（六十个"生肖年"序号）

在干支搭配时候，年月日时各干支之间相生相克的制约关系，成为我国传统的时间生物医学 - "运气学说"、"子午流注"及"天人相应"等理论的有力支柱。

"甲子"的概念是宇宙万物的开始，有着升发的力量和功能；而"癸亥"的理念则代表终结，以寒水冻结内藏来表述。这是古人对宇宙万物运动规律最具科学精神的探索，是古代文化"天人合一"理念的具体产物。

印度上古的天文学也有类似十二地支的观念，只不过他们用十二个动物来表示，随着佛学的融入，中国后来又有用十二生肖代表十二地支的说法。

知识链接 1-8

十二生肖的来历

古时候的文人，为了让平民百姓、目不识丁之人，也能记住自己出生的年号，就使用了最简单的动物纪年法，后来称其为"生肖年"（生肖："生"，出生；"肖"，相似、相像）。生肖的周期为 12 年。每一人在其出生年都有一种动物作为生肖。十二生肖即鼠、牛、虎、兔、龙、蛇、马、羊、猴、鸡、狗、猪是中国民间计算年龄的方法，也是一种古老的纪年法（图 1-6）。

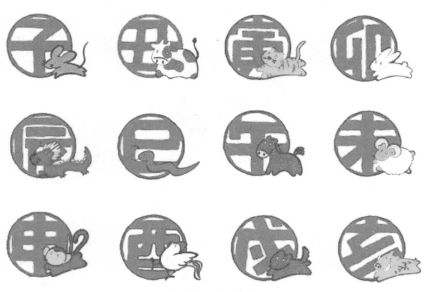

图 1-6　十二生肖

2. 中医四时养生与古代天文学的关系　远古时代人们就已懂得按照大自然的规律作息，即"日出而作，日落而息"。形成了"天人合一"的世界观，认为人的生理节律以及气血运行与自然界事物的运行是同步的，养生保健须遵循天文规律。

人类的生存需要天地之气所提供的物质条件，同时也要需要适应四时阴阳的变化规律。四时养生，即生活中要顺应"春生、夏长、秋收、冬藏"的生物规律。四时对人体的精神、气血、五脏、水液代谢、疾病等方面均有着重要的影响。人体五脏的生理活动，必须适应四时阴阳的变化，才能与外界环境保持协调平衡。例如，春夏之季，气血容易趋向于体表，表现为皮肤松弛，疏泄多汗等，而秋冬阳气收藏，气血容易趋向于脏腑，表现为皮肤致密，少汗多溺等，因此人们在养生时就必须适时变化，顺应自然规律，所谓"春夏养阳，秋冬养阴"。

（二）中医学与古代术数之学

"术数"即数学方法的一种，数学方法被认为是科学知识具备精确性的基本条件。由于在中国古代科技领域内，数学方法的应用与现代科学有着本质的不同，在中国传统文化领域内，不叫数学而叫术数，中国古代的数学曾经处于世界先进水平。

在中医学的经典著作中也有很多数与量的描写。《易经》作为中国文化的源头之一，是一本充满数学符号的著作，其学术体系"生于数，成于数，变通于数"。《易经》中阳爻（—）与阴爻（——）的组合变化，实际上是数学语言的表述。因此，中国古代数学又称为"术数之学"。

在中医学中"象数之学"的运用同样具有上述特征。如《素问·三部九候论》中"天地之至数，始于一，终于九"，这里数字"一"至"九"作为一种名称尺度，是对生命现象加以分类的标志，类似于标签的作用。具体所指为"一者天，两者地，三者人，因而三之，三三者九，以应九野。故人有三部，部有九候，以决死生，以处百病，以调虚实，而除邪疾。"

《素问·五常政大论》中以数字论五行"木，其数八；火，其数七；土，其数五；金，其数九；水，其数六"。《太玄·玄数》中则以数字表示五行、方位及四季，"一、六为水；二、七为火；三、八为木；四、九为金；五、五为土"。此外，还包含了属性、方位、气候、地域等信息，可见，数字成了这些信息的符号。

（三）儒家思想与中医学

儒家是指以孔丘、孟轲、荀况为代表的思想流派，崇尚"礼乐"和"仁义"，提倡"忠恕"和"中庸"之道。政治上主张"德治"和"仁政"，重视伦理道德教育。儒家思想是中华民族传统文化的重要组成部分，对中医的影响主要反映在以下几个方面：

1. 儒家思想促进了中医学核心价值观的形成　首先，儒家的中庸思想是中医学术体系的重要组成部分。从中医理论的构架来看，包含了儒、道、阴阳等诸家思想学说，而儒家的中庸思想影响了中医学价值观和思维模式的形成。其次，儒家的"仁义"、"孝道"，提倡尊重他人，并注重自我修养。这些对中医伦理学、医学社会学和医疗行为规范都产生了积极的影响。第三，儒家主张精学博览，学而不厌、诲人不倦是儒家的优良传统。这种思想影响到中医学领域，促使医家博采众长、精益求精，如张仲景、孙思邈、李时珍等医家用一生追求精深的医理和精湛的医术。

2. 儒家文化从三个方面推动了中医学学术的发展　一是推动中医学教育发展。纵观我国古代的医学教育制度，与儒家的教育体系有着密切的联系。二是丰富中医学理论体系。儒家的《周易》、《论语》、《礼记》中所提出的阴阳、中庸和整体观等，早已成为中医学的重要组成部分。三是儒学使中医形成了独具特色的研究方法和思想方法。儒学重形象思维而轻抽象思维，促使中医从宏观的功能表现来认识人体，逐渐形成以天人相应、取类比象为基础，以整体观念、辨证施治为特征，具有浓厚人文哲学色彩的医学理论体系。

（四）中医学与宗教

中国历史上多种宗教盛行，而其中道教与佛教这两大传统宗教对中国的历史文化以及中医学的发展都有着极为深远的影响。

1. 道教对中医学的影响　道教出现于 1800 年前的东汉时期，是唯一发源于中国的本土宗教。它以鬼神崇拜为基础，以民间各种神秘传说为信仰，以老庄思想中的长生不老和今生幸福为宗旨，并融合了佛教和儒教的教义，吸收了部分儒家和佛教思想，将中国古代哲学、神话和巫术整合为一体。

"道"是道教教义的核心。道家思想认为自然界有一个万事万物都必须遵守的法则，这个法则叫做"道"。天地万物都由"道"而派生，"一生二，二生三，三生万物"；"德"则是这个法则人性、人伦、人情等方面的体现，符合"道"的才叫"德"。人类需遵循"道"的法则。道教认为人"在天曰命，在人曰性"，所以在养生活动中形神并重、性命兼修，强调身体健康和道德修养的双重意义。道教认为人的长寿是由身心健康交互作用而完成的。

古人云"医道同源"，道教中的仪典、练功、炼丹、药食等与中医有着密切的关系，其中道教对对中医贡献最大的为其养生技术，如气功、食疗、性保健、药物等养生技术。

2. 佛教对中医学的影响　主要体现对医德的培养和养生等方面。佛教的教义劝恶从善，强调精神境界的修养，有利于保持良好的精神状态，促进身心健康。僧侣或佛教崇拜者多有长寿之人；佛教中的坐禅类似于气功修炼，所以佛教医书中有关静坐方法和养生关系等方面的论著既是宗教修养形式，也是内功修炼方法，以静坐为特点的禅功在中国气功史上有一定的地位；佛教多数宗派均要求素食，鼓励僧侣艰苦修行，素食有益身心，客观上有食养、食疗之效；寺院作息制度非常严格，诵经、劳作、运动皆有定规，不少寺院有演练巫术以健身护寺的传统，这些活动对健康有利；此外，寺院环境优美，建筑大都高大宽敞，植被繁茂，空气新鲜，有利于健康长寿。可见佛教在道德、精神、心理、气功、食疗、体育、环境、个人卫生等方面的要求对中医养生学的发展也有着积极的影响。

（五）中医学与中国古代军事思想

军事与医学之间有着共通的原理，所谓"用药如用兵"，所以历代医家常常借鉴兵家理论来启发临床思维，为中医学的发展做出了重大的贡献。

《黄帝内经》中对与针刺时机的选择原则的阐述，就是引用《兵法》中的内容，即要根据病邪的形势来"避实就虚"。《灵枢·逆顺》中记载："《兵法》曰：无迎逢逢之气，无击堂堂之阵。"《刺法》曰："无刺熇熇之热，无刺漉漉之汗，无刺浑浑之脉，无刺病与脉相逆者"，在《孙子兵法·军争篇》中可以看到类似的文字。《黄帝内经》借用战争的规律性来说明人体内正邪的斗争，并用以指导针刺。古代医家认为正与邪的较量，如同打仗一样，也表现出一个回合过后，再进行下一个回合的起伏过程。

"用药如用兵"，指战争以对方为敌，医者以病邪为敌。兵家讲战术，重用兵之道，医家论医术，重治疗之法。古代军事理论较好地体现了中国传统思维方式中的"直觉思维"，如"因势利导"、"声东击西"、"避实就虚"、"分兵合击"等。这些中医临床思维与之有着惊人的相似。因此兵家、医家思想的相互通用也就不难理解了，在这一理论的指导下历代医家创造了很多临床奇迹。

----- 知识链接 1-9 --

宋代，有位便秘患者，看遍名医均无效。一位史姓医生用了一味治咳嗽的中药"紫苑"，一会儿大便就通了。其原理就是肺与大肠相表里，该患者的便秘是肺气不降所致，用紫苑通肺气，则秘结自消。中医治则中有"提壶揭盖法"，也是通过调节肺的功能来治疗水肿、小便不通。

《中医美学》有这样一个病例：患者晨起时发现右髋关节弯曲僵硬，不能活动，即使用很大的力量也无法使其活动，遍寻名医，经服药、按摩、推拿、理疗等治疗后均无明显效果。该书作者当时在患者肩关节相应部位施针，针刺入约 2cm 时，患者右腿猛力一伸，跳下地即起，取针后行动如常。

可见中医的临床思维需要和战争一样的出其不意，原理大家都懂，但临床治疗时往往被"常理"所拘束。经常运用军事方面的理论触动僵化的思维，才能灵活自如地运用熟读的理论。

（六）中医学与中国古代地理学

地理与医学的关系十分密切，因为地域不同，地理环境和生活习惯就有差异，时差、温差、降雨量和地貌等方面也有明显的区别。地域是诞生文化的土壤，也是承载文明的摇篮。自然条件的形成受到地理环境的影响，而自然条件对于人的生理、心理、世界观、方法论等有着直接的影响。

中国疆域广阔，具有不同的地貌特征，如平原、山地、丘陵、沙漠、隔壁、高原、岛屿等地形各不相同，自然条件也各不相同，人们的患病和治疗情况也不相同，因此，中医养生防病，治疗康复都要"因地制宜"。《素问·异法方宜论》记载了东、西、南、北、中央的地理风貌、物产民情，及其对人生理、性格与疾病的影响，指出不同的医疗方法，如中国的东部地区易生外科痈疡，应该用手术（砭石）治疗；西部地区，病多生于内脏，应该使用药性猛烈的食物；北部地区，脏腑容易受寒而出现腹胀，应该用灸法治疗；南部地区易患风湿关节病，应该用针刺治疗；中部地区，多患四肢萎软恶寒发热，应该用推拿按摩的方法治疗。

此外，用药剂量、药性的峻猛与平缓也应随地理环境不同，有相应的选择。北方高寒，用药宜重，南方炎热，用药宜轻，西南地区气候潮湿，用附子、细辛如家常便饭，但江南地区气候潮湿，使用附子、细辛便需慎之又慎。此外，不同的地理也能为治疗疾病提供不同的方法，如各地的民间疗法和地方医学等。

----- 知识链接 1-10 --

中国古代地理学的成就

中国古代对各种地理的研究也有很大的成就。地图及地图测绘理论也很早就产生，并留下了相当多的地理文献。公元前 11 世纪到公元前 8 世纪，中国人的地理概念已经相当成熟，已开始用地图来表示地域分布，并运用于国家行政管理。2500 年前成书的《山海经》描述了我国古代地理、历史、神话、民族、动植物、矿产、医学、宗教等多方面的内容。这本书以山脉为标志，系统描述了全国地理。书中列出 460 多座山名，260 多条河名，记录了 140 多种植物和 112 种动物，书中还有大量的矿物记载，是世界上最早的矿物文献。

公元 6 世纪初的《水经注》是一部以水系为纲领和坐标全面记述全国地理情况的综合性

地理著作，记述了全国 1252 条河流，对这些河川的流域地区从地理现状到历史事迹都选择典型事例做了记录。

17 世纪初明代地理学家徐霞客，自 22 岁起就以惊人的毅力从事科学的地理考察和探险旅行，前后达 30 余年之久，足迹遍及大半个中国，著有《徐霞客游记》。徐霞客是世界上最早提出分水岭、流域面积的科学家之一。他在世界上第一个提出了长江的流域面积比黄河的流域面积大一倍。他也是世界上最早广泛而系统地对岩溶地貌进行科学考察的科学家，亲身探查和描述过 300 多个洞穴……这些成就使徐霞客在科学文化史上声名卓著，成为近代地理学的创建人之一。

四、中西医学的异同与融合

（一）中西医学对疾病的认识方法的异同

中西医学的根本区别，首先是认识方法上的区别。中医是人们的感觉器官直接观察自然现象和人体现象，从具体形象到抽象思维，又从抽象思维推导未知的哲学认识方法。西医则是建立在分析方法上的实验科学。西医学的实验分析认识方法和中医学的系统思维认识方法，是揭示人体的不同的医学理论，使人体的多方面内容得以展现，使人们能够全面认识人体的生理现象。

1. 中医的认识侧重功能关系　中医从观察人的生命现象入手，在人的自然整体层面把握功能变化的规律，并不过分关注内部结构的规律。《素问·五常政大论》云："气始生而生化，气散而有形，气布而藩育，气终而象变，其致一也。"中医认为，人的有形之体是在气的运化过程中形成的，气的运化是人的基本生命功能，生命是人在自然中与各种因素综合作用下的一种生命功能状态。人体气的变化过程表现出来的现象，反映了人体的功能状态，所谓"有诸内，必形诸外"。

中医的藏象学说以"象"的变化为依据，建立了一个独特的以功能联系为基础的人体系。"象"，形象也。藏居于内，形见于外。藏象学说描述的脏与脏之间的相生相克关系、腑与腑之间的传导关系、脏与腑之间的表里关系、内脏与五官之间的开窍关系、脏腑与经络之间的从属关系等，并不特指某一特定的实体器官功能和活动，而是由外在之"象"推知的人体功能系统间的关系。美国的弗里乔夫·卡普拉指出："中国的关于身体的概念始终以功能为主，并且着重考虑各部分之间的关系，而不重视其精确的结构。"中医观察研究的是功能的变化规律。

中医在认识和治疗疾病中都是以功能为基础的。中医认为疾病就是阴阳失调、气机失常造成的脏腑气血功能异常，并非必须有器质性的病变。中医的治疗也是以功能调理为基础，强调人体内在的生化，助内在生生不息的气机。药物或其他治疗手段往往并不直接作用于疾病靶点，而是通过调节机体的功能状态，使阴阳消长升降出入保持平衡，维持健康状态。当然，中医也认识到功能性的异常也是器质性病变的前奏，"大凡形质之失宜，莫不由气行之失序"，调整功能状态也是对器质性病变的一种预防手段。

2. 西医的认识侧重实体结构　1543 年，比利时的维萨利发表的《人体的构造》标志西医学的现代发展的历程的开始。西医学从形态结构研究入手，逐步建立了以形态结构为基础的西医学科体系。从人体到组织、细胞、分子直到基因等对形态结构的认识不断走向微观、精细，试图在基因甚至更微观的层面揭示生命的本质。

西医学以形态结构为基础的，按在结构上的连贯性和相似性把人体器官与组织分成几大系统，对人的生理与病理的研究也在结构的基础上展开，对疾病的认识也纳入了以形态结构为坐标的框架体系中，对疾病的认识的焦点集中在解剖形态的器质性变化，注重局部定位，注重病变的病理解剖根据。因此，器质性病变成为西医的主要关注对象，功能的病变放在次要和从属的地位，认为器质性病变是疾病的普遍的、基本的形态，甚至有学者认为人的任何功能性的变化都可以在身上找到器质性的变化的根据。

（二）中医学独特的思维模式

由于思维方式的差别，很多人在初学中医时感到非常困难。然而，如果实现了思维方式的转换或者将两种思维方式融会贯通，那么学习中医就是会变得非常有乐趣。影响到中医思维方式的因素非常多，但归根结底，其基本范畴在于"象"和"意"。中医学的主导思维方式是直觉思维，即采用取象比类、审证求因，辩证推理等思维方法，注重事物表象和本质的直接联系和动态把握。强调"取象比类"、"圆机活法"的思维方式，即以辩证逻辑为主的思维方式。然而，在中医方法论中，观察与思维、感性与理性并非截然分离的，而是融为一体的。感性与理想的合一即"悟性"，即所谓"直觉"。因此，中医思维的结果既是具体的，又是抽象的，具有形象生动、灵活自然的特点。

1. 取象比类的思维方法　"象"的概念出自《易经》。"圣人有以见天下之赜而拟诸其形容，象其物宜，是故谓之象"（《系辞上》）；"易者，象也，象也着，像也"（《系辞下》）。中医从医学的角度给"象"做出了定义："有诸内，必形诸外"。"脏腑藏于内，必象形于外"，五脏六腑虽然藏于内部，但它们的功能、特性却能被观察到，人们可以从观察到的功能特点，推测脏腑的实质，所以中医的脏腑理论称作藏象学说。

中医"唯象"方法是依靠对完整的人体进行观察、比较、分析，研究其生理、病理、治疗规律，建立在人体内部与外部的规律性联系的基础上，是一种简洁的、通过内外联系原理把握对象的方法，属于整体系统方法。在原理上，"唯象方法"接近于控制论的"黑箱方法"。"唯象方法"反映了人体的整体和动态特征以及整体与局部的和谐统一。

中医学四诊的方法，是局部的"象"反映整体变化这一思维方法的临床运用，是依靠医生的感觉器官对患者生命信息进行观察。常用的局部诊法有脉诊、面诊、耳诊、舌诊、小儿指纹等。这些诊法的原理，即"脏腑藏于内，必象形于外"，外表的局部变化，反映着整体的功能，因此这些被人们作为诊断或治疗的局部，就是整体的"象"。

中医"天人相应"理论，将人与自然界的诸多现象进行类比，如人体气血运行和自然界海水潮汐运行相类似，也会受到日月、寒温、昼夜的影响。这种类比强调的是人体与大自然在运动规律方面的统一，古人将人体这一"小宇宙"与大自然这一"大宇宙"加以类比，从对大自然的欣赏和理解中，寻找对人体科学的认识途径。

（1）将社会现象与人体功能做相似性的联系：《素问·灵兰秘典论》将脏腑功能与官职的相似性做了类比联系：心者，君主之官；肺者，相傅之官；肝者，将军之官；脾胃者，仓廪之官。这是因为这些脏腑的功能特点与这些管阶职能特征有相似之处。这种相似性的联系还表现在方剂的组成中药物的君臣佐使。

（2）将自然物与人体解剖、生理做相似性比较：《素问·五脏生成篇》将人体经脉内气血运行状态与大海潮汐消长相类比；《脉经》据月亮的圆缺周期与妇女经水来潮的规律之间的相似性，把这种生理现象命名为"月经"；《中藏经》把肺的形状比作"五脏六腑之华盖，以覆诸脏"，肺的内部则"虚如蜂巢，下无透窍，吸之则满，呼之则虚"，再如人体很多穴位也是按照其部位特征与自然物的相似性来命名的,如"大陵穴"如山之突起、"太渊穴"凹如山谷。

(3)对致病因素与病理结果进行相似性类比:中医认为自然界的因素是人体生存所必需的,但超出常度即转化为致病因素。病因作用于人体后,往往表现为与病因性质相类似的病理结果,如水湿有下流、重浊的特点,而人体受到湿邪侵犯后也表现为下注、重浊的特点,如水肿、身重、乏力、头重如裹等。同理,"火"有炎上、耗津的特点,人受暑热后则表现为发热,面红,口干,尿少等炎上、耗津的特点。

2. 司外揣内的方法　司外揣内,是指通过观察事物外在的表象,来推测事物内部变化的一种方法,是中医学认识方法、实践方法、哲学方法的基础。

在漫长的生活实践中,古人发现人体外部表象与内部脏腑、器官的变化存在着相应的关系,所谓"有诸内,必形诸外"。《灵枢·外揣》中以日光照射出现影子,敲击锣鼓就会发出响声等事实为例,来说明事物的现象和本质之间存在着因果联系,既可以从结果来找原因,也可以从原因来推测结果。

司外揣内的方法与现代控制论的"黑箱"理论类似,即不打开黑箱,只通过对"黑箱"输入信息,观察反馈出的信息,比较研究输入、输出信息的异同就可测知黑箱内部情况,并把握其运动变化的规律。由于这一方法没有干扰和破坏对象本身的各种联系,观察到的是对象固有的特性和变化,因此,这一方法在研究许多复杂现象,特别是对生命过程的研究方面具有许多其他方法所无法比拟的优越性。

(三)中医学认识治疗疾病的基本特点

1. 中医学辨证论治的思想　辨证论治就是按照中医理论,运用望、闻、问、切等各种诊断方法获得患者信息,并根据这些信息,结合患者的生理特点、生活习惯以及气候、地理环境等因素进行综合分析,辨别不同的证候、研究其致病原因,进而确定恰当的治疗方法的思维过程。

----- 知识链接 1-11 ---

三国的时候,府吏倪寻和李延去找华佗看病,两人都是头痛发热,华佗给二人诊断后说:"倪寻应当用下泄的方法治疗,而李延应当用发汗的方法治疗。"有人不解,华佗说"倪寻外实,邪气滞留体内,就好比山间积水,需要用下的方法来疏导;李延内实,内实就容易实火上冲,就好像地气郁结,需要用发汗的方法来发散。"于是就给二人开了不同的方子,次日两人的病情都有所好转。

---

2. "治病求本"的基本原则　中医在治疗中治病求本的原则是区别于西医的最鲜明的特征。《素问·刺法》曰:"正气存内,邪不可干"。"正气"指机体自身的抗病能力,包括自身的组织结构、物质和功能活动。"邪气"泛指各种致病因素。疾病发生发展取决于正邪斗争的结果,"正气"充沛,是抵御疾病发生的内在根据。"治病求本"就是要抓住疾病过程中"邪"、"正"斗争中矛盾的关键因素,鼓舞"正气",通过提高人体自身的抗病与修复能力来达到治疗的目的。中医学"治病求本"的原则贯穿于预防、保健、治疗等各个领域。

3. 调整阴阳平衡的治疗原则　中医认为疾病是由于人体阴阳动态平衡失调,出现了对外界环境变化的不适应、形神失秩、脏腑功能失调等。《素问·生气通天论》"阴平阳秘,精神乃治;阴阳离决,精气乃绝"。《灵枢·根结》说"调阴与阳,精神乃光"。《素问·至真要大论》指出,治疗要"谨察阴阳所在而调之,以平为期"。更明确指出"寒者热之,热者寒之,温者清之，清者温之，散者收之，抑者散之，燥者润之，急者缓之，坚者软之，脆者坚之，强者泻之，各安其气，必清必静，则病气衰去，归其所宗，此治之大体也"。中医的治疗是以调、养为主。调，就是调和，调整。养，就是补、泄、疏、通。中医运用中草药、针灸等手段，调和人体的气血阴阳，调整人体各个脏腑的生理功能，使人体的各脏腑功能协调平衡，从内在提高机体的抵抗力，清除疾病在人体内赖以产生和存在的土壤。可见注重调整，以促使机体恢复到阴阳的动态平衡是中医治疗的根本原则。

（四）中西医学融合发展趋势

中医学正在融入当代文化、科学、技术的大背景，其现实的价值、发展的优势和潜力更为凸显。"按照中医药自身发展规律，满足时代发展需求，充分利用现代科学技术，继承和发扬优势和特色，使中医学从理论到实践都产生新的变革和升华，成为具有当代科学水平的医学理论体系"。

西方耗散结构理论的创始人普里高津指出："中国传统的学术思想是着重于研究整体性和自然性，研究协调与协和"。现代新科学的发展，近十年物理和数学的研究，如托姆的突变理论、重正化群、分支理论等，都更符合中国的哲学理想。德国汉学家 Porker 认为"中医是感应综合性科学，西医是因果分析性科学，中西医学都能够从现实的完全不同的方面提供同样确实的和有意义的资料，就像两个登山队，一个从南坡，一个从北坡，通过不同途径同样可到峰顶一样，但两种方法各有局限性，应该互相补充"。

中西医学在相当长的时期内，将在相互交流、渗透、补充、结合的过程中，沿着自己的轨迹继续发展。世界科技史学家李约瑟博士认为，"越具有生物学特点的科学，其形成世界自然科学统一体这一过程所需要的时间就越长"。相信有着同一研究对象的中西医学，经过数代人的不懈努力，中西医学能在彼此交融发展中达到还原论与整体论的辩证统一，建立在功能、结构与代谢相统一的关于人类健康与疾病的新医学体系。

（马雪玲）

第二节　中医护理学发展简史

中医护理学的形成和发展，经历了漫长的历史阶段。自古以来，中医治病都是集医、药、护为一身，在历史上没有形成中医护理专门学科，但是我国传统医药学中一直都包含有丰富的护理内容，中医护理学的理论和技术内容散见于历代各种医学著作中。

一、古代中医护理学

（一）战国至东汉时期（公元前 475—公元 220 年）

《黄帝内经》是我国现存最早，比较全面系统阐述中医学理论体系的古典医学巨著，包括《素问》和《灵枢》两部分，系统阐述了人体生理、病理以及疾病的诊断、治疗和预防等内容，形成了中医学独特的理论体系，为中医学理论和临床的形成和发展奠定了坚实的基础。在中医护理学方面，论述了病证护理、饮食护理、生活起居护理、情志护理、养生康复护理、服药护理以及针灸、推拿、导引、热熨、洗药等护理技术，因此《内经》奠定了中医护理学的基础。如在生活起居护理方面，《素问·上古天真论》指出："法于阴阳，和于数术，饮食有节，起居有常，不妄劳作。"指出要遵循自然界的阴阳变化规律办事，要按时起卧，劳逸适度。这不仅是养生防病之道，也是日常生活自我调护之理。《内经》之"顺四时而适寒暑"理论，指出了四时养生起居的规律，也是人与天地相应的整体观。对五脏病证的护理，《内经》指出"病在脾……禁温食饱食、湿地濡衣"，"病在肺……禁寒饮食、寒衣"等。在饮食护理方面，如在五脏病变饮食的禁忌中指出"肝病禁辛、心病禁咸、脾病禁酸、肾病禁甘、肺病禁苦"。《内经》在情志护理上也予以高度重视，认为这关系到疾病的发生、发展及预后，强调不良情志刺激可导致人体气血失调，脏腑功能紊乱，而诱发或加重病情，如"怒则气上"、"喜则气缓"、"悲则气消"、"恐则气下"、"惊则气乱"、"思则气结"等。此外，《内经》记载的中医特殊护理疗法，包括针灸、导引、推拿、热熨等，至今仍在临床护理中继续使用。

东汉末年著名医学家张仲景的《伤寒杂病论》，是我国最有影响的一部临床医学巨著。它总结了东汉以前众多医家的临床经验，不仅奠定了中医辨证论治的理论体系，还论述了对疾病的辨证施护的理论和措施，为临床辨证施护开创了先河。在护理技术方面，《伤寒杂病论》较详细地论述了熏洗法、烟熏法、坐浴法、点烙法、溃脚法等。特别是张仲景首创了药物灌肠法，如用"蜜煎导方"及猪胆汁灌肠法，充分反映东汉时期的护理发展水平。在急救护理方面提出了对自缢者的抢救，具体方法与现代人工呼吸法极其相似。在服药护理方面，《伤寒杂病论》对煎药方法、服药注意事项、观察服药后反应及饮食宜忌均有详细记载。如此之类的护理要求，在大青龙汤、五苓散、十枣汤、大承气汤、甘草附子汤、防己黄芪汤等方后注中有详细记载，还告诫应"如法将息"。如《伤寒论》桂枝汤方后注明在煎煮时应"以水七升，微火煮取三升，去渣，适寒温，服一升"，而服药后又应"啜热稀粥一升余，以助药力"，并还应"温覆令一时许，遍身漐漐微似有汗者益佳"。认为出汗，"不可令如水流漓，病必不除"。且在服药后的饮食禁忌方面主张服桂枝汤后要"禁生冷、粘滑、肉面、五辛、酒酪、臭恶等物"。《伤寒杂病论》在饮食护理上，也有专篇论述。如对禽兽鱼虫及果实菜谷的禁忌，指出了五脏病食忌、四时食忌、冷热食忌、妊娠食忌等。明确指出了饮食也应辨证，所谓"所食之味，有与病相宜，有与身为害，若得宜则益体，害则成疾"。在饮食卫生上，已明确告诫："秽饭、馁肉、臭鱼、食之皆伤人"，"梅多食，坏人齿"，"猪肉落水浮者，不可食"，"肉中有米点者，不可食"等。在治疗与护理上，《伤寒杂病论》强调有病早治早防和防止疾病传变发展的观点，如"见肝之病，知肝传脾，当先实脾"等预防医学的思想。

华佗是后汉三国时期的名医，是我国外科和医疗体育的奠基人，他吸取了前人"导引"的精华，模仿虎、鹿、熊、猿、鸟等禽兽的运动姿态，创造了"五禽戏"。他认为人体健康，应"欲得劳动，但不当使极耳，动摇则谷得消，血脉流通，病不得生，譬如户枢不朽也"。"五禽戏"可以帮助消化，疏通气血，增强体质，减少疾病，是我国医疗、护理、体育三位一体的世界最早的健身保健方法。华佗的另一伟大贡献是发明了麻沸散并作为全身麻醉剂应用在外科手术中，对外科学的发展做出了贡献。在手术治疗过程中指导弟子或家属做了大量护理工作，可以说是我国最早的外科护理专家。

（二）魏晋南北朝时期（公元220—581年）

晋代王叔和在其所著《脉经》中将脉象名称规范化，归纳为二十四脉，深入阐述了脉理，并比较了脏腑各部的生理、病理脉象，分析了各种杂病及小儿、妇女的脉证，明确提出了切脉独取寸口及左右手六部分配脏腑的理论，使诊脉法成为护理临床观察病情时的重要手段。

东晋葛洪所著《肘后备急方》集中医急救、传染病及内、外、妇、五官、精神、骨伤各科之大成。在书中提出的各科急诊诊治中，已广泛涉及了护理要求。如明确提出外伤大出血患者，应禁食水及刺激性食物，患者宜安静，避免活动和情绪波动。又如在"治卒大腹水病方"中说："勿食盐、常食小豆饭，饮小豆汁，鲤鱼佳也。"该书还记有世界上关于天花的最早记载。

南北朝时期我国现存最早的一部外科专著《刘涓子鬼遗方》中记载，对腹部外伤肠管脱出者，还纳时要注意保持环境卫生、安静。还应注意外敷药的干湿，干后应当立即更换，这都是护理中值得注意的问题。

（三）隋唐五代时期（公元581—960年）

隋朝名医巢元方等所著的《诸病源候论》中有各种疾病的病因、病理、症状、诊断、预防和护理的论述，并有大量的养生导引方法。例如在"消渴候"中记有："此肥美之所发，此人必数食甘美而多肥也。"提出消渴病与过食肥甘美食有关。在外科方面，介绍了外科肠吻合术后的饮食护理。在妇科护理方面，北齐徐之才的"十月养胎法"，强调了妇女妊娠期间的饮食起居和情志调养，这对于保护孕妇和胎儿身心健康，防止流产具有积极的作用。还介绍了乳痈的护理方法"手助捻去其汁，并令旁人助嗍饮"，以使淤积的乳汁排出，而使乳痈消散。这一护理方法一直沿用至今。在儿科护理方面，主张应经常在和暖无风的时候抱小儿于阳光中嬉戏，可使孩子身体健康，耐受风寒，不易得病。

唐代孙思邈的《千金要方》中，详细地论述了临床各科的护理及食疗、养生等内容，并高度重视妇女与儿童的保健和治疗，并把饮食疗法放在药疗之上。该书在各种疾病的诊疗中，既有药疗方，又有食疗方，如目不明者用动物肝脏，防治脚气病用谷白皮煎汤煮粥，用瓜蒌治疗糖尿病等。对消渴病的护理提出"所慎者有三：一饮酒，二房事，三咸食及面"的主张，强调了饮食护理对消渴病的重要。在护理操作技术上，孙思邈首创了用细葱管进行导尿，比法国人发明的橡皮管导尿术要早1200多年。他的预防为主的思想亦十分鲜明，主张"上医医未病之病"，教导人们"常习不唾地"，还提出"凡衣服、巾、栉、枕、镜不宜与人同之"以预防传染病。该书在"大医习业"与"大医精诚"两篇文章中，专论医德。他强调医家的医德，对病者要不分贫富贵贱、一视同仁，治病要严肃认真、全心全意；告诫医家不可以医疗技术作为获取钱财的手段。在医疗作风方面，须有德有体，仪表要端庄，举止要检点，要有社会责任感。

唐代另一著名医家王焘编撰的一部综合性巨著《外台秘要》，论述了伤寒、肺结核、疟疾、天花、霍乱等传染病的病情观察、饮食护理和生活起居等护理措施。如对肺痨患者的病情观察，指出患者午后有可能出现潮热、盗汗、面部潮红，若日益消瘦、大便赤黑色或出现腹水，则是病情加重的象征。该书还详细论述了对黄疸病的病情观察，提出："每日小便里浸少许帛，各书记日，色渐退白则瘥。"另外，还注意到了消渴患者的尿是甜的，对消渴病治疗采用饮食疗法和饮食起居的禁忌等。

（四）宋金元时期（公元960—1368年）

宋代以后，由于造纸业和印刷术的发展，为医药学著作的整理和推广创造了有利条件，医家百家争鸣，各抒己见。

著名的金元四大家，如李杲创立了脾胃学说，重视对脾胃的调养和护理。提出了一系列护理脾胃的主张，如："方怒不可食"，"勿困中饮食，食后少动作"，重视饮食、劳倦、情志三者的护理。在其《脾胃论》一书中，涉及脾胃护理的就有"用药宜禁论"、"安养心神调治脾胃论"等篇著。其重视饮食起居的调理，提出了温食、减食、养食等食养事宜。刘河间倡导火热论，主张"六气皆能化火"说，在治疗中主寒凉清热，后人称其为"寒凉派"。张子和则认为"病由邪生，攻邪已病"，弘扬"汗、吐、下"三法，而成"攻邪派"之代表。朱丹溪创立了滋阴学说，认为"阳常有余，阴常不足"，建立了滋阴降火护理法则，提出了许多宝贵的保健护理要求，如提出幼年时不宜过于饱暖；青年当晚婚以待阴气长成。朱氏还非常重视老年人的护理与保健以及小儿的身心护养。

《本草衍义》一书中，记有食盐与疾病的关系，认为"水肿者宜全禁之"。这与现代护理学的饮食调护中水肿者应吃无盐或低盐饮食是一致的。

陈自明的《妇人大全良方》论述了孕妇妊娠按月份服药方法、产前、产后护理以及食忌和孕妇药忌。

齐德之的《外科精义》中有专篇论述护理。首先提出病室环境宜安静以及"只可方便省问，不可久坐多言，劳倦患者"的探视制度。

金元时期医学家重视养生保健和饮食调护，《饮膳正要》一书中提出了养生避忌、妊娠食忌、乳母食忌、饮食避忌以及各种珍奇食品的食用食谱。记载了大量医疗、保健饮食，包括汤煎、食疗、植物食品等。继承了我国古代食、养、医结合的传统，全书总结并发展了饮食护理中的宝贵经验。该书对每种食品都同时注意到了它的食用、养生与医疗的关系。如用苦豆汤"补下元，理腰膝，温中顺气"；用生地黄鸡"治腰背疼痛，骨髓虚损，身重气乏"；用鲫鱼羹"治脾胃虚弱，泄泻久不瘥者"等。这些食物可使人强壮身体，延年益寿，是预防和治疗疾病的良药，又是鲜美可口的佳肴。该书对饮食卫生提出了护理要求，提倡："先饥后食，勿令过饱"；"不可饱食而卧，尤其夜间不可多食"；"勿食不洁或变质之物"；饮酒适量，"不可大醉"；注意口腔卫生，"食毕宜用温水漱口，睡前刷牙"等。

（五）明清时期（公元 1368—1840 年）

明代在科学技术与文化上有较大的发展，取得多方面突出的成就，出现了很多有重大意义的医学发明与创造，中医护理学也得到进一步发展，并取得了突出的成就。

吴又可在其所著的《温疫论》中，指出引起"疫病"的特殊病因是"戾气"，传染途径是自口鼻而入，无论老少强弱，触之皆病。书中记载了鼠疫、天花、白喉等传染病发病的特点、治疗与护理疫病的原则和方法。在治疗与护理的基本原则上，认为应以"客邪贵乎早逐"，而"早逐"主张早用攻下祛邪法，而祛邪必须"要识人之虚实，度邪之轻重，察病之缓急"；在护理方面详细论述了温疫病的护理要求，如在对温疫病的饮食护理方面，认为温为阳邪，易于伤津耗液，对如何及时补充津液，提出"大渴思饮冰水及冷饮，无论四时，皆可量与"，但"能饮一升，止与半升，宁使少顷再饮"，而对内热烦渴者，应给"梨汁、藕汁、蔗浆、西瓜皆可备不时之需"，用以清热止渴生津。

明代著名医药学家李时珍所著《本草纲目》，是一部重要的药物学巨著。李时珍亲自采药、炮炙，不但为患者看病还为患者煎药、喂药，并指导患者家属或弟子对患者实施护理。

名医张景岳在《景岳全书》中写道："凡伤寒饮食有宜忌者，……不欲食，不可强食，强食则助邪。"说明饮食护理的重要性。当时对瘟疫是传染性疾病已有明确的认识，如名医胡正心说"凡患瘟疫之家，将初患者之衣于甑上蒸过，则一家不得染"，明确指出传染患者的衣服要用蒸汽消毒法处理。

明代冷谦在《修龄要旨》一书中提出的"养生十六宜"，即发宜多梳、面宜多擦、目宜常运、耳宜常弹、舌宜抵腭、齿宜数叩、津宜数咽、浊宜常呵、背宜常暖、胸宜常护、腹宜常摩、谷道宜常撮、肢节宜常摇、皮肤宜常干沐浴、大小便宜闭口勿言，可谓养生术的经验之谈，至今对护理和养生有着重要的指导价值。

在清代，鸦片战争以后，大量西方医学的涌入，冲击了中医药学的发展。由于当时战争频繁，疫病流行，温病学说逐渐形成。如名医叶天士的《温热论》系统阐明了温病发生、发展的规律，提出了温病卫、气、营、血四个阶段辨证论治与辨证施护的纲领。其中，提出对于温病孕妇以"井底泥或蓝布浸冷覆盖腹上"。对老年病的防护强调颐养，主张饮食当"薄味"，力戒"酒肉厚味"；在情志方面主张"务宜怡悦开怀"，"戒嗔怒"；在病情观察方面主张温热病要注意观察舌、齿，辨斑疹，而且还指出了在观察舌象、判断病情、推测预后的同时，还应做好口腔护理。还提出"食物自适者即胃喜为补"的观点，主张使用质重味厚的血肉有情之品。

清代大疫流行频繁，对疫病的预防，除让健康者预服药物外，也非常重视采取隔离消毒的措施，如《治疫全书》说："毋近患者床榻，染其秽污；毋凭死者尺棺，触其恶臭；毋食病家时菜；毋拾死人衣物。"

清代名医钱襄的中医护理学专著《侍疾要语》，记载了饮食护理、生活起居护理和老年患者的护理，其中记录了十位百岁老人延年益寿、防病抗老经验的"十叟长寿歌"，认为要长寿就应该注意起居、饮食、锻炼和情志修养。

二、现代中医护理学

随着科学技术的发展，中医药学近几十年也逐步走向科学化、现代化。中医学和中药学既继承中医传统方法，也结合现代化诊断手段和先进的诊疗设备，更加完善了中医诊断和治疗疾病的方法，提高了中医治疗效果。现代化的中医医院相继建成，并开始了严格的医护分工。在综合性医院的中医病房及各中医院，涌现出一支中医护理专业队伍。

中医护理学也在此形势下发展，并日益成熟和完善。20世纪60年代初，中医护理培训班在南京首次举办，1959年南京出版第一部系统中医护理专著《中医护病学》，标志着中医护理学已走向新时代。1984年6月在南京召开了中华护理学会中医、中西医结合护理学术会议，会上成立了中华护理学会中医、中西医结合护理学术委员会。从此中医护理学逐步发展并日渐成熟，各种中医护理学书籍相继问世。1996—2001年学苑出版社正式出版了5本系列高等中医院校中医护理学教材，分别是《中医护理学基础》、《中医内科护理学》、《中医儿科护理学》、《中医外科护理学》和《中医妇科护理学》，为当时全国唯一一套正式出版的中医护理高等教育系列教材。2005年，国家中医药管理局委托全国中医药高等教育学会规划、组织编写了21门"新世纪全国高等中医药院校护理专业规划教材"，并由中国中医药出版社出版。

目前，中医护理队伍正在发展壮大，涌现出一大批富有献身精神、具有高中级职称的专业技术人才。中医护理的科学研究工作也有了新的进展，学术研究氛围日益浓厚，学术水平也不断提高。中医护理学术骨干主持各种有关中医护理科研课题，深入探讨中医护理学的发展，使中医护理理论更加系统、完善，逐渐形成一个独立、完整、系统的科学理论体系。

具有中医特色的护理教育事业也迅速发展，多层次、多渠道、多形式的中医特色护理教育体系正在全国范围内逐步形成。硕士、本科、高职、中专、业余、函授、短期培训等各类中医特色护理教育，培养出符合临床需求的各类中医护理人才。

1977年以来，中华护理学会和各地分会先后恢复学术活动，多次召开护理学术交流会，举办各种不同类型专题学习班和研讨班等。1980年以后，国际学术交流活动日益增多。2002年全国中医药高等教育学会护理教育研究会成立，并积极开展中医特色护理教育的学术活动。中医护理学的发展，日益受到国际护理界的重视。许多国家的护理代表团先后来参观或考察中医护理工作，不仅增进了国际学术交流，开阔了视野，活跃了学术气氛，而且扩大了中医护理事业在国际上的影响。

（马雪玲）

第二章
中医护理学基础

第一节 中医基础理论

中医护理学的理论基础是来自于中医学基础理论。本章节主要介绍中医基础理论中的阴阳、五行和藏象学说，并简要介绍其在护理学中的指导意义和应用。阴阳、五行学说属于中医哲学基础，而藏象学说等属于中医的生理认识。

中医基础理论的框架还包括病因病机、治则治法等内容。这些内容属于中医学的病理认识，在分疾病种类的护理章节中将提及。完整中医基础理论理论内容请参看相应教材。

一、阴 阳 学 说

（一）阴阳的基本含义

"阴阳"最初的涵义是指日光的向背，朝向日光则为阳，背向日光则为阴。之后"阴阳"的涵义逐渐得到引申，如向日光处温暖、明亮；背日光处寒冷、晦暗。于是古人就以光明、黑暗、温暖、寒冷分阴阳。如此不断引申，几乎把自然界所有的事物和现象都划分为阴与阳两个方面。于是"阴阳"变为一个概括自然界相互关联的事物和现象对立双方的抽象概念。

一般地说，凡是温热的、明亮的、运动的、外在的、上升的、兴奋的、机能亢进的、强大的、功能的都属于阳；反之，寒冷的、晦暗的、静止的、内在的、下降的、抑制的、机能衰退的、弱小的、物质的都属于阴。甚至把构成宇宙间万物的"气"也分为阴和阳，即清轻者为阳，重浊者为阴。由于气的运动变化是事物运动变化的总根源，因而人们又逐渐把阴阳与事物的运动变化联系起来，认为一切自然现象的变化都是阴阳消长的结果，也因此赋予了阴阳学说更为丰富的内涵。阴阳属性分类举例参见表2-1。

阴阳学说认为，自然界的一切相互关联事物和现象都存在着互相对立的阴阳两个方面。阴阳的相互对立，是说阴阳性质的相反，这种相反特性主要表现在它们之间的互相制约、互相斗争上。如温热可以驱散寒冷，冰冷可以降低高温。事物的变化和发展也正是阴阳之间相互对立和制约的结果。如夏季阳气隆盛，但夏至以后阴气渐生，用以制约炎热的阳气；冬季阴寒盛，但冬至以后阳气渐复，用以制约严寒的阴气，这样便产生了体现对立双方在制约关系中力量消长变化的寒、热、温、凉四季。

同时，阴阳之间又是相互依存。阴阳双方均以对方的存在为自身存在的前提和条件。阴阳所代表的性质或状态，如天与地、上与下、动与静、寒与热、虚与实等，不仅互相排斥，而且互为存在的条件。阳根于阴，阴根于阳，无阳则阴无以生，无阴则阳无以化。阳蕴含于阴之中，阴蕴含于阳之中。阴阳一分为二，又合二为一，对立又统一。一方的不足，也会导致对方的亏虚。所谓"孤阴不生，独阳不长"。

表 2-1 阴阳属性划分举例

分类	阳	阴
时间	白昼	夜晚
空间	天	地
季节	春,夏	秋,冬
温度	热	寒
重量	轻	重
速度	快	慢
运动	向上,向外,明显的	向下,向内,隐匿的
亮度	明亮	黑暗
性别	雄性	雌性
组织器官	皮毛	筋骨
疾病进程	急性	慢性

（二）阴阳的相互作用和关系

阴阳对立的双方,存在着互相依存的关系,阴阳两个方面,既互相对立,又互相依存,双方互为存在的条件和依据,任何一方都不能脱离另一方而单独存在。如上为阳,下为阴。没有上,也就无所谓下;没有下,也就无所谓上。热为阳,寒为阴。没有热,就无所谓寒;没有寒,也就无所谓热。非但如此,它们在一定条件下还可以向着各自相反的方向转化,即阴可转化为阳,阳也可以转化为阴。阴阳互相转化是有条件的,一般表示事物发展的物极阶段,即所谓"物极必反"。阴阳的转化,大多数也是一个由量变到质变的发展过程,而阴阳消长是一量变过程,是阴阳转化质变过程的准备阶段。其消长变化示意参见图 2-1。

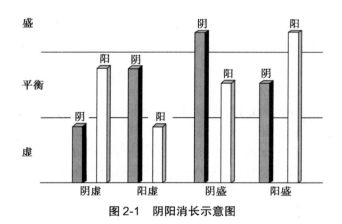

图 2-1 阴阳消长示意图

阴阳之间的这种对立制约、消长平衡、互根互用、相互转化的关系,为中医学理论提供了极为充分的思维方法,如人体的形态结构、生理现象、病理变化等,都可用阴阳来概括。

诊断为阳盛的人会有阳性症状比如:高热,烦躁,面红,脉数,苔黄。因为阳盛则热。出现阳热,则阴液也会受损,故而患者会出现口干、口渴、舌干的症状。其他典型表现参见表 2-2。

表 2-2　阴阳盛衰典型表现

	典型表现
阳盛	发热，恶热，口渴喜冷饮，面红，烦躁，痰黄，尿赤，便秘，舌红，苔黄，脉数
阴盛	畏寒，口不渴，喜热饮，痰液清稀，便溏，面白，舌淡，苔白，脉迟紧
阳虚	喜温，肢冷，面白，自汗，疲倦，气短，便溏，舌淡胖，苔白，脉沉迟弱
阴虚	口渴，口干，咽干，五心烦热，午后潮热，盗汗，舌红少苔，脉细数

因为个体的差异，在临床中每个患者又各自有不同的辨证。即便是一个患者，随着疾病发展、生活方式或者环境的改变，相应的诊断也会发生改变。而阴阳的诊断是基于患者某个特定时期所有症状体征的综合分析。

（三）阴阳学说在中医护理学中的应用

阴阳失调是疾病发生、发展的根本原因，所以调整阴阳、补其不足、泻其有余、恢复阴阳的相对平衡，就是疾病治疗与护理的基本原则。

1. 阴阳偏盛的治则　阴阳偏盛，即阴或阳的过盛有余，多为邪气有余的病证。

由于阳盛则热，阳盛则阴病，阳热盛易于损耗阴液。阳盛则热属实热证，宜用寒凉药以制其阳，治热以寒，即"热者寒之"。

阴盛则寒，阴盛则阳病，阴寒盛易于损伤阳气。阴盛则寒属实寒证，宜用温热药以制其阴，治寒以热，即"寒者热之"。

2. 阴阳偏衰的治则　阴阳偏衰，即阴或阳虚损不足，或为阴虚，或为阳虚，可直接采取滋阴或温阳之法。

如果阴虚不能制阳而致阳偏亢者，属虚热证，一般不能用寒凉药直折其热，须用滋阴壮水法，以抑制阳亢热盛，即"壮水之主，以制阳光"。

如果阳虚不能制阴而导致阴偏盛者，属虚寒证，更不宜用辛温发散药以散阴寒，须"益火之源，以消阴翳"。

在治疗阴阳偏衰时，根据阴阳互用的原理，还可考虑"阴中求阳，阳中求阴"之法，即在用温阳药时兼用滋阴药，在用滋阴药时加用补阳药，以发挥阴阳互用的生化作用。

二、五 行 学 说

五行学说，是运用木、火、土、金、水五种物质的运动变化规律，阐释宇宙事物的相互联系和运动变化的古代哲学理论。

古代自然哲学的五行学说渗透到中医学，与医学理论和实践相结合，以五行的运动规律阐释人体生理、病理及其与外在环境的相互联系，进而指导临床诊断、治疗与护理，从而形成了中医独特的五行学说。

（一）五行的基本含义

五，指木、火、土、金、水五种物质。行，意为运动变化、运行不息。五行，即木、火、土、金、水五种物质的运动变化和相互作用。

在长期生活实践中，人们认识到木、火、土、金、水五种物质是人类生活中不可或缺的物质，故称其为"五材"。五行学说是在"五材"说的基础上，将五种物质的属性加以抽象描述，用以说明自然界一切事物和现象之间相生、相克的运动变化的一门学说。

中医学运用五行特性、归类以及生克规律，来概括脏腑组织的功能属性，阐释五脏系统的内在联系,借以说明人体的生理、病理及其与外在环境的相互关系等,从而指导辨证论治,达到预防和治疗疾病的目的。

（二）五行特性和五行归类

1. 五行特性 是古人在对木、火、土、金、水五种物质的朴素认识基础上,进行抽象升华而逐渐形成的理论含义。主要用于分析各种事物的五行属性和研究事物之间的相互联系。对五行特性的认识已超越了五种具体物质的本身,而具有更为抽象、广泛的涵义。

木的特性:古人称"木曰曲直"。曲直,是指树木的枝干能曲能直,向上向外舒展。因而引申为具有生长、升发、条达舒畅等作用或性质的事物,均归属于木。

火的特性:古人称"火曰炎上"。炎上,是指火具有温热、上升的特性。因而引申为具有温热、升腾等作用或性质的事物,均归属于火。

土的特性:古人称"土爰稼穑"。"爰"通"曰"。稼穑,是指土地可播种和收获农作物。因而引申为具有生化、承载、受纳等作用或性质的事物,均归属于土。

金的特性:古人称"金曰从革"。从革,是指金可顺从人意,改变其状。因而引申为具有清洁、肃降、收敛等作用或性质的事物,均归属于金。

水的特性:古人称"水曰润下"。润下,是指水具有滋润和向下的特性。因而引申为具有寒凉、滋润、向下运行等作用或性质的事物,均归属于水。

2. 五行归类 五行学说是以五行的特性来推演和归类事物的五行属性。事物的五行属性并不等同于木、火、土、金、水五类物质本身,而是将事物的性质和作用,与五行的特性相类比,从而得出事物的五行属性。例如:与木的特性相类似的事物,则归属于木;与火的特性相类似的事物,则归属于火。再例如:东方为日出之地,富有生机,与木的升发、生长特性相类,故归属于木;南方气候炎热,植物繁茂,与火的炎上特性相类,故归属于火。

五行学说对事物属性的推演归类以天人相应为指导原则,以五行为中心,以空间结构的五方、时间结构的五季、人体结构的五脏为基本框架,将自然界的各种事物和现象及人体的生理病理现象按其属性进行归纳,见表2-3。

表 2-3 五行归类表

自然界							五行	人体							
五音	五味	五色	五化	五气	五季	五方		五脏	五腑	五体	五华	五志	五官	五液	五脉
角	酸	青	生	风	春	东	木	肝	胆	筋	爪	怒	目	泪	弦
徵	苦	赤	长	暑	夏	南	火	心	小肠	脉	面	喜	舌	汗	洪
宫	甘	黄	化	湿	长夏	中	土	脾	胃	肉	唇	思	口	涎	缓
商	辛	白	收	燥	秋	西	金	肺	大肠	皮	毛	悲	鼻	涕	浮
羽	咸	黑	藏	寒	冬	北	水	肾	膀胱	骨	发	恐	耳	唾	沉

由此可见,根据五行特性,自然界千变万化的事物和现象均可归结为木、火、土、金、水的五行系统,人体的各种组织和功能也可归结为以五脏为中心的五个生理系统。

（三）五行学说在中医护理学中的应用

1. 确定疾病治则与治法 根据相生规律确定的治则是补母和泻子,治法主要有滋水涵木、金水相生、培土生金、益火补土等。根据相克规律确定的治则包括抑强和扶弱,治法主要有抑木扶土、培土制水、佐金平木、泻南补北等。

2. 控制疾病传变　中医学运用五行生克乘侮关系，既可推断和概括疾病的传变规律，又可确定预防性治疗措施。例如：肝病容易传脾，治疗时可以先健脾，防止肝病传脾。

3. 指导精神疗法　精神疗法主要适用于情志失调病证。中医学运用五行生克乘侮关系，以悲、恐、怒、喜、思的五情配五脏，利用五行相互制约的关系达到疾病治疗的目的。例如：悲为肺志，属金；怒为肝志，属木。金克木，故悲能胜怒。

五行生克规律对疾病治疗与护理具有一定的指导意义，但并非适用于所有的病证，临床上必须根据具体情况灵活运用。

三、藏 象 学 说

藏，是指藏于体内的脏腑组织器官；象，是指表现于外的生理、病理现象。

藏象学说中的脏腑，不完全等同于现代解剖学中的脏器。藏象学说中的脏腑，不单纯是一个形态器官，而主要是指一个功能活动系统。

根据内脏的功能特点，可分为脏、腑、奇恒之腑。脏，即心、肺、脾、肝、肾，合称为五脏。其共同的生理功能是化生和贮藏精气，特点是藏而不泻，满而不实。腑，即胆、胃、大肠、小肠、三焦、膀胱，合称为六腑，其共同的生理功能是受盛和传化水谷，特点是泻而不藏，实而不满。奇恒之腑，即脑、髓、骨、脉、胆、女子胞（子宫）。因其功能似脏，主贮藏精气，而形态似腑，为中空器官，有异于正常的五脏、六腑，故称奇恒之腑。本节只论述五脏和六腑。

（一）心与小肠

1. 心　心的生理功能主要是主血脉和主藏神。心与小肠通过经脉相互络属，构成表里关系。心为"君主之官"，"五脏六腑之大主"，在人体生命活动中起主宰作用。

（1）心的主要生理功能

1）主血脉：心主血脉，指心脏具有生成血液并推动血液在经脉内运行的生理功能。

①心主生血：血液主要由营气和津液所化生，而营气和津液在化生血液过程中需要心阳的温煦和气化才能化赤为血液。

②心主行血：指心气具有推动血液在血脉内运行的作用。心脏与血脉形成一个密闭循环的系统，血液在血脉中正常运行依赖于心气的推动作用。心气充沛，心主血脉功能正常，则面色红润而有光泽，脉搏节律均匀、和缓有力。反之，心气不足可见心慌心悸、面色无华、脉虚无力，甚则气滞血瘀，而见心前区憋闷刺痛、面色灰暗、唇舌青紫、脉搏节律不整等。

2）主藏神：心主藏神，指心具有主宰人的精神、意识、思维活动以及人体生命活动的作用。

心主藏神功能正常，则精神振作、神志清晰、思维敏捷，对外界信息的反应灵敏。反之，如心血虚，血不养心，可见心悸、健忘、失眠、多梦；痰迷心窍，可见神昏、痴呆、举止失常；痰火扰心，则可见躁狂，甚至影响他脏而危及生命。

心主藏神与心主血脉的生理功能密切相关。血液是神志活动的物质基础，精神活动能调节和影响血液循环。如果心主血脉功能失常，如血虚、血热等，常可出现神志的改变；若心神不安，也可引起血行不畅。

（2）心与志、液、体和窍的关系

1）在志为喜：喜乐愉悦，一般说来，属于良性的刺激，有助于心主血脉等生理功能。但喜乐过度，则又可使心神受伤，神志涣散而不能集中或内守，甚则出现喜笑不休，精神失常等神志病变。

2）在液为汗：汗为津液所化生，血与津液又同出水谷精气之源，且互生互化，津液渗入脉内可生成血液，血液渗出脉外则化为津液，故有"血汗同源"之说；而血又为心所主，心血充盈，津液充足，汗化有源，心又主藏神，汗液生成排泄受心神的调节。

3）在体合脉，其华在面：在体合脉即全身的血脉都属于心。若心气旺盛，则脉搏和缓有力、节律均匀；如心气虚损，则见脉搏细弱无力。其华在面，指心的生理功能正常与否，反映于面部的色泽变化。若心气旺盛，血脉充盈，则面部红润而有光泽；如心气虚损，则面色白甚或滞暗；若心血虚少，则可见面色苍白无华；心血瘀阻，则可见面色青紫等。

4）在窍为舌：心开窍于舌，是指舌为心之外候。如心的功能正常，则舌体红活荣润、柔软灵活、味觉灵敏、语言流利。心主血脉功能异常，心阳不足，可见舌质淡白胖嫩；心阴血不足，则舌质红绛瘦瘪；心火上炎则可见舌红，甚则生疮；心血瘀阻，则可见舌质暗紫，或有瘀斑；心主神志的功能异常，则可见舌卷、舌强、语謇或失语等症。

2. 小肠 小肠位于腹腔，其上端与胃相通，下端与大肠相连，小肠的生理功能主要有主受盛与化物、泌别清浊。

（1）主受盛与化物：是指小肠接受经胃下传的食糜而盛纳之，食糜在小肠内停留一定的时间，以便进一步充分地消化和吸收。若小肠的受盛功能失常，则可见腹部胀闷疼痛，如化物功能失常，可致消化不良、腹泻，甚则完谷不化等。

（2）泌别清浊：是指小肠能将经胃下降到小肠的食物，分为水谷精微及食物残渣两部分，吸收水谷精微并把食物残渣下降到大肠，在吸收水谷精微同时也吸收大量水分，并把废液下输膀胱。

小肠泌别清浊功能正常，则清浊各走其道。如小肠泌别清浊失常，则见大便稀薄、小便短少等症。

（二）肺与大肠

1. 肺 肺生理功能主要是主气，主宣发和肃降，通调水道，肺朝百脉、主治节。肺与大肠通过经脉相互络属，构成表里关系。肺在五脏中位置最高，故有"华盖"之称。肺叶娇嫩，易受外邪，故又有"娇脏"之称。

（1）肺的主要生理功能

1）肺主气：肺主气，即指全身的气均由肺来主持管理。肺主气包括主呼吸之气与主一身之气两方面。

①主呼吸之气：是指肺具有呼出体内浊气，吸入自然界清气，实现人体内外气体交换，从而维持人体新陈代谢顺利进行的作用。

②主一身之气：是指肺有主持、调节全身各脏腑经络之气生成和运行的作用。肺主一身之气主要体现于以下两个方面：

一是气的生成方面，主要是宗气的生成。宗气的生成主要来源于肺吸入的自然界清气和脾胃运化来的水谷精微之气，两者结合而产生宗气并积聚于胸中。宗气的主要功能是上出喉咙助肺以司呼吸，贯注心脉助心以行气血。肺通过宗气的生成起到了主一身之气的作用。

二是肺能调节全身的气机。肺的呼吸运动，即气的升降出入运动，而气的升降出入运动即气机。因此，肺有节律的一呼一吸，对全身之气的升降出入运动起着重要的调节作用。

一般来说，肺主气的生理功能失常，一方面表现为呼吸功能失常，如呼吸无力，动则气喘，或咳喘胸闷等症；另一方面则表现为主一身之气功能失常，可见身倦乏力，语声低微，血运不畅及或水液代谢障碍等病变。

2）主宣发和肃降：所谓肺主宣发，是指肺气具有向上、向外升宣布散的生理功能；所谓肺主肃降，即指肺气具有向下通降和使呼吸道保持洁净的生理功能。

肺主宣发的功能主要体现于三个方面：一是排出浊气，完成气体交换；二是宣发卫气，温养肌肤，抵御外邪，调节腠理之开合，控制汗液的排出；三是将脾胃运化来的水谷精微及津液布散于周身，润泽皮毛。因此，肺气失宣可见咳喘、畏寒，或自汗、易感外邪，或痰饮、颜面周身水肿等。

肺主肃降亦体现于三个方面：一是吸入自然界的清气。二是将脾传输至肺的水谷精微和津液向下、向内布散，以濡润脏腑组织。肃降作用还可把代谢后的水液下输到膀胱生成尿液排出到体外，还有利于大肠传导糟粕。三是肃清呼吸道的痰浊等异物，保持呼吸道的洁净、通畅。因此，肺主肃降的生理功能失常，可出现呼吸急促表浅、胸闷、咳喘，或小便不利、痰饮水肿，或便秘等。

在正常生理情况下，肺气的宣发和肃降相互依存，相互制约，能宣能降，则肺呼吸平稳自如。在病理情况下两者的功能失去协调，即可出现"肺气失宣"或"肺失肃降"等病变，临床可见胸闷、咳嗽及喘息、痰饮等病证。

3）通调水道：肺主通调水道，是指肺的宣发和肃降对人体水液代谢具有疏通和调节作用。肺气宣发，可将人体的津液布散于皮毛周身，还能布散卫气，主司腠理开合，将代谢后的水液，通过汗孔排出于体外，同时，肺的呼气还可带走一部分水分。肺气肃降，不但可使津液向下布散，还可将代谢后的水液经肾的气化作用下输到膀胱，生成尿液排出于体外，同时，肺的肃降，推动大肠的传导，通过大便排出一部分水液。可见肺通调水道功能正常，机体水液代谢才能正常。如果肺通调水道功能失调，可导致水液代谢障碍，出现痰饮停滞等病理变化。

4）肺朝百脉、主治节：肺朝百脉，是指全身的血液，都通过经脉聚会于肺。通过肺的呼浊吸清，进行气体交换，再通过肺宣发和肃降、助心行血，可将富含养分的血液经过百脉输送到全身。治节，即治理调节。肺主治节是指肺辅助心脏治理调节全身气、血、津液及脏腑生理功能的作用。因此，肺气充沛，全身的气血生成和运行顺畅。反之，肺气虚衰，不能辅助心脏以行气血，血液运行迟滞，则可见胸闷心悸、唇青舌紫等气虚血瘀之象。

（2）肺与志、液、体和窍的关系

1）在志为悲（忧）：悲哀和忧伤使气不断地消耗，即所谓"悲则气消"。由于肺主气，所以过度悲忧易于伤肺，出现呼吸气短等肺气不足之象。反之，在肺虚时，人体对外来非良性刺激的耐受性就会下降，从而易于产生悲忧的情绪变化。

2）在液为涕：涕为鼻腔分泌液，而肺开窍于鼻。肺中精气充足，涕液润泽鼻窍而不外流，并能防御外邪，有利于肺的呼吸。如风寒犯肺，则鼻流清涕；风热犯肺，则鼻流黄稠涕；燥邪伤肺，则鼻干而无涕。

3）在体合皮，其华在毛：皮毛，为一身之表。肺气具有宣发卫气和轻清之气输布到体表等生理功能，起到温养肌肤、润泽皮毛，分泌汗液、调节体温，抵御外邪等生理功能，故肺与皮毛联系密切。肺气充足，则皮肤致密，毫毛光泽，抗御外邪侵袭的能力亦较强；反之，肺气虚损，宣发卫气和输精于皮毛的功能减弱，则卫表不固，抗御外邪侵袭之能力低下，出现多汗或自汗，易于感冒，或皮毛憔悴枯槁等病理表现。

4）在窍为鼻：肺气宣畅，则鼻的通气和嗅觉功能正常，表现为鼻窍通利，嗅觉灵敏。反之,肺气失宣,可见鼻塞、流涕、喷嚏等。由于肺开窍于鼻,故外邪侵袭,也常从口鼻而入,引发肺的病变。

2. 大肠　大肠的主要生理功能是传导糟粕。大肠接受小肠泌别清浊后的糟粕,并吸收多余水分后化为粪便排出体外。若大肠传导功能正常,则大便的质、量、次数正常,若大肠吸收水分过多,则大便干结而致便秘;反之,可见腹泻,大便稀溏。

(三)脾与胃

脾主要生理功能是主运化、主升清、主统血。脾与胃通过经脉相互络属,构成表里关系。脾将水谷化为精微,为人出生后的生命活动和气血生成奠定基础,故称为"后天之本"、"气血生化之源"。

1. 脾

(1)脾的主要生理功能

1)主运化:是指脾具有消化吸收食物中的水谷精微并将其传输至全身的生理功能。脾的运化功能包括运化水谷和运化水液两个方面。

①运化水谷:指脾对食物的消化、吸收和运化作用。食物的消化虽然在胃肠进行,但必须依赖于脾的运化,才能把饮食水谷消化成精微物质。同样,精微物质亦要靠脾的运化,才能被吸收,并传输到各脏腑组织器官。脾的运化水谷功能旺盛,全赖于脾气,只有在脾气强健的情况下,水谷精微才得以正常的消化吸收,为化生精、气、血、津液提供足够的养料,从而使人体脏腑、经络、四肢百骸,以及皮毛筋肉等得到充分的营养。若脾气虚损,运化水谷的功能减退,则可出现腹胀、便溏、食欲缺乏,甚则倦怠乏力,面黄肌瘦等气血生化不足的症状。

②运化水液:是指脾对水液的吸收、传输功能。包括两个方面:一是摄入到人体内的水液,需经过脾的运化传输,气化成津液,布达周身脏腑组织器官,发挥其滋润、濡养作用;二是经过代谢后的水液,亦要经过脾传输,而至肺、肾,通过肺、肾的气化作用,化为汗、尿等而排出体外,以维持人体水液代谢的协调平衡。脾气充足,即可保证运化水液功能的正常发挥,又可防止水、湿、痰、饮等病理产物的产生。如果脾气虚,运化水液功能减退,则水液停滞于局部,即可产生痰饮、湿浊、水肿等病变。

2)主升清:是指脾具有把水谷精微上输于心、肺、头目及维持人体脏器位置恒定的生理功能。脾主升清的功能主要体现在以下两个方面:

①将水谷精微上输于心肺头目:脾主升清可将水谷精微上输于心肺头目,以滋养清窍,并通过心肺的作用化生气血,以营养周身。若脾不升清,可见面色无华、头晕目眩、腹胀、慢性泄泻等症。

②维持内脏位置的相对恒定:内脏之所以能保持其位置的相对恒定,是有赖于脾气主升清的作用。如果脾气虚损,不能升清反而下陷,则可导致人体内脏下垂,如胃下垂、子宫脱垂、久泻脱肛等。

3)主统血:是指脾具有统摄血液在经脉内运行,防止逸出脉外的功能。脾气强健,统摄有权,血液才不会逸出于脉外而致出血;反之,脾的运化功能减退,则气血虚亏,气的固摄功能减退,则导致出血。

(2)脾与志、液、体和窍的关系

1)在志为思:思虑过度,导致气滞与气结,影响脾的运化和升清功能,出现食欲缺乏,脘腹胀闷,头目眩晕等症,即所谓"思则气结"。

2）在液为涎：涎为口津，是唾液中较清稀的部分。脾的运化和升清功能正常，则津液上行于口，但不溢出于口外而为涎，有助于食物的吞咽和消化。若脾胃不和，则导致涎液分泌急剧增加，出现口涎自出等现象。

3）在体合肌肉、主四肢：脾气健运，气血生化有源，才能保持肌肉丰满，四肢健壮有力。若脾失健运，气血化源不足，肌肉失养，则可致肌肉瘦削无力，甚至痿软不用。

4）在窍为口、其华在唇：脾气强健，则饮食、口味、唇色才能正常。若脾失健运，则可见食欲缺乏、口淡无味、口腻、口甜等异常感觉，或唇色异常，如青紫、苍白无华等。

2. 胃　胃的生理功能主要有受纳、腐熟水谷、主通降，以降为和。

（1）受纳、腐熟水谷：是指胃有接受和容纳食物，并初步消化，使水谷变成食糜，有利于进一步消化吸收的生理功能。如胃受纳、腐熟水谷正常，则食欲正常；如胃的受纳、腐熟功能失常，则表现为食欲缺乏、胃脘部胀满疼痛、饮食停滞，或吞酸嘈杂、消谷善饥等。

（2）主通降：是指胃有通利下降的生理功能及特性，以通降为正常。食物经过胃的受纳腐熟并保留一定时间后，必须下降到小肠，泌别清浊，其清者，经脾的运化输布周身，浊者继续下降到大肠，形成糟粕排出到体外。若胃的通降功能失常，胃失和降，可见脘腹胀满或疼痛、口臭、大便秘结等症；胃气不降，反而上逆，则可见恶心、呕吐、嗳腐吞酸及呃逆等症。

（四）肝与胆

肝脏主要生理功能是主疏泄、主藏血。肝与胆通过经脉相互络属，构成表里关系。肝性主升、主动，喜条达而恶抑郁，故有"刚脏"之称。

1. 肝

（1）肝的主要生理功能

1）主疏泄：指肝脏可以疏通调节人体气的作用，进而促进血液运行和津液代谢、调节脾胃运化、胆汁分泌与排泄、情志活动，以及男子排精和女子行经等，具体表现在以下几个方面：

①调畅气机：肝的疏泄功能正常，则人体气机调畅，气血和调，经脉通利，各脏腑组织器官的功能正常、协调。若肝主疏泄功能减退，导致人体气机阻滞不畅，则出现胸胁、两乳或少腹胀闷疼痛、情志郁闷及血或津液运动障碍等病理现象；肝的疏泄功能太过，可出现头胀头痛、面红目赤、心烦易怒，甚则呕血、咯血等。

②促进血液运行和津液输布代谢：气行则血行，气滞则血瘀；气行则水行，气滞则水停。而肝主疏泄，能调畅气机。肝主疏泄的生理功能正常，气机调畅，则血与津液运行通利。反之，肝气郁滞，则可导致血及津液的病变，如气滞日久，可形成血瘀，或肿块；血随气逆，则可致吐血、咯血，甚则猝然昏倒、不省人事。若肝失疏泄，气的升降出入障碍，则导致水湿停留于人体，生成水、湿、痰、饮等病理产物。

③促进脾胃的运化：一方面，肝主疏泄的功能正常，脾胃才能升清降浊有序，食物方能得以正常的消化吸收和排泄。肝失疏泄，脾胃升降失司，而致食物的消化吸收及排泄异常。如肝气失疏泄，影响脾的升清功能，则见眩晕，腹泻等症；影响胃的受纳与腐熟功能，则见呕逆嗳气、脘腹胀满、便秘等症。另一方面，肝主疏泄正常，肝脏生成、分泌胆汁，以助消化则正常；如肝失疏泄，则胆汁生成排泄障碍，可见胁肋胀满疼痛、口苦、纳食不化等症。若胆汁外溢于皮肤，则可见黄疸等病证。

④调畅情志：如果肝气升发太过，可见急躁易怒、头胀头痛等症。若肝气疏泄功能不及，肝气郁结，可见情绪低沉、抑郁寡欢、多疑善虑等症。

⑤调节男子排精和妇女行经：肝的疏泄功能正常，气机调畅，则男子排精通畅、有度，女子月经正常通畅；反之，肝的疏泄功能失常，气机不畅，则男子排精失畅、无度，女子月经不调，经行不畅。

2）主藏血：是指肝脏具有贮藏血液、调节血量和防止出血的生理功能。表现在三个方面：一是肝脏贮藏一定的血量，以涵敛肝阳，防止其生发太过；二是肝脏根据机体需要，调节血量分配，人动则血运于诸经，人静则血归于肝脏；三是肝藏血的功能有助于血液收摄在血脉之中，可以防止出血。因此，肝不藏血既可见肝血虚少的目暗昏花、筋脉拘急、妇女月经量少、闭经等，还可见肝阳生发太过的急躁易怒等，又可见各种出血证。

（2）肝与志、液、体和窍的关系

1）在志为怒：一方面，怒可以伤肝，导致疏泄失常，肝气亢奋，血随气涌，可见面红目赤，甚则可见吐血、衄血、猝然昏倒、不省人事。另一方面，肝失疏泄，也可致情志失常，表现为情绪抑郁，或急躁易怒。

2）在液为泪：肝之气血调和，则泪液濡润目而不外溢。反之，如肝阴血不足，则两目干涩；如肝经风热，则可见两目红赤，羞光流泪；肝经湿热，则可见目眵增多等症。

3）在体合筋，其华在爪：中医的"筋"包括韧带和肌腱等结构。如肝血虚少，血不养筋，可见肢体麻木、屈伸不利，甚则手足震颤；若热邪燔灼肝经，劫夺肝阴，筋脉失养，则可见四肢抽搐、颈项强直、角弓反张等动风之象。

4）在窍为目：若肝之阴血不足，则可见两目干涩，视物昏花或夜盲；肝火上炎，则可见两目红肿热痛；肝阴虚而阳亢，可见头晕目眩。

2. 胆 胆的生理功能主要是贮藏和排泄胆汁。肝疏泄正常，胆汁生成、排泄正常，水谷消化吸收则正常。如肝疏泄功能失常，胆汁不能正常生成和排泄，则可见胁痛腹胀、食欲缺乏、恶心、呕吐；胆汁上逆，则可见口苦、呕吐黄绿苦水等；若胆汁外溢肌肤，则见身、面、目俱黄的黄疸症。

（五）肾与膀胱

1. 肾 肾主要生理功能是肾主藏精，肾主水液，肾主纳气。肾与膀胱通过经脉相互络属，构成表里关系。肾藏先天之精，为生命之源，故称为"先天之本"。

（1）肾的主要生理功能

1）肾主藏精：指肾对精气具有闭藏作用，可使肾中精气不无故流失，从而发挥促进人体生长、发育与生殖并调控全身各脏腑生理活动的作用。肾为封藏之本，主藏精。肾所藏的精，包括"先天之精"和部分"后天之精"。先天之精，来源于父母的生殖之精，与生俱来，是构成胚胎发育的原始物质，又称为"生殖之精"。后天之精，来源于脾胃运化生成的精微物质，藏于五脏六腑，又称为"脏腑之精"。各脏腑之精在完成各脏腑生理功能后多余的部分输送至肾，以充养"先天之精"。"先天之精"和"后天之精"互相融合构成"肾精"。"肾精"是化生肾气的物质基础。肾中精气的生理功能主要是促进人体的生长、发育和生殖，并调控全身各脏腑生理活动。人的整个生、长、壮、老、已的生命过程，都由肾中精气的盛衰主管和调节。肾中精气旺盛，人的生长、发育和生殖能力较强；肾中精气虚衰，在幼年，可见小儿发育障碍；在成年人，可见早衰现象，还可致性功能减退、闭经、不孕等。因此，保养肾中精气，对养生保健、预防早衰、延年益寿具有重要意义。

肾精化为肾气，肾气又可分为肾阴、肾阳两个方面的生理效应。肾阴具有凉润、宁静、抑制等作用，肾阳具有温煦、推动、兴奋等作用。肾阴、肾阳相互制约、相互协调，共同维持并调控着各脏腑阴阳的平衡。若肾阴虚，则现五心烦热、腰膝酸软、耳鸣、眩晕、遗精、舌红少津等症；若肾阳虚，则见形寒肢冷、腰膝酸困、冷痛、小便清长、或不利、或遗尿、性欲低下、水肿、舌质淡等症。

2）肾主水液：是指肾中精气具有主持和调节体内津液的输布和排泄，维持津液代谢平衡的作用。在整个水液代谢过程中，涉及多个脏腑一系列活动，而肾中精气起着主持和调节作用。如果肾中精气的蒸腾气化功能失常，可引起小便不利、水肿、遗尿、尿失禁等病理变化。

3）肾主纳气：是指肾有摄纳肺所吸入的清气，保持呼吸深度的生理功能。人体的呼吸虽然由肺来主司，但肺所吸入的清气，必须下达到肾，靠肾的封藏作用才能摄纳潜藏，保持呼吸深度。故有"肺为气之主，肾为气之根，肺主出气，肾主纳气"的说法。肾中精气充盛，摄纳有权，则呼吸均匀和调；反之，肾中精气不足，摄纳无权，则肺气上浮而不下行，可出现呼吸表浅，动则气喘，呼多吸少或呼吸困难等症。

（2）肾与志、液、体和窍的关系

1）在志为恐：恐则气下，肾气不能向上布散而下泄，则出现二便失禁等。

2）在液为唾：若唾多或久唾，则易耗伤肾中精气。所以，养生家以舌抵上腭，待津唾满口后，咽之以养肾精，称此法为"饮玉浆"。

3）在体为骨，生髓，其华在发：肾精充盛，骨髓充足，骨骼得养，则骨坚劲有力，牙齿坚固，故又称"齿为骨之余"。若肾精不足，骨髓空虚，骨骼失养，在小儿可见生长发育迟缓、骨软无力、囟门迟闭；在成人可见腰膝酸软、足痿不能行走；在老年人则易发生骨折、牙齿松动。

肾其华在发，肾气强盛，则头发浓密乌黑而有光泽；肾气衰弱，头发花白脱落，失去光泽。

4）在窍为耳及二阴：肾精充足，髓海得养，则耳的听觉功能正常；肾中精气虚衰，髓海空虚，则可见听力减退，或见耳鸣、耳聋。

二阴，即前阴和后阴。前阴具有排尿及生殖功能；后阴是排泄粪便的通道。人的生殖功能依赖于肾中精气的充盛，而尿液和粪便的排泄也与肾的气化密切相关，故有"肾司二便"、"肾开窍于二阴"的说法。

2. 膀胱 膀胱的主要生理功能为贮尿和排尿。肾气充足，膀胱开合有度；若肾气虚，气化失常，引起膀胱的气化不利，则可见排尿不畅，甚或癃闭；若肾气虚，固摄失常，引起膀胱失于约束，则可见小便频数、量多、遗尿或尿失禁。

（六）心包与三焦

1. 心包 心包是心脏外面的包膜，其功能为保护心脏，代心受邪。藏象学说认为心为君主之官，邪不能犯，所以外邪侵犯到人体的心时，首先侵犯心包络，其临床表现主要是藏神的功能的异常。如在外感温热病中，因温热之邪内陷，出现神昏、高热、谵语、妄言等心神受扰的病态时，称为"热入心包"。实际上，心包受邪所出现的病变与心是一致的，所以在辨证治疗上也大体相同。

2. 三焦 三焦为六腑之一，是上、中、下三焦的合称。关于"焦"的含义，历代医家认识不一。有认为"焦"为体内脏器是有形之物。有认为"焦"指能腐熟水谷变化的功能。有认为"焦"谓人体有上、中、下三节段也。

《内经》不但首先提出三焦的名称，并作为六腑之一，与心包相为表里，同时还论述了三焦的部位和功能。由于《内经》对三焦的某些具体概念的论述不够明确，而且《难经》又提出三焦的"有名无形"说，使后世医家众说纷纭。而争论的焦点是在有无实质形体的问题上但对三焦的生理功能的认识都是一致的。认为三焦的主要生理功能为：一是主持诸气，二是水液运行的道路。

1）总司全身的气机和气化：三焦是气升降出入的通道，也是气化的场所。也就是说，气的运行于周身脏腑，是通过三焦的通道来实现的，故三焦有主总司气机和气化的功能。

2）为水液运行的通道：三焦有疏通水道、运行水液的作用，是人体水液升降出入的道路。

（七）脏腑辨证与中医护理

脏腑是构成人体的一个密切联系的有机整体。五脏之间有生克乘侮的关系，脏腑之间有表里的联系，经络将人体五脏六腑、四肢百骸、五官九窍、皮肉筋脉等联结为一个有机的统一整体。

脏腑辨证，是脏腑功能失调发生的病理变化反映于临床的不同证候。脏腑辨证就是以脏腑为纲，根据各个脏腑不同的生理功能和病理变化对疾病进行辨证，是明确病变部位及性质的辨证方法。脏腑辨证是中医内科疾病辨证论治的核心，也是中医辨证护理的基本要素。

以上基础理论部分内容是指导中医护理学实践的理论基础。中医护理学以中医理论为指导，以整体护理、辨证施护为特色，包括预防、保健、护理和康复等多个环节的护理知识和技能，具有独特的临床特色和辅助疗效。

（李晓莉）

第二节　经　络　腧　穴

一、经　　络

（一）经络的概念

经络是运行气血、联系脏腑和体表、沟通全身各部的通路。经，有"路径"、"通道"的意思，就是纵行的主线，是经络系统中的主干，深而在里，贯通上下，沟通内外；络，有"网络"的意思，是经络别出的细小分支，浅而在表，纵横交错，网络全身。

（二）经络系统的组成

经络系统由经脉、络脉和连属于体表的经筋和皮部组成。经脉主要包括十二经脉、奇经八脉和十二经别，络脉包括十五络脉和网络周身、难计其数的浮络、孙络等（图2-2）。

1. 十二经脉　十二经脉是经络系统的主体，在内属于脏腑，在外联络四肢、头面和躯干，是气血运行的主要通道。十二经脉也称十二正经，包括手三阴经、手三阳经、足三阳经、足三阴经。

十二经脉有一定的起止、循行部位和交接顺序，在肢体的分布和走向有一定的规律，与体内脏腑有直接的络属关系，相互之间有表里关系。

（1）十二经脉的名称及含义：十二经脉的名称由手足、阴阳和脏腑三部分组成（表2-4）。手足，表示经脉的外行路线分别分布于上肢和下肢，行于上肢的称为手经，行于下肢的称为足经。阴阳，表示经脉的阴阳属性和阴气阳气的多少，阴经循行于肢体内侧，阳经循行于肢体外侧。阴气最盛为太阴，其次为少阴，再次为厥阴；阳气最盛为阳明，其次为太阳，再次为少阳。脏腑，表示经脉所连属的脏腑。

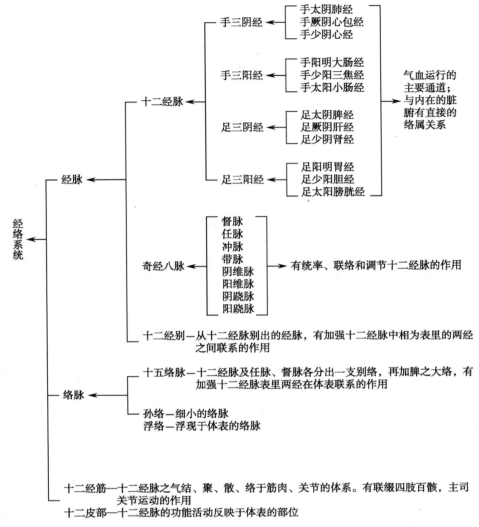

图2-2　经络系统简表

表2-4　十二经脉名称分类表

	阴经（属脏）	阳经（属腑）	循行部位（阴经行内侧、阳经行外侧）	
手	太阴肺经	阳明大肠经	上肢	前缘
	厥阴心包经	少阳三焦经		中线
	少阴心经	太阳小肠经		后缘
足	太阴脾经	阳明胃经	下肢	前缘
	厥阴肝经	少阳胆经		中线
	少阴肾经	太阳膀胱经		后缘

（2）十二经脉在体表的分布：十二经脉在体表左右成对分布于头面、躯干和四肢，称为外行部分。

经络腧穴分布定位的方位术语与现代解剖学不完全相同。比如：将上肢的掌侧称为内侧，上肢的背侧称为外侧；将下肢向正中线的一侧称为内侧，远离正中线的一侧称为外侧。

十二经脉在体表的分布大多是纵行的。除足阳明胃经外，阴经均行于四肢内侧及躯干的胸腹面，阳经均行于四肢外侧及躯干的背面。手经行于上肢，足经行于下肢。

在四肢部，阴经分布在内侧面，阳经分布在外侧面，内侧分三阴，外侧分三阳。上肢内侧为太阴经在前，厥阴经在中，少阴经在后；上肢外侧为阳明经在前，少阳经在中，太阳经在后；下肢内侧，内踝尖上8寸以下为厥阴经在前，太阴经在中，少阴经在后；内踝尖上8寸以上则太阴经在前，厥阴经在中，少阴经在后；下肢外侧为阳明经在前，少阳经在中，太阳经在后。

在头面部，阳明经行于面部；太阳经行于面颊部、头顶及头后部；少阳经行于头侧部。诸阴经并不都是皆到颈部、胸中而还，其中手少阴心经、足厥阴肝经均上达目系，足厥阴肝经与督脉会于头顶部，足少阴肾经上抵舌根，足太阴脾经连舌本、散舌下，均行达头面的深部或巅顶。

在躯干部，手三阳经行于肩胛部；足三阳经则阳明经行于前（胸、腹面）；太阳经行于后（背面）；少阳经行于侧面。手三阴经均从腋下走出，足三阴经均行于腹面。

（3）十二经脉的表里关系：十二经脉内属于脏腑，阴经属脏络腑，阳经属腑络脏，组合成六对表里相合关系。即：手太阳小肠经与手少阴心经相表里；手少阳三焦经与手厥阴心包经相表里；手阳明大肠经与手太阴肺经相表里；足太阳膀胱经与足少阴肾经相表里；足少阳胆经与足厥阴肝经相表里；足阳明胃经与足太阴脾经相表里。十二经脉的表里关系还通过经别和络脉的表里沟通而得到加强。

（4）十二经脉的走向与交接规律：十二经脉的走向是：手三阴经从胸腔内脏走向手指端，与手三阳经交会；手三阳经，从手指走向头面部，与足三阳经交会；足三阳经，从头面部走向足趾端，与足三阴经交会；足三阴经，从足趾走向腹部和胸部，在胸部内脏与手三阴经交会。如此，手经交于手，足经交于足，阳经交于头，阴经交于胸腹内脏，十二经脉就构成了"阴阳相贯，如环无端"的循环路径（图2-3）。

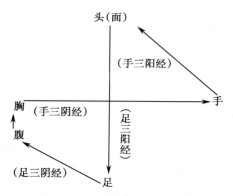

图2-3　十二经脉走向交接规律

十二经脉的交接有三种方式：

1）相为表里的阴经与阳经在四肢末端交接。相为表里的阴经与阳经共六对，都在四肢末端交接。其中相为表里的手三阴经与手三阳经交接在上肢末端，相为表里的足三阳经和足三阴经交接在下肢末端。

2）同名手足阳经在头面部交接。同名的手足阳经有三对，都在头面部交接。如手阳明大肠经与足阳明胃经交接于鼻翼旁，手太阳小肠经与足太阳膀胱经交接于目内眦，手少阳三焦经与足少阳胆经交接于目外眦。

　　3）足手阴经在胸部交接。足手阴经，又称"异名经"，也有3对，交接部位皆在胸部内脏。如足太阴脾经与手少阴心经交接于心中；足少阴肾经与手厥阴心包经交接于胸中；足厥阴肝经与手太阴肺经交接于肺中。

　　（5）十二经脉流注次序：十二经脉是人体气血运行的主要通道，它们首尾相贯、依次衔接，因而脉中气血的运行也是循经脉依次传注的。

　　由于全身气血皆由脾胃运化的水谷之精化生，故十二经脉气血的流注从起于中焦的手太阴肺经开始，依次传至足厥阴肝经，然后再传手太阴肺经，首尾相贯，如环无端（图2-4）。

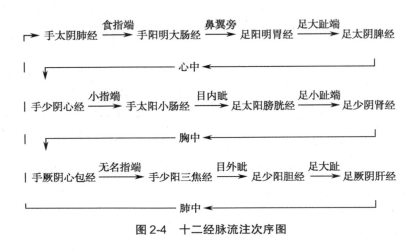

图2-4　十二经脉流注次序图

　　2. 奇经八脉　奇经八脉包括任脉、督脉、冲脉、带脉、阴维脉、阳维脉、阴跷脉、阳跷脉。奇经八脉与十二经脉不同，与体内脏腑没有直接的络属关系，相互之间也没有表里关系，故称为"奇经"。有统率、联络和调节十二经脉中气血的作用。

　　3. 十二经别　十二经别是从十二经脉别出的正经，属于经脉范围。它们分别起自四肢，循行于体腔脏腑深部，上出于颈项浅部。阳经的经别从本经别出而循行体内后，仍回到本经；阴经的经别从本经别出而循行体内后，却与相为表里的阳经相合。十二经别的作用，主要是加强十二经脉中相为表里的两经之间的联系，由于它通达某些正经未循行到的器官与形体部位，因此能补正经的不足。

　　4. 十五络脉　十二经脉在四肢部各分出一条络脉，加上躯干后的督脉络、躯干前的任脉络以及躯干侧的脾的大络，称为"十五络脉"。十五络脉的主要功能是加强相为表里的两条经脉之间在体表的联系，通达某些正经所没有到达的部位，可补正经的不足，还具有统领周身阴阳诸络的作用。

　　此外，从络脉分出、浮行于浅表的络脉称为"浮络"，其分布广泛，没有定位，起着沟通经脉，输达肌表的作用。最细小的络脉称为"孙络"，孙络分布全身，难计其数。

　　5. 十二经筋　十二经筋是十二经脉的气"结、聚、散、络"于筋肉、关节的体系，其分布范围与十二经脉大体一致，也分成手足三阴三阳。经筋均起于四肢末端，结聚于骨骼和关节部位，有的进入胸腹腔，但不像经脉那样属脏腑。经筋有联缀四肢百骸、主司关节运动的作用。

6. 十二皮部　十二皮部是指与十二经脉相应的皮肤部分，是十二经脉在体表的功能活动部位，也是络脉的气血散布所在。皮部具有抗御外邪、反映病证和协助诊断的作用。

二、腧　穴

（一）腧穴的概念

腧，意为转输、输注；穴，有孔、隙之意。腧穴是人体脏腑经络的气血输注于体表的特殊部位。

腧穴既是疾病的反应部位，又是针刺、穴位按压、拔罐、艾灸等方法的施术部位。腧穴与经络、脏腑密切相关，刺激腧穴可以促进脏腑气血运行，调和机体阴阳平衡，达到疾病预防和治疗作用。

（二）腧穴的分类

腧穴通常分为经穴、奇穴、阿是穴三大类。

1. 经穴　指分布于十二经脉以及任、督二脉的腧穴，总称"十四经穴"，共计 361 个。经穴都有具体的穴名和固定的位置，分布在十四经循行路线上，有明确的针灸主治证。

2. 奇穴　指未归入十四经穴范围，但是既有明确位置、又有固定穴位名称和治疗作用的腧穴，又称"经外奇穴"。奇穴的主治范围比较单一，多数对某些病证有特殊的治疗作用，如四缝穴治小儿疳积等，多为经验穴。

3. 阿是穴　指没有固定位置和具体名称，只是以压痛点或病变局部或其他反应点作为针灸施术的部位，又称"不定穴"。阿是穴大多位于病变附近，针刺后可疏通经气，达到治疗作用。

（三）腧穴的主治作用

腧穴是气血输注的部位，也是邪气所侵犯的部位，又是针灸防治疾病的刺激点，有接受刺激、防治疾病的作用。通过针刺、穴位按压、艾灸等对腧穴的刺激，可以通经络、调气血、平衡阴阳、调和脏腑，达到扶正祛邪的治疗目的。腧穴的主治作用主要表现在以下三个方面。

1. 近治作用　指每一个腧穴都能治疗其所在部位及临近部位的病证。近治作用又称为局部作用，是经穴、奇穴、阿是穴共同具有的特点。例如：眼区的睛明、承泣、四白各穴都能治疗眼病。

2. 远治作用　指某些腧穴不仅能治局部病证，而且能治本经循行所到达的远隔部位的病证，又称为循经作用。远治作用是十二经脉位于四肢肘、膝关节以下的腧穴的主治特点。例如：合谷穴，不仅能治疗上肢病证，而且还能治疗颈部和头面部病证。

3. 特殊作用　除近治作用、远治作用之外，腧穴还具有双向调整、整体调整和相对特异治疗的作用。

（1）双向调整作用：指针刺某些腧穴对机体的不同状态，可以起到双向的良性调整作用。例如：天枢穴，便秘时针刺可通便，泄泻时针刺可止泻。

（2）整体调整作用：指针刺某些腧穴可以起到调治全身性病证的作用。这些腧穴多见于手足阳明经穴和任督二脉经穴。

（3）相对特异治疗作用：指有些腧穴的治疗作用具有相对的特异性。例如：阑尾穴可治阑尾炎。

（四）腧穴的定位方法

腧穴的定位法，指确定腧穴位置的方法，又称为取穴法。常见的方法有体表解剖标志定位法、骨度分寸定位法、手指同身寸定位法三种。

1. 体表解剖标志定位法　是以人体体表解剖标志作为依据来确定穴位位置的方法，又称为自然标志定位法。体表解剖标志可分为固定标志和活动标志两类。

（1）固定标志定位法：指利用五官、毛发、爪甲、乳头、脐窝、骨节凹凸、肌肉隆起等固定标志来取穴的方法。例如：两眉之间取穴印堂。

（2）活动标志定位法：指利用关节、肌肉、皮肤随活动而出现的孔隙、凹陷、皱纹等活动标志来取穴的方法。例如：张口取穴听宫、听会；曲池宜屈肘于肘横纹头处取之。

2. 骨度分寸定位法　指以两骨节之间的长度为主要标志测量人体周身各部的大小、长短，并依据该尺寸按比例折算作为确定穴位标准的方法，又可称为骨度法。现将人体周身各部骨度分寸列表、图示说明如下（表2-5，图2-5）。

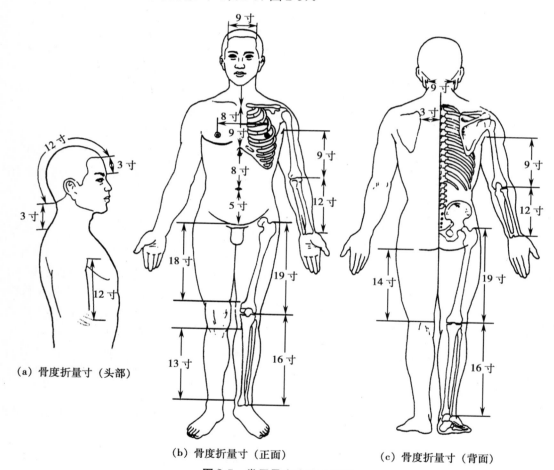

（a）骨度折量寸（头部）　　（b）骨度折量寸（正面）　　（c）骨度折量寸（背面）

图 2-5　常用骨度分寸示意图

Fig. 2-5　Bone-length proportional measurement

3. 手指同身寸定位法　指以患者本人的手指为尺寸折量标准来量取穴位的方法，又可称为"手指比量法"和"指寸法"。常用的手指同身寸有以下三种：

（1）中指同身寸：以患者的中指中节屈曲时，内侧两端横纹间距离作为1寸量取穴位（图2-6）。

（2）拇指同身寸：以患者的拇指骨关节的横纹宽度作为1寸量取穴位（图2-7）。

表2-5 常用骨度表

部位	起止点	折量寸	度量法	说明
头部	前发际至后发际	12寸	直	如前发际不明,从眉心至大椎穴作18寸,眉心至前发际3寸,大椎穴至后发际3寸
	前额两发角之间	9寸	横	用于量头部的横寸
	耳后两完骨(乳突)之间	9寸	横	
胸腹部	天突至歧骨(胸剑联合)	9寸	直	胸部与胁肋部取穴直寸,一般根据肋骨计算,每一肋骨折作1.6寸(天突穴至璇玑穴可作1寸,璇玑穴至中庭穴,各穴间可作1.6寸计算)
	歧骨至脐中	8寸	直	
	脐中至横骨上廉(耻骨联合上缘)	5寸	直	
	两乳头之间	8寸	横	胸腹部取穴横寸,可根据两乳头间的距离折量,女性可用锁骨中线代替
背腰部	大椎以下至尾骶	21椎	直	背腰部腧穴以脊椎棘突作为定位标志
	两肩胛骨脊柱缘之间	6寸	横	一般两肩胛骨下角连线平第7胸椎棘突;两髂嵴连线平第4腰椎棘突身侧部
	腋以下至季胁	12寸	直	季胁此指第11肋端下方
	季胁以下至髀枢	9寸	直	髀枢指股骨大转子高点
上肢部	腋前纹头(腋前皱襞)至肘横纹	9寸	直	用于手三阴、手三阳经的骨度分寸
	肘横纹至腕横纹	12寸	直	
下肢部	横骨上廉至内辅骨上廉	18寸	直	内辅骨上廉指股骨内侧踝上缘
	内辅骨下廉至内踝尖	13寸	直	内辅骨下廉指胫骨内侧踝下缘,内踝尖指内踝向内的凸起处
	髀枢至膝中	19寸	直	
	膝中至外踝尖	16寸	直	臀横纹至膝中,可作14寸折量
	外踝尖至足底	3寸	直	膝中的水平线,前平膝盖下缘,后平腘横纹,屈膝时可平犊鼻穴

(3)横指同身寸:令患者食指、中指、无名指、小指四指并拢,以中指中节近端横纹为标准,四指宽度为3寸量取穴位(图2-8)。

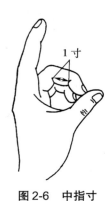

图2-6 中指寸
Fig 2-6 Middle finger measurement

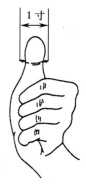

图2-7 拇指寸
Fig 2-7 Thumb measurement

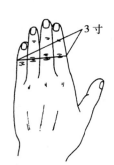

图2-8 横指寸
Fig 2-8 Four-finger measurement

总 论

（五）常用腧穴

每个腧穴都有较为广泛的主治范围，常用穴位的定位主治及穴位按压手法见表2-6。

表2-6 常用穴位表

经络	穴名	位置	主治	穴位按压手法
手太阴肺经	尺泽	肘横纹中，肱二头肌腱桡侧	肘臂挛痛、咳喘、胸胁胀痛、小儿惊风	按法、揉法、拿法、点法
	孔最	在尺泽与太渊连线上，腕横纹上7寸	咳嗽、咯血、音哑、咽喉痛、肘臂痛	按法、揉法、拿法、点法
	列缺	桡骨茎突上方，腕横纹上1.5寸	咳嗽、气急、头项强痛、牙痛	一指禅推法、按法、揉法
	太渊	腕横纹桡侧端，桡动脉桡侧凹陷中	咳嗽、气喘、乳胀、咽喉痛、手腕痛	按法、揉法、掐法
	鱼际	第一掌骨中点，赤白肉际	胸背痛、头痛、眩晕、喉痛、发热恶寒	按法、揉法、掐法
	少商	拇指桡侧指甲角旁约0.1寸	中风昏仆、手指挛痛、小儿惊风	掐法
手阳明大肠经	合谷	手背，第一、二掌骨之间，约平第二掌骨中点处	头痛、牙痛、发热、喉痛、指挛、臂痛、口眼㖞斜	拿法、按法、点法、揉法
	手三里	曲池穴下2寸	肘挛、屈伸不利、手臂麻木酸痛	拿法、按法、点法、一指禅推法
	曲池	屈肘，当肘横纹外端凹陷中	发热、高血压、手臂肿痛、肘痛、上肢瘫痪	拿法、按法、揉法
	肩髃	肩峰前下方，举臂时呈凹陷处	肩膀痛、肩关节活动障碍、偏瘫	按法、揉法
	迎香	鼻翼旁0.5寸，鼻唇沟中	鼻炎、鼻塞、口眼㖞斜	擦法、按法、揉法
足阳明胃经	四白	目正视，瞳孔直下，当眶下孔凹陷中	口眼㖞斜、目赤痛痒	按法、揉法、点法
	地仓	口角旁0.4寸	流涎、口眼㖞斜	按法、揉法、点法
	下关	颧弓与下颌切迹之间的凹陷中，合口有孔，张口即闭	面瘫、牙痛	按法、揉法
	头维	额角发际直上0.5寸	头痛	摩法、按法、揉法、扫散法
	天枢	脐旁2寸	腹泻、便秘、腹痛、月经不调	揉法、摩法、一指禅推法
	足三里	犊鼻穴下3寸，胫骨前棘外一横指处	腹痛、腹泻、便秘、下肢冷麻、高血压	按法、揉法、点法、一指禅推法
	丰隆	外膝眼与外侧踝尖连线中点	头痛、咳嗽、肢肿、便秘、狂痛、下肢痿痹	按法、揉法
足太阴脾经	三阴交	内踝上3寸，胫骨内侧面的中央	失眠、腹胀纳呆、遗尿、小便不利、妇科病	按法、点法、揉法、拿法
	地机	阴陵泉下3寸	腹痛、泄泻、水肿、小便不利、遗精	拿法、按法、揉法、点法
	阴陵泉	胫骨内侧髁下缘凹陷中	膝关节酸痛、小便不利	拿法、按法、揉法、点法
	血海	髌骨内上方2寸	月经不调、膝痛	拿法、按法、揉法、点法
	大横	脐中旁开4寸	虚寒泻痢、大便秘结、小腹痛	摩法、揉法、按法

44

续表

经络	穴名	位置	主治	穴位按压手法
手少阴心经	极泉	腋窝正中	胸闷胁痛,臂肘冷麻	拿法、拨法
	少海	屈肘,当肘横纹尺侧端凹陷中	肘关节痛、手颤肘挛	拿法、拨法
	通里	神门穴上1寸	心悸、怔忡、头晕、咽痛、暴喑、舌强不语、腕臂痛	掐法、按法、揉法
	神门	腕横纹尺侧端,尺侧腕屈肌腱的桡侧凹陷中	惊悸、怔忡、失眠、健忘	按法、揉法、掐法
手太阳小肠经	少泽	小指尺侧指甲角一旁约0.1寸	发热、中风昏迷、乳少、咽喉肿痛	掐法
	后溪	第五掌指关节后尺侧、横纹头赤白肉	头项强痛、耳聋、咽痛、齿痛、目翳、肘臂挛痛	掐法
	肩贞	腋后纹头上1寸	肩关节酸痛、活动不便、上肢瘫痪	拿法、按法、揉法、㨰法
	天宗	肩胛骨冈下窝的中央	肩背酸痛、肩关节活动不便、项强	按法、点法、揉法、㨰法
足太阳膀胱经	睛明	目内眦旁0.1寸	眼病	点法、揉法
	攒竹	眉头凹陷中	头痛失眠、眉棱骨痛、目赤痛	点法、揉法
	天柱	后发际正中直上0.5寸(哑门穴),旁开1.3寸,当斜方肌外缘凹陷中	头痛、项强、鼻塞、肩背痛	拿法、揉法、点法、按法
	大杼	第一胸椎棘突下,旁开1.5寸	发热,咳嗽、项强、肩脚酸痛	点法、按法、揉法、㨰法
	风门	第二胸椎棘突下,旁开1.5寸	伤风、咳嗽、项强、腰背痛	㨰法、按法、点法、揉法、一指禅推法、拨法
	肺俞	第三胸椎棘突下,旁开1.5寸	咳嗽气喘、胸闷、背肌劳损	㨰法、按法、点法、揉法、一指禅推法、拨法
	心俞	第五胸椎棘突下,旁开1.5寸	失眠,心悸	㨰法、按法、点法、揉法、一指禅推法、拨法
	膈俞	第七胸椎棘突下,旁开1.5寸	呕吐、噎嗝气喘、咳嗽、盗汗	㨰法、按法、点法、揉法、一指禅推法、拨法
	肝俞	第九胸椎棘突下,旁开1.5寸	胁肋痛、肝炎、目疾	㨰法、按法、点法、揉法、一指禅推法、拨法
	胆俞	第十胸椎棘突下,旁开1.5寸	胁肋痛、口苦、黄疸	㨰法、按法、点法、揉法、一指禅推法、拨法
	脾俞	第十一胸椎棘突下,旁开1.5寸	胃脘胀痛、消化不良、小儿慢惊风证	㨰法、按法、点法、揉法、一指禅推法、拨法
	胃俞	第十二胸椎棘突下,旁开1.5寸	胃病、小儿吐乳、消化不良	㨰法、按法、点法、揉法、一指禅推法、拨法
	三焦俞	第一腰椎棘突下,旁开1.5寸	肠鸣、腹胀、呕吐、腰背强痛	㨰法、按法、点法、揉法、一指禅推法、拨法
	肾俞	第二腰椎棘突下,旁开1.5寸	肾虚、腰痛、遗精、月经不调	㨰法、按法、点法、揉法、一指禅推法、拨法
	气海俞	第三腰椎棘突下旁开1.5寸	腰痛	㨰法、按法、点法、揉法、一指禅推法、拨法

经络	穴名	位置	主治	穴位按压手法
足太阳膀胱经	大肠俞	第四腰椎棘突下,旁开1.5寸	腰腿痛、腰肌劳损、肠炎	㨰法、按法、点法、揉法、一指禅推法、拨法
	关元俞	第五腰椎棘突下,旁开1.5寸	腰痛、泄泻	㨰法、按法、点法、揉法、一指禅推法、拨法
	八髎	在第一、二、三、四骶后孔中(分别为上髎、次髎、中髎、下髎)	腰腿痛、泌尿生殖系疾患	按法、点法、揉法、擦法
	秩边	第4骶椎棘突下,旁开3寸	腰臀痛、下肢痿痹、小便不利、便秘	㨰法、按法、点法、揉法
	殷门	臀沟中央下6寸	坐骨神经痛、下肢瘫痪、腰背痛	㨰法、按法、点法、揉法、拍法
	昆仑	外踝与跟腱之间凹陷中	头痛、项强、腰痛、踝关节扭伤	按法、拿法、点法
	申脉	外踝下缘凹陷中	癫狂痫、腰腿酸痛	掐法、点法、按法
足少阴肾经	涌泉	足底中、足趾跖屈时呈凹陷处	偏头痛、高血压、小儿发热	擦法、按法、揉法、点法
	太溪	内踝与跟腱之间凹陷中	喉痛、齿痛、不寐、遗精、阳痿、月经不调	拿法、按法、揉法、点法
	照海	内踝下缘凹陷中	月经不调	按法、揉法、点法
手厥阴心包经	内关	腕横纹上2寸,掌长肌腱与桡侧腕屈肌腱之间	胃痛、呕吐、心悸、精神失常	按法、点法、揉法、拿法
	大陵	腕横纹中央,掌长肌腱与桡侧腕屈肌腱之间	心痛、心悸、胃痛、呕吐、癫痫、胸胁痛	按法、点法、揉法、拿法
	劳宫	手掌心横纹中,第二、三掌骨之间	心悸、颤抖	按法、点法、揉法、擦法
手少阳三焦经	中渚	握拳第四、五掌骨小头后缘之间凹陷中	偏头痛、掌指痛屈伸不利、肘臂痛	点法、按法、揉法
	阳池	腕背横纹中、指总伸肌腱尺侧缘凹陷中	肩臂痛、腕痛、疟疾、消渴、耳聋	点法、按法、揉法
	外关	腕背横纹上2寸,桡骨与尺骨之间	头痛、肘臂手指痛、屈伸不利	点法、按法、揉法
	肩髎	肩峰外下方,肩髃穴后寸许凹陷中	肩臂酸痛、肩关节活动不便	㨰法、点法、按法、揉法
足少阳胆经	风池	胸锁乳突肌与斜方肌之间,平风府穴(后发际正中直上1寸)	偏正头痛、感冒项强	按法、揉法、拿法、一指禅推法
	肩井	大椎穴与肩峰连线的中点	项强、肩背痛、手臂上举不便	拿法、㨰法、一指禅推法、按法、揉法
	环跳	股骨大转子与骶裂孔连线的外1/3与内2/3交界处	腰腿痛、偏瘫	㨰法、点法、按法、揉法
	风市	大腿外侧中间,腘横纹水平线上7寸	偏瘫、膝关节酸痛	㨰法、点法、按法、揉法
	阳陵泉	腓骨小头前下方凹陷中	膝关节酸痛、胁肋痛	拨法、点法、按法、揉法
	光明	外踝上5寸,腓骨前缘	膝痛、下肢疾痹、目痛、夜盲、乳胀	拨法、点法、按法、揉法

经络	穴名	位置	主治	穴位按压手法
足少阳胆经	丘墟	外踝前下方，趾长伸肌腱外侧凹陷中	踝关节痛、胸胁痛	按法、揉法
	足临泣	足背，第四、五趾间缝纹端上1.5寸	瘰疬、胁肋痛、足跗肿痛、足趾挛痛	掐法、按法、揉法
足厥阴肝经	太冲	足背，第一、二跖骨底之间凹陷中	头痛、眩晕、高血压、小儿惊风	掐法、按法、揉法
	蠡沟	内踝上5寸，胫骨内侧面的中央	小便不利、月经不调、足胫痿痹	按法、揉法、一指禅推法
	章门	第十一肋端	胸胁痛、胸闷	摩法、按法、揉法
	期门	乳头直下、第六肋间隙	胸胁痛	摩法、按法、揉法
任脉	关元	脐下3寸，前正中线上	腹痛、痛经、遗尿	一指禅推法、摩法、按法、揉法
	气海	脐下1.5寸	腹痛、月经不调、遗尿	一指禅推法、摩法、按法、揉法
	中脘	脐上4寸	胃痛、腹胀、呕吐、消化不良	一指禅推法、摩法、按法、揉法
	膻中	前正中线，平第四肋间隙处	咳喘、胸闷、胸痛	一指禅推法、摩法、按法、揉法
督脉	长强	尾骨尖下0.5寸	腹泻、便秘、脱肛	按法、揉法
	命门	第二腰椎棘突下	腰脊疼痛	按法、揉法、一指禅推法
	大椎	第七颈椎棘突下	感冒、发热、落枕	按法、揉法、一指禅推法、擦法
	风府	后发际正中直上1寸	头痛、项强	按法、揉法、一指禅推法
	百会	后发际正中直上7寸	头痛、头晕、昏厥、高血压、脱肛	按法、揉法、一指禅推法
	人中	人中沟正中线上1/3与下2/3交界处	惊风、口眼㖞斜	掐法
经外奇穴	印堂	两眉头连线的中点	头痛、鼻炎、失眠	摩法、一指禅推法、按法、揉法
	太阳	眉梢与目外眦之间向后约1寸处凹陷中	头痛、感冒、眼病	摩法、一指禅推法、按法、揉法
	鱼腰	眉毛的中点	眉棱骨痛、目赤肿痛、眼睑颤动	摩法、一指禅推法、按法、揉法
	腰眼	第四腰椎棘突下，旁开3.5寸凹陷处	腰扭伤、腰背酸楚	擦法、按法、揉法、擦法
	夹脊	第一胸椎至第五腰椎，各椎棘突下旁开0.5寸	脊柱疼痛强直、脏腑疾患及强壮作用	擦法、按法、揉法、擦法、拨法
	十宣	十手指尖端，距指甲0.1寸	昏厥	掐法
	鹤顶	髌骨上缘正中凹陷处	膝关节肿痛	按法、揉法、点法
	阑尾	足三里穴下约2寸处	阑尾炎、腹痛	按法、揉法、点法
	胆囊	阳陵泉直下1寸	胆绞痛	按法、揉法、点法

（马良宵）

第三节　中医护理的基本特点

中医护理学秉承了中医学整体观念和辨证论治的基本特点，在长期的医疗和护理实践中，经现代中医护理人员进一步的继承和发扬，形成了中医护理的基本特点，即整体观念和辨证施护。

一、整　体　观　念

中医护理学整体观念是将其研究对象"人"看作一个有机整体，同时认为人与自然环境、社会环境也是一个密切相关的整体。

（一）人体是一个有机的整体

中医学认为人体是以五脏为中心，配以六腑，通过经络系统的联络作用，把五体、官窍、四肢百骸等全身组织器官联结成一个有机的整体，并通过精、气、血、津液的作用，完成人体统一协调的功能活动。而人体患病时，体内的各个部分亦相互影响。如肾虚，不但肾本身的功能减退，肾开窍于耳，故也会影响到耳，出现听力下降、耳鸣、耳聋；肾与膀胱相表里，同样也会影响膀胱功能，使膀胱固摄无力，则见尿频、遗尿等；肾主骨，还可影响骨骼，如老年患者多见骨质疏松，易于发生骨折。因而在中医护理实践中，可以通过观察官窍、形体、舌脉等外在的变化，来了解脏腑、气血等内在的病变。

（二）人与环境的密切联系

1. 人与自然环境的统一性　人类生活在自然界中，自然界存在着人类赖以生存的必要条件。同时，自然界的变化又可以直接或间接地影响到人体，人体就会产生相应的生理和病理性反应。如不同季节、昼夜、地理环境等对人体的影响。

季节对人体的影响非常明显。一年四季有春温、夏热、长夏湿、秋燥、冬寒的气候变化，人体也会发生相应的适应性变化。如春夏季节，阳气发泄，气血趋向于表，表现为皮肤松弛，汗出较多而排尿偏少；秋冬季节，阳气收敛，气血趋向于里，表现为皮肤致密，汗出偏少而排尿较多。脉象也随季节变化而发生适应性变化，春夏脉象多浮大，秋冬脉象多沉小。

昼夜晨昏对人体也有影响。昼夜晨昏的交替是自然界阴阳消长变化的一种表现，人的气血阴阳也会随着昼夜晨昏的变化而进行相应调节。如随着清晨太阳升起，人的阳气随之而升；中午阳气隆盛，生理功能加强；夜晚阳气收敛，适宜休息，恢复精力。

此外，地理环境也影响人的生理功能。如中国江南地势低，气候温暖而湿润，故人的腠理多疏松；北方地势高，气候寒冷干燥，故人的腠理多致密。

2. 人与社会环境关系密切　人是社会的组成要素，人能影响社会，社会环境的变化对人的生理、心理、病理亦会带来相应的影响。社会环境中存在很多影响人类精神和心理的因素，而人的精神心理活动与生理互为影响。如怒伤肝，喜伤心、思伤脾等。中医护理学强调形与神俱、形神相依、形神互动，重视人与社会的和谐统一。

（三）中医整体护理

整体观念贯穿于中医学的所有领域，在中医护理学中也得到了很大的发挥，中医整体护理就是整体观念在临床护理中应用的最好体现。中医整体护理是指在观察判断病情和护理疾病时，应注意把人体的局部病变与机体整体病理变化统一起来，重视外界环境对人的影响,根据四时气候、地理环境、一天中昼夜晨昏变化和社会变化等各方面的因素,制订适宜的护理计划。

二、辨 证 施 护

辨证施护由辨证和施护两部分组成。所谓辨证就是将四诊(望、闻、问、切)所收集的有关病史、症状、体征,通过综合分析,辨清疾病的原因、性质、部位及邪正关系,进而概括、判断疾病的证候属性。施护,则是根据辨证的结果,确立相应的护理原则和方法,制定出护理计划和具体的护理措施,对患者实施护理。辨证是施护的前提与依据,施护是护理疾病的手段和方法,通过施护的效果可以检验辨证的正确与否。

辨证施护时要正确看待症、证之间的关系。"症"包括症状和体征,如头痛、恶寒、咳嗽、面赤、舌红等;而"证"是机体在疾病发展过程中某一阶段的病理概括,包括病因、病变部位、病性及邪正关系。辨证则着眼于"证"的分辨。如感冒分为风寒证、风热证。只有把感冒所表现的"证"是风寒证还是风热证辨别清楚,才能确定施护的方法。若属风寒感冒,采取避风寒、保暖的护理措施,室温宜偏高,饮食上给予豆豉汤、生姜、红糖等辛温解表之品。若属风热感冒者,则室温宜低,宜进食绿豆汤、西瓜、苦瓜等清热生津之品。

在临床辨证施护时,能够辨证地看待病和证的关系。既可见到同一种病包括几种不同的证,又看到不同的病在其发展过程中可以出现同一种证,在调护时需采用"同病异护"和"异病同护"的方法。

"同病异护"是指同一种病,由于发病的时间、地区以及患者机体反应性不同,或处在不同的发展阶段,所表现的证候不同,施护的方法亦各异。如感冒有风寒感冒和暑湿感冒的不同,在调护方法上有辛温解表和祛暑化湿的区别。

"异病同护"是指不同的病,在其发展过程中,出现了性质相同的证候,因而可采用同样的施护方法。例如胃下垂、久泻脱肛、子宫下垂为不同疾病,但如均表现为中气下陷证,则均可采用提升中气的护理方法。具体措施如嘱患者注意休息,避免过劳,以培育中气;给予茯苓粥、薏仁粥等健脾益气之品;针刺百会、关元以补中益气。

由此可见,中医护理不仅重视疾病的异同,更注重病机的区别和证的不同。相同的病机和证,可采用基本相同的护理方法;不同的病机和证要采用不同的施护措施。这种针对疾病发展过程中不同性质的矛盾用不同的护理方法解决的原则,就是辨证施护的实质所在。

第四节　中医护理的基本原则

中医护理基本原则是中医护理人员在护理疾病时必须遵守的法则,是中医学"治则"在护理学中的延伸。中医护理基本原则是以辨证为前提和基础,根据辨证的结果,确定正确的护理原则,并在护理原则指导下制订出针对证侯的具体调护方法。中医护理基本原则对于临床各科病证的护理,具有普遍的指导意义。

一、扶 正 祛 邪

疾病的发生、发展过程,是正气与邪气矛盾双方斗争的过程。正胜于邪则病退,邪胜于正则病进。因此治疗和护理疾病的一个基本原则就是扶助正气,祛除邪气,改变邪正双方的力量对比,使疾病早日痊愈,机体早日康复。

扶正是运用药物、饮食、锻炼、针灸、推拿等方法，以增强体质，提高机体的抗病能力，从而达到扶助正气，祛除邪气，保持和恢复健康的目的。适用于以正虚为主的病证。祛邪是运用药物、针灸、拔罐等方法祛除病邪，达到恢复正气的目的。适用于以邪实为主的病证。

在护理实践中往往要根据正邪的相互消长和盛衰情况，区分单纯扶正法、祛邪法或先扶正后祛邪，或先祛邪后扶正，或两者同时进行。一般来说，扶正法适用于单纯正虚而无外邪者；祛邪法适用于单纯邪盛而正气不虚者；先扶正后祛邪适用于正虚而邪不盛者；先祛邪后扶正适用于邪盛正虚不甚者；扶正祛邪同时进行适用于正虚邪实的患者。

二、护　病　求　本

在疾病发生发展的过程中，病情变化多端，多数疾病临床表现和其疾病本质基本一致，但有些疾病出现某些和本质相矛盾，甚至相反的临床表现，即在证候上出现假象，因此护理人员必须从复杂的因素中找出疾病的本质，并给予恰当的护理。

护病求本是指在护理患者时必须寻求其疾病的根本原因，并采取有针对性的护理措施，这是辨证施护的根本原则。

（一）正护法

正护法又称为逆护法，是指疾病的临床表现与其疾病性质相一致情况下，逆其证候性质和表象而护理的方法。

根据临床症状和体征，判断疾病的寒热虚实，然后采取"寒则热之"、"热则寒之"、"虚则补之"、"实则泻之"等护理方法。如寒邪所致的寒证，其疾病的临床表现和本质均为寒性病证，在护理上宜采用温热护理法，如病室温度宜稍高，使患者感到温暖舒适；中药宜温热服用；给予温热饮食，忌生冷性凉的食品。而热证患者则应采用与寒证患者相反的护理方法。

（二）反护法

反护法又称为从护法，是指当疾病的临床表现与其本质不一致情况下，顺从疾病外在表现的假象而护理的方法。

由于某些严重的、复杂的疾患，其临床表现与疾病本质不相符，因而在护理时应透过假象辨明真伪，治其本质。常用的反护法主要有以下四种：

1. **热因热用**　是指采用温热性质的药物及方法治疗护理具有假热征象的病证。适用于真寒假热证，即阴寒内盛，格阳于外，此时患者虽有四肢厥逆、脉微欲绝等真寒的表现，又反见身热、面赤等假热之象，所以在护理时应以温热法护其真寒，如给予温热性食物、汤药宜温服、室温宜偏高、注意保暖等以治其真寒，假热的症状则会自然消失。

2. **寒因寒用**　是指采用寒凉性质的药物及方法治疗护理具有假寒征象的病证。适用于真热假寒证，如某些外感热病，在其里热盛极之时，由于阳盛格阴，此时患者常表现出壮热、口渴喜冷饮、小便短赤等里热征象，但同时又出现四肢厥冷、脉沉等假寒之象，所以在护理时应以寒凉法护其真热，如给予清凉饮料、汤药宜凉服、室温宜偏凉等以治其真热，假寒之象也会随之消失。

3. **塞因塞用**　是指使用补益的药物和方法治疗护理具有闭塞不通症状的虚证。适用于真虚假实证，如脾气虚，虚则脾运化无力，出现脘腹胀满、纳呆，但无水湿或食积留滞，所以在护理时宜用健脾益气，以补开塞的护法，饮食上给予山药粥、大枣粥等补中气，并配合针灸、推拿等疗法，以加强药效和振奋脾气，脾气健运则腹胀自消。

4. 通因通用　是指使用具有通利作用的药物及方法治疗护理具有通泄症状的实证。适用于真实假虚证，如食积停滞、胃肠失调所导致的腹泻，则不仅不能使用止泻药，而应用消食导滞法以去其积滞，病邪祛除，通泄的症状自然会停止。

三、标 本 缓 急

标和本是相对的概念。标是指疾病的现象，本是指疾病的本质。在中医学中，标和本有多种含义：从正邪关系来分，正气为本，邪气为标；从疾病本身来分，病因为本，症状为标；从疾病新旧来分，旧病为本，新病为标；从发病先后来分，先病为本，后病为标；从疾病部位来分，内脏为本，体表为标；等等。只有掌握疾病的标与本，才能分清主次，选择适宜的护理方法。而疾病是一个千变万化的复杂过程，常有标本主次的不同，因此在临床护理中对疾病标和本的护理要视情况而定，可根据标本缓急决定护理方案。

（一）急则护其标

急则护其标是指标病甚急，如不及时解决，即将危及生命或影响本病总体治疗和护理时所采取的方法。如溃疡病患者，当出现呕血、便血时，首先应先止血以治标，待血止后，病情有所缓解，再针对病因以治其本病。

（二）缓则护其本

缓则护其本是指在标证不急，症状及病势较缓的情况下，针对疾病本质所采取的护理方法。如虚劳内伤的阴虚发热，发热是标，阴虚是本，在发热不甚，症状不急时，护理上采用滋阴护本法，当阴虚平复后发热症状即可缓解。

（三）标本兼护

标本兼护是指在标病、本病俱急并重的情况下，在护病求本的同时，亦兼顾标病的护理方法。如气虚患者又复感外邪而感冒，气虚不足以战胜外邪，气虚为本，外邪为标，单纯祛邪又恐进一步损伤正气，此时即应扶正祛邪，标本同护。

四、调 整 阴 阳

阴阳的相对平衡维持着人体正常的生命活动过程，当这种平衡被打破，人体就会出现阴阳的偏盛偏衰。因此在治疗和护理疾病时，应协调阴阳，补偏救弊，恢复阴阳相对平衡的状态，促进其阴平阳秘。

调整阴阳，是指纠正疾病过程中机体阴阳的偏盛偏衰，损其有余而补其不足，恢复和重建人体阴阳的相对平衡。

（一）损其有余

损其有余是指阴或阳一方偏盛有余的病证，应当采用"实则泻之"的方法治疗护理。如阳偏盛表现出的阳盛而阴相对未虚的实热证，应采用"热者寒之"清泻阳热的方法治疗护理。护理措施是病室宜凉爽通风；服药温度宜凉服；避免情绪过激；饮食上辅以西瓜汁、梨汁、绿豆等清热生津之品，共泻阳热之火。

（二）补其不足

补其不足是指阴或阳偏衰不足的病证，应当用"虚则补之"的方法来治疗护理。若阴虚不能制阳，常表现为阴虚阳亢的虚热证，则应滋阴以制阳，如保持病室内凉爽通风，在饮食护理上给予银耳、百合、甲鱼等滋阴清热之品养阴生津；若阳虚不能制阴，常表现为阳虚阴盛的虚寒证，则应补阳以制阴，如保持病室温暖，给予补阳制阴的饮食；若阴阳两虚，则应阴阳双补。由于阴阳是互助互用的，在调整阴阳时，应注意"阳中求阴"或"阴中求阳"，即在补阴时适当顾及补阳，补阳时适当顾及补阴。

五、三 因 制 宜

三因制宜是指护理患者时应因时、因地、因人而采取适宜的护理方法。由于四时气候、地域环境、患病个体（性别、年龄、体质、生活习惯）等因素，对于疾病的发生、发展变化与转归都有着不同程度的影响，因此，在护理中除了掌握一般护理原则外，还要根据具体情况做出具体分析，灵活对待，制定出适宜的调护方案。

（一）因时制宜

因时制宜是指根据不同季节气候特点而确定相应护理措施的原则。四时气候变化，对人体生理功能、病理变化均有一定影响，而反常的气候更是诱发疾病的重要条件。如春夏季节，阳气升发，人体腠理开泄，服解表药后不宜覆盖衣被或饮热饮，以免开泄太过，耗伤津液；秋冬季节，人体腠理致密，阳气内敛，感受风寒时，服解表药宜热服，注意防寒保暖，还可饮热饮以助药力。另外，因时制宜还应注意某些季节性好发病，如痹证、哮喘、中风等，做好预防护理。

（二）因地制宜

因地制宜是指根据不同地区的地理环境及其生活习惯特点而确定相应护理措施的原则。地理环境、生活习惯的不同直接影响到人体的生理、病理变化，在治疗与护理疾病时要充分考虑地理因素的影响。如中国西北地区，气候寒冷，干燥少雨，病多风寒，宜用温热药，而寒凉之剂就必须慎用；而中国东南地区，气候潮湿温暖，病多温热、湿热，在护理上宜用清凉与化湿法，温热之剂必须慎用。

（三）因人制宜

因人制宜是指根据患者的年龄、性别、体质等不同特点而制定相应护理措施的原则。不同年龄的生理状况和气血盈亏各不同，如老年人气血虚亏，生理功能减退，患病多虚，虚证宜补；小儿生机旺盛，但气血未充，脏腑娇嫩，易寒易热，易虚易实，病情变化较快，慎用补益，用药量宜轻。此外，男女性别不同，各有其生理特点，如女性有经、带、胎、产等生理变化，护理中应予以注意一些药物禁忌。由于人的体质不但有强弱，而且还有偏寒偏热之差异，如一般素体阳虚者，应注意避寒保暖，予以滋补温热食物，慎用寒凉之品；素体阴虚内热之体，注意居室要清凉，通风良好，并给予清补生津滋阴食品，慎用温热之品。

三因制宜的原则，充分体现了中医护理学的整体观念在护理实践应用中的原则性和灵活性。只有全面地看问题，具体情况具体分析，才能更有效地实施适宜的护理措施。

六、预 防 护 理

中医学对疾病的预防自古以来就给予高度重视，《素问·四气调神大论》中指出："是故圣人不治已病治未病，不治已乱治未乱，此之谓也。夫病已成而后药之，乱已成而后治之，譬犹渴而穿井，斗而铸锥，不亦晚乎！"。预防保健是中医学理论体系中重要的组成部分。预防护理是在中医基本理论指导下，采取一定的措施，以防止疾病的发生、发展、传变或复发。"治未病"包括未病先防和既病防变两个方面。

（一）未病先防

未病先防是指在疾病未发生之前，做好各种预防措施以防止疾病的发生。疾病的发生关系到正邪两方面因素,邪气侵入是发病的外在条件,而正气不足是疾病发生的内在因素,因此未病先防,应在防止病邪侵害的同时,注重提高人体正气,增强抗病能力。

1. 护正气以抵外邪 《素问·刺法论》中指出:"正气存内,邪不可干。"正气充足,阴阳气血旺盛,脏腑功能健全,机体抗病能力强,故调养正气是提高抗病能力的关键。

(1)适时起居,劳逸结合:根据四时气候变化合理安排作息时间,养成规律的起居习惯,提高对自然界环境变化的适应能力。同时注意劳逸适度,量力而行,则能保养神气,使人体精神充沛,生命力旺盛;反之,起居无常,过度劳逸,日久则神气衰败,机体抗病能力下降,易于患病。

(2)调理饮食,顾护脾胃:脾为后天之本,气血生化之源,对饮食进行消化、吸收并输布其精微物质,而饮食所化生的水谷精微是生成气血的物质基础。若气血充足,正气旺盛,则机体不易被邪气侵袭而发病。中医护理强调饮食有节,是指饮食要适宜、规律,即要寒热调和、五味均衡,不可偏食;食量适中,不可过饱、过饥;饮食要因人因时而异;要注意饮食卫生,防止"病从口入"等。若饮食不节,食饮无度,将导致疾病的发生。

(3)调摄精神,锻炼形体:人的精神情志活动是以精、气、血、津液为物质基础,与脏腑的功能活动、气血运行等密切相关。如愉快的情绪使人体的气机调畅,气血平和,则脏腑功能协调,正气充盛,抗病能力强,可预防疾病的发生;而抑郁的情绪可以导致人体气滞血瘀,功能紊乱,抗病能力下降。故中医护理中强调精神调养,做到"恬淡虚无,真气从之",从而达到"精神内守,病安从来"的养生目的。体育锻炼也是促进人体健康的一项重要措施,中国古代医家发明了多种健身术,如太极拳、五禽戏、八段锦等。通过合理的运动,不仅能促进血脉流通、关节灵活,而且可使气机调畅,从而增强机体的抗病能力,防止和减少疾病的发生。形神统一,则身体健康。

(4)药物预防,保精抗衰:通过人工免疫的方法能够增强体质,预防某些疾病的发生。中国古人发明了"人痘接种法",用于预防天花,是我国对世界预防医学做出的贡献。近年来运用中草药预防疾病已引起人们的重视,如用板蓝根、贯众或大青叶等预防流感;用马齿苋预防痢疾;用茵陈、栀子预防肝炎等,都有较好的预防效果。此外由于人体的生长发育以及衰老程度与肾中精气的盛衰有着直接的关系,如肾的精气充足,则精神旺盛,身体健康,延年益寿。护肾保精可通过节欲保精,食疗保肾、药物调补、按摩固肾以及运动保健等方法,达到养护肾精,增强抗病能力的目的。

2. 避虚邪以安其正 病邪疫毒是导致疾病发生的重要条件,因此未病先防除了要养护人体的正气以外,还应注意避免病邪的侵害。《素问·上古天真论》中指出:"虚邪贼风,避之有时。"顺应四时气候的变化,春夏之时调养阳气,秋冬之时保养阴精,使肌腠紧致,卫气固密,邪气无隙可乘。在气候反常或遇到传染病流行之时,要避免接触,做好隔离,防止环境、水源和食物等被污染。此外在日常生活中注意防止外伤、虫兽咬伤等。

(二)既病防变

既病防变是指在发生疾病以后要早期诊断、早期治疗,防止疾病的进一步发展与传变。护理工作的重点是观察病情变化,给予及时的护理。

1. 观察病情,早期诊治 疾病初期,病情较轻,病位表浅,正气未衰,如果积极治疗,较易治愈。《素问·阴阳应象大论》中指出:"故邪风之至,疾如风雨,故善治者治皮毛,其次治肌肤,其次治筋脉,其次治六腑,其次治五脏。治五脏者半生半死也。"因此护士应通过对病情的观察和综合分析,判断疾病的证候属性,为医生的早期诊断、及时治疗提供可靠的依据,防止疾病的进一步发展和变化。

　　2. 及时护理,防止传变　《金匮要略·脏腑经络先后病脉证》中指出:"夫治未病者,见肝之病,知肝传脾,当先实脾。"在临床护理工作中,要密切观察患者病情变化,掌握其疾病发生发展和传变的规律,实施预见性治疗与护理,阻断其病传途径,先安未受邪之地,防止疾病的发展与传变。

(杨晓玮)

各　论

第三章

中医护理常用方法与技术

第一节　耳穴压丸法

耳穴压丸法是在耳穴表面贴敷圆形、坚硬而表面光滑的小颗粒，如王不留行籽、小磁珠等，通过在敷贴处按压耳穴以加强刺激来防治疾病的一种方法。其治疗范围较广，操作简便安全，副作用少，运用非常广泛。

一、耳廓表面解剖

耳廓的表面解剖见图 3-1。

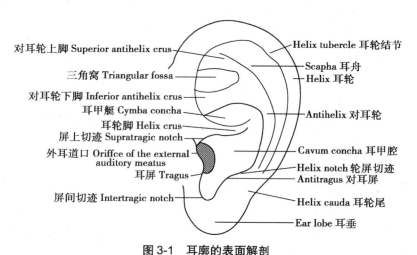

对耳轮上脚 Superior antihelix crus
三角窝 Triangular fossa
对耳轮下脚 Inferior antihelix crus
耳甲艇 Cymba concha
耳轮脚 Helix crus
屏上切迹 Supratragic notch
外耳道口 Oriffce of the external auditory meatus
耳屏 Tragus
屏间切迹 Intertragic notch

Helix tubercle 耳轮结节
Scapha 耳舟
Helix 耳轮
Antihelix 对耳轮
Cavum concha 耳甲腔
Helix notch 轮屏切迹
Antitragus 对耳屏
Helix cauda 耳轮尾
Ear lobe 耳垂

图 3-1　耳廓的表面解剖
Fig. 3-1　Anatomy of the front surface of the auricle

耳轮　耳廓卷曲的游离部分。

耳轮结节　耳轮外上部的膨大部分。

耳轮尾　耳轮向下移行于耳垂的部分。

耳轮脚　耳轮深入耳甲的部分。

对耳轮　与耳轮相对呈 Y 字形的隆起部，由对耳轮体、对耳轮上脚和对耳轮下脚三部分组成。

对耳轮体　对耳轮向下部呈上下走向的主体部分。

对耳轮上脚　对耳轮向上分支的部分。

对耳轮下脚　对耳轮向下分支的部分。

三角窝　对耳轮上、下脚与相应耳轮之间的三角形凹窝。

耳舟　耳轮与对耳轮之间的凹沟。

耳屏　耳廓前方呈瓣状的隆起。

屏上切迹　耳屏与耳轮之间的凹陷处。

对耳屏　耳垂上方、与耳屏相对的瓣状隆起。

屏间切迹　耳屏与对耳屏之间的凹陷处。

轮屏切迹　对耳轮与对耳屏之间的凹陷处。

耳垂　耳廓下部无软骨的部分。

耳甲　部分耳轮和对耳轮、对耳屏及外耳门之间的凹窝。由耳甲艇、耳甲腔两部分组成。

耳甲腔　耳轮脚以下的耳甲部。

耳甲艇　耳轮脚以上的耳甲部。

外耳门　耳甲腔前方的孔窍。

二、耳穴的分布

耳穴是指分布在耳廓上的一些特定穴位。人体的内脏或躯体发生病变时，往往在耳廓的相应部位出现压痛敏感、皮肤电特异性改变和变形、变色等反应。参考这些现象来诊断疾病，并通过刺激这些部位可防治疾病。

耳穴在耳廓的分布有一定的规律，根据形如胚胎的耳穴分布图看到：与头面相应的穴位在耳垂，与上肢相应的穴位居耳舟，与下肢相应的穴位在对耳轮上下脚，与胸腔内脏相应的穴位集中在耳甲腔，与腹腔内脏相应的耳穴分布在耳甲艇，与脊柱和躯干相应的耳穴分布在对耳轮上，与盆腔相应的耳穴分布在三角窝，与消化道相应的耳穴分布在耳轮脚周围，与泌尿道相应的耳穴分布在耳轮下脚与耳甲艇交界处（图3-2）。

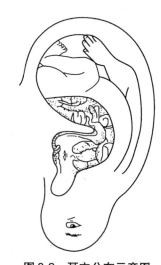

图3-2　耳穴分布示意图

Fig. 3-2　Distribution of the auricular points

三、耳穴的部位和主治

耳穴的部位见图3-3（a）、（b）。

（一）耳轮穴位

将耳轮分为12个区。耳轮脚为耳轮1区。耳轮脚切迹到对耳轮下脚上缘之间的耳轮分为3等份，自下向上依次为耳轮2区、3区、4区；对耳轮下脚上缘到对耳轮上脚前缘之间的耳轮为耳轮5区；对耳轮上脚缘到耳尖之间的耳轮为耳轮6区；耳尖到耳轮结节上缘为耳轮7区；耳轮结节上缘到耳轮结节下缘为耳轮8区。耳轮结节下缘到轮垂切迹之间的耳轮分为4等份，自上而下依次为耳轮9区、10区、11区和12区（表3-1）。

（二）耳舟穴位

将耳舟分为6等份，自上而下依次为耳舟1区、2区、3区、4区、5区、6区（表3-2）。

表 3-1 耳轮穴位部位及主治

穴名	部位	主治
耳中	在耳轮脚处,即耳轮1区	呃逆、荨麻疹、皮肤瘙痒症、小儿遗尿、出血性疾病
直肠	在耳轮脚棘前上方的耳轮处,即耳轮2区	便秘、腹泻、脱肛、痔疮
尿道	在直肠上方的耳轮处,即耳轮3区	尿频、尿急、尿痛、尿潴留
外生殖器	在对耳轮下脚前方的耳轮处,即耳轮4区	睾丸炎、附睾炎、外阴瘙痒症
肛门	在三角窝前方的耳轮处,即耳轮5区	痔疮、肛裂
耳尖	在耳郭向前对折的上部尖端处,即耳轮6、7区交界处	发热、高血压、急性结膜炎、麦粒肿、牙痛、失眠
结节	在耳轮结节处,即耳轮8区	头晕、头痛、高血压
轮1	在耳轮结节下方的耳轮处,即耳轮9区	发热、扁桃体炎、上呼吸道感染
轮2	在轮1区下方的耳轮处,即耳轮10区	发热、扁桃体炎、上呼吸道感染
轮3	在轮2区下方的耳轮处,即耳轮11区	发热、扁桃体炎、上呼吸道感染
轮4	在轮3区下方的耳轮处,即耳轮12区	发热、扁桃体炎、上呼吸道感染

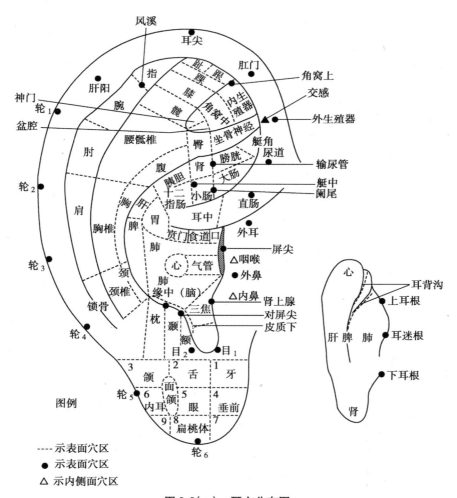

图 3-3(a) 耳穴分布图

Fig. 3-3(a) Locations of the auricular points

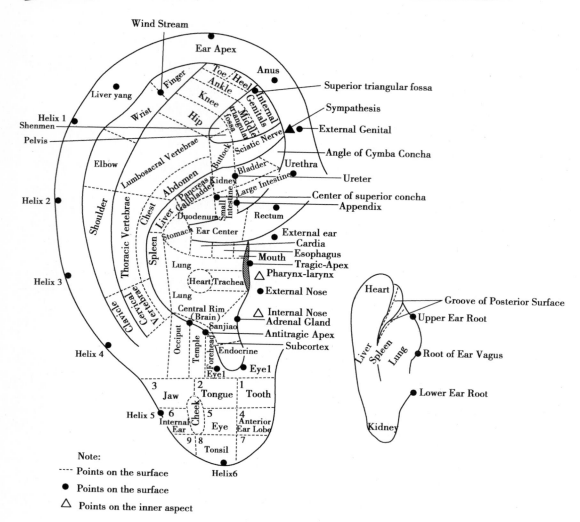

图 3-3（b）　耳穴分布图

Fig. 3-3（b）　Locations of the auricular points

表 3-2　耳舟穴位部位及主治

穴名	部位	主治
指	在耳舟上方处，即耳舟 1 区	甲沟炎、手指麻木和疼痛
腕	在指区的下方处，即耳舟 2 区	腕部疼痛
风溪	在耳轮结节前方，指区与腕区之间，即耳舟 1、2 区交界处	荨麻疹、皮肤瘙痒症、过敏性鼻炎
肘	在腕区的下方处，即耳舟 3 区	肱骨外上髁炎、肘部疼痛
肩	在肘区的下方处，即耳舟 4、5 区	肩关节周围炎、肩部疼痛
锁骨	在肩区的下方处，即耳舟 6 区	肩关节周围炎

（三）对耳轮穴位

将对耳轮分为 13 区。对耳轮上脚分为上、中、下 3 等份；下 1/3 为对耳轮 5 区，中 1/3 为对耳轮 4 区；再将上 1/3 分为上、下 2 等份，下 1/2 为对耳轮 3 区，再将上 1/2 分为前后 2 等份，后 1/2 为对耳轮 2 区，前 1/2 为对耳轮 1 区。对耳轮下脚分为前、中、后 3 等份，中、前

2/3 为对耳轮 6 区，后 1/3 为对耳轮 7 区。对耳轮体从对耳轮上、下脚分叉处至轮屏切迹分为 5 等份，再沿对耳轮耳甲缘将对耳轮体分为前 1/4 和后 3/4 两部分，前上 2/5 为对耳轮 8 区，后上 2/5 为对耳轮 9 区，前中 2/5 为对耳轮 10 区，后中 2/5 为对耳轮 11 区，前下 1/5 为对耳轮 12 区，后下 1/5 为对耳轮 13 区（表 3-3）。

表3-3　对耳轮穴位部位及主治

穴名	部位	主治
跟	在对耳轮上脚前上部，即对耳轮 1 区	足跟痛
趾	在耳尖下方的对耳轮上脚后上部，即对耳轮 2 区	甲沟炎、趾部疼痛
踝	在趾、跟区下方处，即对耳轮 3 区	踝关节扭伤
膝	在对耳轮上脚中 1/3 处，即对耳轮 4 区	膝关节疼痛、坐骨神经痛
髋	在对耳轮上脚的下 1/3 处，即对耳轮 5 区	髋关节疼痛、坐骨神经痛、腰骶部疼痛
坐骨神经	在对耳轮下脚的前 2/3 处，即对耳轮 6 区	坐骨神经痛、下肢瘫痪
交感	在对耳轮下脚末端与耳轮内缘相交处，即对耳轮 6 区前端	胃肠痉挛、心绞痛、胆绞痛、输尿管结石、自主神经功能紊乱
臀	在对耳轮下脚的后 1/3 处，即对耳轮 7 区	坐骨神经痛、臀筋膜炎
腹	在对耳轮体前部上 2/5 处，即对耳轮 8 区	腹痛、腹胀、腹泻、急性腰扭伤、痛经、产后宫缩痛
腰骶椎	在腹区后方，即对耳轮 9 区	腰骶部疼痛
胸	在对耳轮体前部中 2/5 处，即对耳轮 10 区	胸胁疼痛、肋间神经痛、胸闷、乳腺炎
胸椎	在胸区后方，即对耳轮 11 区	胸痛、经前乳房胀痛、乳腺炎、产后泌乳不足
颈	在对耳轮体前部下 1/5 处，即对耳轮 12 区	落枕、颈椎疼痛
颈椎	在颈区后方，即对耳轮 13 区	落枕、颈椎综合征

（四）三角窝穴位

将三角窝分为 5 区。三角窝由耳轮内缘至对耳轮上、下脚分叉处分为前、中、后 3 等份，中 1/3 为三角窝 3 区；再将前 1/3 分为上、中、下 3 等份，上 1/3 为三角窝 1 区，中、下 2/3 为三角窝 2 区；再将后 1/3 分为上、下 2 等份，上 1/2 为三角窝 4 区，下 1/2 为三角窝 5 区（表 3-4）。

表3-4　三角窝穴位部位及主治

穴名	部位	主治
角窝上	在三角窝前 1/3 的上部，即三角窝 1 区	高血压
内生殖器	在三角窝前 1/3 的下部，即三角窝 2 区	痛经、月经不调、白带过多、功能性子宫出血、阳痿、遗精、早泄
角窝中	在三角窝中 1/3 处，即三角窝 3 区	哮喘
神门	在三角窝后 1/3 的上部，即三角窝 4 区	失眠、多梦、戒断综合征、癫痫、高血压、神经衰弱、痛证
盆腔	在三角窝后 1/3 的下部，即三角窝 5 区	盆腔炎、附件炎

（五）耳屏穴位

将耳屏分成 4 区。耳屏外侧面分为上、下 2 等份，上部为耳屏 1 区，下部为耳屏 2 区。将耳屏内侧面分为上、下 2 等份，上部为耳屏 3 区，下部为耳屏 4 区（表 3-5）。

表 3-5 耳屏穴位部位及主治

穴名	部位	主治
上屏	在耳屏外侧面上 1/2 处,即耳屏 1 区	咽炎、鼻炎、单纯性肥胖
下屏	在耳屏外侧面下 1/2 处,即耳屏 2 区	鼻炎、鼻塞、单纯性肥胖
外耳	在屏上切迹前方近耳轮部,即耳屏 1 区上缘处	外耳道炎、中耳炎、耳鸣
屏尖	在耳屏游离缘上部尖端,即耳屏 1 区后缘处	发热、牙痛、斜视
外鼻	在耳屏外侧面中部,即耳屏 1、2 区之间	鼻前庭炎、鼻炎
肾上腺	在耳屏游离缘下部尖端,即耳屏 2 区后缘处	低血压、风湿性关节炎、腮腺炎、眩晕、哮喘、休克、过敏性疾病
咽喉	在耳屏内侧面上 1/2 处,即耳屏 3 区	声音嘶哑、咽炎、扁桃体炎
内鼻	在耳屏内侧面下 1/2 处,即耳屏 4 区	鼻炎、上颌窦炎、鼻衄
屏间前	在屏间切迹前方耳屏最下部,即耳屏 2 区下缘处	咽炎、口腔炎、眼病

（六）对耳屏穴位

将对耳屏分为 4 区。由对屏尖及对屏尖至轮屏切迹连线之中点,分别向耳垂上线作两条垂线,将对耳屏外侧面及其后部分成前、中、后 3 区,前为对耳屏 1 区、中为对耳屏 2 区、后为对耳屏 3 区。对耳屏内侧面为对耳屏 4 区（表 3-6）。

表 3-6 对耳屏穴位部位及主治

穴名	部位	主治
额	在对耳屏外侧面的前部,即对耳屏 1 区	前额痛、头晕、失眠、多梦
屏间后	在屏间切迹后方对耳屏前下部,即对耳屏 1 区下缘处	额窦炎、眼病
颞	在对耳屏外侧面的中部,即对耳屏 2 区	偏头痛、头晕
枕	在对耳屏外侧面的后部,即对耳屏 3 区	头晕、头痛、癫痫、哮喘、神经衰弱
皮质下	在对耳屏内侧面,即对耳屏 4 区	痛症、神经衰弱、假性近视、失眠
对屏尖	在对耳屏游离缘的尖端,即对耳屏 1、2、4 区交点处	哮喘、腮腺炎、睾丸炎、附睾炎、神经性皮炎
缘中	在对耳屏游离缘上,对屏尖与轮屏切迹之中点处,即对耳屏 2、3、4 区交点处	遗尿、内耳性眩晕、尿崩症、功能性子宫出血
脑干	在轮屏切迹处,即对耳屏 3、4 区之间	眩晕、后头痛、假性近视

（七）耳甲穴位

将耳甲用标志点、线分为 18 个区。在耳轮的内缘上,设耳轮脚切迹至对耳轮下脚间中、上 1/3 交界处为 A 点;在耳甲内,由耳轮脚消失处向后作一水平线与对耳轮耳甲缘相交,设交点为 D 点;设耳轮脚消失处至 D 点连线中、后 1/3 交界处为 B 点;设外耳道口后缘上 1/4 与下 3/4 交界处为 C 点;从 A 点向 B 点作一条与对耳轮耳甲艇缘弧度大体相仿的曲线;从 B 点向 C 点作一条与耳轮脚下缘弧度大体相仿的曲线（图 3-4）。

将 BC 线前段与耳轮脚下缘间分成 3 等份,前 1/3 为耳甲 1 区,中 1/3 为耳甲 2 区,后 1/3 为耳甲 3 区。ABC 线前方,耳轮脚消失处为耳甲 4 区。将 AB 线前段与耳轮脚上缘及部分耳轮内缘间分成 3 等份,后 1/3 为 5 区,中 1/3 为 6 区,前 1/3 为 7 区。

将对耳轮下脚下缘前、中 1/3 交界处与 A 点连线,该线前方的耳甲艇部为耳甲 8 区。将 AB 线前段与对耳轮下脚下缘间耳甲 8 区以后的部分,分为前、后 2 等份,前 1/2 为耳甲 9

区,后 1/2 为耳甲 10 区。在 AB 线后段上方的耳甲艇部,将耳甲 10 区后缘与 BD 线之间分成上、下 2 等份,上 1/2 为耳甲 11 区,下 1/2 为耳甲 12 区。由轮屏切迹至 B 点作连线,该线后方、BD 线下方的耳甲腔部为耳甲 13 区。以耳甲腔中央为圆心,圆心与 BC 线间距离的 1/2 为半径作圆,该圆形区域为耳甲 15 区。过 15 区最高点及最低点分别向外耳门后壁作两条切线,切线间为耳甲 16 区。15、16 区周围为耳甲 14 区。将外耳门的最低点与对耳屏耳甲缘中点相连,再将该线以下的耳甲腔部分为上、下 2 等份,上 1/2 为耳甲 17 区,下 1/2 为耳甲 18 区(表 3-7)。

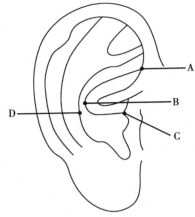

图 3-4 耳廓标志点线示意图
Fig. 3-4 Marker points and lines on the auricle

表 3-7 耳甲穴位部位及主治

穴名	部位	主治
口	在耳轮脚下方前 1/3 处,即耳甲 1 区	面瘫、口腔炎、胆囊炎、胆石症、戒断综合征、牙周炎、舌炎
食道	在耳轮脚下方中 1/3 处,即耳甲 2 区	食管炎、食管痉挛
贲门	在耳轮脚下方后 1/3 处,即耳甲 3 区	贲门痉挛、神经性呕吐
胃	在耳轮脚消失处,即耳甲 4 区	胃痉挛、胃炎、胃溃疡、消化不良、恶心呕吐、前额痛、牙痛、失眠
十二指肠	在耳轮脚及部分耳轮与 AB 线之间的后 1/3 处,即耳甲 5 区	十二指肠溃疡、胆囊炎、胆石症、幽门痉挛、腹胀、腹泻、腹痛
小肠	在耳轮脚及部分耳轮与 AB 线之间的中 1/3 处,即耳甲 6 区	消化不良、腹痛、腹胀、心动过速
大肠	在耳轮脚及部分耳轮与 AB 线之间的前 1/3 处,即耳甲 7 区	腹泻、便秘、咳嗽、牙痛、痤疮
阑尾	在小肠区与大肠区之间,即耳甲 6、7 区交界处	单纯性阑尾炎、腹泻
艇角	在对耳轮下脚下方前部,即耳甲 8 区	前列腺炎、尿道炎
膀胱	在对耳轮下脚下方中部,即耳甲 9 区	膀胱炎、遗尿、尿潴留、腰痛、坐骨神经痛、后头痛
肾	在对耳轮下脚下方后部,即耳甲 10 区	腰痛、耳鸣、神经衰弱、肾盂肾炎、遗尿、遗精、阳痿、早泄、哮喘、月经不调
输尿管	在肾区与膀胱区之间,即耳甲 9、10 区交界处	输尿管结石绞痛
胰胆	在耳甲艇的后上部,即耳甲 11 区	胆囊炎、胆石症、胆道蛔虫症、偏头痛、带状疱疹、中耳炎、耳鸣、急性胰腺炎
肝	在耳甲艇的后下部,即耳甲 12 区	胁痛、眩晕、经前期紧张症、月经不调、更年期综合征、高血压、近视、单纯性青光眼
艇中	在小肠区与肾区之间,即耳甲 6、10 区交界处	腹痛、腹胀、胆道蛔虫症
脾	在 BD 线下方,耳甲腔的后上部,即耳甲 13 区	腹胀、腹泻、便秘、食欲缺乏、功能性子宫出血、白带过多、内耳性眩晕

续表

穴名	部位	主治
心	在耳甲腔正中凹陷处，即耳甲15区	心动过速、心律不齐、心绞痛、无脉症、神经衰弱、癔病、口舌生疮
气管	在心区与外耳门之间，即耳甲16区	哮喘、支气管炎
肺	在心、气管区周围处，即耳甲14区	咳嗽、胸闷、声音嘶哑、皮肤瘙痒症、荨麻疹、便秘、戒断综合征
三焦	在外耳门后下，肺与内分泌区之间，即耳甲17区	便秘、腹胀、上肢外侧疼痛
内分泌	在屏间切迹内，耳甲腔的前下部，即耳甲18区	痛经、月经不调、更年期综合征、痤疮、甲状腺功能减退或亢进症

（八）耳垂穴位

将耳垂分为9区。在耳垂上线至耳垂下缘最低点之间划两条等距离平行线，于上平行线上引两条垂直等份线，将耳垂分为9个区，上部由前到后依次为耳垂1区、2区、3区；中部由前到后依次为耳垂4区、5区、6区；下部由前到后依次为耳垂7区、8区、9区（表3-8）。

表3-8　耳垂穴位部位及主治

穴名	部位	主治
牙	在耳垂正面前上部，即耳垂1区	牙痛、牙周炎、低血压
舌	在耳垂正面中上部，即耳垂2区	舌炎、口腔炎
颌	在耳垂正面后上部，即耳垂3区	牙痛、颞颌关节功能紊乱症
垂前	在耳垂正面前中部，即耳垂4区	神经衰弱、牙痛
眼	在耳垂正面中央部，即耳垂5区	急性结膜炎、电光性眼炎、麦粒肿、近视
内耳	在耳垂正面后中部，即耳垂6区	内耳性眩晕症、耳鸣、听力减退、中耳炎
面颊	在耳垂正面与内耳区之间，即耳垂5、6区交界处	面瘫、三叉神经痛、痤疮、扁平疣、面肌痉挛、腮腺炎
扁桃体	在耳垂正面下部，即耳垂7、8、9区	扁桃体炎、咽炎

（九）耳背穴位

将耳背分为5区。分别过对耳轮上、下脚分叉处耳背对应点和轮屏切迹耳背对应点作两条水平线，将耳背分为上、中、下3部，上部为耳背1区，下部为耳背5区，再将中部分为内、中、外3等份，内1/3为耳背2区、中1/3为耳背3区、外1/3为耳背4区（表3-9）。

表3-9　耳背穴位部位及主治

穴名	部位	主治
耳背心	在耳背上部，即耳背1区	心悸、失眠、多梦
耳背肺	在耳背中内部，即耳背2区	哮喘、皮肤瘙痒症
耳背脾	在耳背中央部，即耳背3区	胃痛、消化不良、食欲缺乏
耳背肝	在耳背中外部，即耳背4区	胆囊炎、胆石症、胁痛
耳背肾	在耳背下部，即耳背5区	头痛、头晕、神经衰弱
耳背沟	在对耳轮沟和对耳轮上、下脚沟处	高血压、皮肤瘙痒症

（十）耳根穴位

表 3-10　耳根穴位部位及主治

穴名	部位	主治
上耳根	在耳根最上处	鼻衄
耳迷根	在耳轮脚后沟的耳根处	胆囊炎、胆石症、腹痛、腹泻、鼻塞、心动过速
下耳根	在耳根最下处	低血压、下肢瘫痪、小儿麻痹后遗症

四、耳穴压丸法的临床应用

（一）适应证

疼痛性疾病：如各种扭挫伤、头痛和神经性疼痛等。

炎性疾病及传染病：如急慢性结肠炎、牙周炎、咽喉炎、扁桃体炎、胆囊炎、流感、百日咳、菌痢、腮腺炎等。

功能紊乱和变态反应性疾病：如眩晕综合征、高血压、心律不齐、神经衰弱、荨麻疹、哮喘、鼻炎、紫癜等。

内分泌代谢紊乱性疾病：甲状腺功能亢进或低下、糖尿病、肥胖症、更年期综合征等。

其他：耳穴可以催乳、催产，预防和治疗输血、输液反应，同时还有美容、戒烟、戒毒、延缓衰老、预防保健等作用。

（二）选穴原则

按相应部位取穴：当机体患病时，在耳廓的相应部位上有一定的敏感点，它便是本病的首选穴位。如胃痛，取"胃"穴等。

按脏腑辨证取穴：根据脏腑学说的理论，按各脏腑的生理功能和病理反应进行辨证取穴。如脱发，取"肾"穴；皮肤病，取"肺"、"大肠"穴等。

按经络辨证取穴：根据十二经脉循行和其病候选取穴位。如坐骨神经痛，取"膀胱"或"胰胆"穴；牙痛，取"大肠"穴等。

按现代医学理论取穴：如炎性疾病、哮喘，取"肾上腺"穴；疼痛、炎症，取"神门、皮质下"穴；月经不调，取"内分泌"穴。

按临床经验取穴：临床实践发现有些耳穴具有治疗本部位以外疾病的作用，如"外生殖器"穴可以治疗腰腿痛，目赤肿痛取"耳尖"放血。

（三）操作方法

1. 耳穴探查

望诊：当人体脏腑或四肢躯干有病时，可以在耳廓的一定部位出现各种阳性反应，如变形、变色、丘疹、脱屑、结节、充血、凹陷、小水疱等。

压痛：在患者耳廓病变的相应部位，用探针、火柴梗或毫针柄等，用轻、慢、均匀的压力寻找压痛点。

测定电阻改变：通常用电阻测定仪测定皮肤电阻的良导点，低电阻点的耳穴可反映在仪器的显示屏、指示灯或声音的改变。

2. 选穴　诊断明确后，根据耳穴的选穴原则或用以上耳穴探查方法在耳廓上所获得阳性反应点，确立处方。

3. 消毒　耳穴用 75% 乙醇常规消毒。

4. 压丸　压丸所选材料多用王不留行籽、小磁珠等。先将其贴在 0.5cm × 0.5cm 小方块胶布中央，然后一手捏住耳廓，另一手用探棒按压耳穴，寻找敏感点，再将小丸贴敷于耳穴上，并给予适当按压，使耳廓有发热、胀痛感。主要贴压患病侧耳穴，也可双侧同时贴压或交替贴压。一般每天患者可自行按压 2~4 次，贴好的耳豆可保留 3~5 天，复诊时按病情酌情增减或更换穴位。

5. 注意事项

（1）使用中应防止胶布潮湿或污染，以免引起皮肤炎症。对胶布过敏的病人改用其他耳穴刺激方法。

（2）为避免耳廓皮肤损伤，不宜上下或环形揉动贴压的耳穴。

（3）耳廓皮肤有炎性病变、冻疮等不宜采用此法。

（4）有习惯性流产的孕妇和严重心脏病患者禁用此法。

（5）对扭伤和有运动障碍的患者，按压后宜适当活动患部，有助于提高疗效。

第二节　推　拿　法

推拿法是操作者用手或肢体其他部分刺激治疗部位和活动肢体的规范化技巧动作。由于刺激方式、强度、时间的不同，形成了不同的手法，如推法、按法、揉法等，这些基本手法是推拿手法的主要组成部分。两个以上基本手法结合起来操作形成复合手法，如按揉法、推摩法等。推拿法具有疏通经络、行气活血、滑利关节、调节脏腑功能等作用。

一、推拿法的适应证

成人推拿手法适用于：骨伤科病证，如落枕、颈椎病、急性腰扭伤、慢性腰肌劳损、肩周炎、腰椎间盘突出症等；慢性软组织劳损；急性软组织损伤；内科病证，如便秘、腹泻、高血压、头痛等；妇科病证，如痛经、月经不调；五官科病证，如牙痛、耳聋。儿科推拿手法适用于咳嗽、发热、哮喘、呕吐、厌食、便秘等病证。

二、推拿手法的基本要求

手法的基本要求是：持久、有力、均匀、柔和、深透。"持久"要求手法操作能持续一定的时间，且动作规范不变形；"有力"要求手法必须具有恰当的力量，力量的大小应根据患者的体质、病情和治疗部位的不同进行调整，切忌使用拙力、暴力；"均匀"要求手法动作有节奏性，速度、压力在一定范围内维持恒定；"柔和"要求手法轻柔缓和，不能生硬粗暴；"深透"要求手法作用达到组织深层。只有符合持久、有力、均匀、柔和要求的手法才能深透。成功的手法应以柔为先、和为贵。

三、成人常用推拿手法

（一）一指禅推法

以拇指指端或罗纹面着力，前臂摆动，使所产生的力通过拇指持续不断的作用于施术部位或穴位上，称为一指禅推法。

【操作方法】术者手握空拳，腕掌悬屈，拇指自然伸直，盖住拳眼，用拇指指端或末节罗纹面着力于体表上,沉肩、垂肘、悬腕,运用前臂的主动摆动带动腕部的横向摆动及拇指关节的屈伸活动,使力轻重交替、持续不断地作用于经络穴位上,频率每分钟120~160次。

【动作要领】

(1)沉肩:肩关节放松,肩胛骨自然下沉,保持腋下空松,能容纳一拳的距离,不要耸肩用力。

(2)垂肘:肘关节自然下垂,略低于腕部。肘部不要向外支起,亦不宜过度内收。

(3)悬腕:腕关节屈曲,自然悬垂,在保持腕关节放松的基础上,尽可能屈腕至90°。

(4)指实:拇指指端或罗纹面自然着实,吸定于施术部位或穴位上,但不可拙力下压。

(5)掌虚:除拇指外的其余四指及手掌放松,握虚拳,做到蓄力于掌,发力于指。

(6)紧推慢移:紧推是一指禅推法的摆动频率相对较快,维持在每分钟120~160次;慢移是拇指指端或罗纹面在吸定于体表的基础上,可沿经络或特定的路径缓慢移动,同时不可滑动或摩擦。

【注意事项】

(1)操作时宜气定神敛,心神和宁,专注于手法操作。姿势端正,要领正确,使手法形神俱备。

(2)一指禅推法有拇指指间关节屈伸和不屈伸两种不同术式。若术者拇指指间关节较僵硬,活动范围较小或治疗时需要较柔和的刺激,可采用屈伸拇指指间关节的操作;若术者拇指指间关节较柔软,宜选用不屈伸拇指指间关节的操作。

(3)在体表操作时应遵循"推经络,走穴道"的原则,循经取穴施治。

(二)㨰法

以尺侧手背为接触面,前臂摆动带动腕关节屈伸,手背在体表施术部位滚动,称为㨰法。

【操作方法】

术者拇指自然伸直,手握空拳,小指、无名指的掌指关节自然屈曲约90°,其余手指掌指关节屈曲角度依次减小,使手背沿掌横弓排列成弧面,以手掌背部近小指侧部分贴附于治疗部位上,前臂主动摆动,带动腕关节较大幅度的屈伸和前臂旋转的协同运动,使手背尺侧在治疗部位上做持续不断的来回滚动,摆动频率每分钟120次左右。

【动作要领】

(1)沉肩,垂肘,肘关节自然屈曲140°,距胸壁一拳左右,松腕,手握空拳,小指至食指掌指关节屈曲角度依次减小,手背呈弧形,吸定于治疗部位。

(2)腕关节屈伸幅度要在120°左右,即外摆时屈腕约80°,回摆时伸腕约40°,使手掌背部分的二分之一面积依次接触治疗部位。外摆的同时前臂外旋,回摆时前臂内旋。

(3)刺激轻重交替,前滚同回滚时着力重轻之比为3:1,即"滚三回一"。

(4)㨰法在体表移动时应在吸定的基础上,保持手法的固有频率,移动速度不宜过快。

(5)㨰法在临床应用时经常配合患者肢体的被动运动,可在一手㨰法同时,另一手协同肢体做被动运动,两手要协调,被动运动要"轻巧、短促、随发随收"。

【注意事项】

(1)㨰法操作应尽量做到腕关节最大幅度的屈伸,避免出现前臂旋转为主、腕关节屈伸幅度不足的错误方式。

(2)㨰法宜吸定,不宜拖动、跳动或旋转摆动,避免出现手背与体表的撞击感。

(3)避免在脊椎棘突或其他各部位关节的骨突处施术,以免给患者带来不适感。

（三）揉法

以指、掌的某一部位着力吸定于体表上，带动该处的皮下组织做轻柔缓和的环旋揉动，称为揉法，是推拿常用手法之一。根据操作时接触面的不同可分为掌根揉法、鱼际揉法和指揉法。

【操作方法】

（1）掌根揉法：术者以掌根部分着力，手指自然弯曲，腕关节略背伸，肘关节微屈作为支点，前臂做主动摆动，带动掌根在治疗部位揉动，频率为每分钟120～160次。

（2）鱼际揉法：术者以手掌鱼际部着力，腕关节微屈120°～140°，以肘关节为支点，前臂做主动摆动，带动鱼际在治疗部位揉动摆动，频率每分钟120～160次。

（3）拇指揉法：以拇指罗纹面着力，其余手指扶持于合适部位，腕关节微屈或伸直，前臂做小幅度摆动，带动拇指在施术部位上做环转运动，频率为每分钟120～160次。

（4）中指揉法：以中指罗纹面着力，中指指间关节伸直，掌指关节微屈，以肘关节为支点，前臂作小幅度主动运动，带动中指罗纹面在施术部位做环转运动，频率为每分钟120～160次。

以食指或食、中、无名指并拢做指揉法分别称为食指揉法和三指揉法，操作要领同中指揉法。

【动作要领】

（1）要做到沉肩、垂肘、腕关节放松，以前臂小幅度的主动摆动，通过腕关节传递，带动接触部位回转运动。

（2）操作时要带动皮下组织一起运动，动作要灵活协调而有节律。

（3）所施压力要适中，以受术者感到舒适为度。

【注意事项】

（1）操作时，接触部位不可和体表之间有相对摩擦运动。

（2）功力要通过放松的腕关节传递，注意在做指揉法的时候，腕关节应在放松的基础上，保持一定的紧张度，不可使腕关节过分僵硬。

（四）摩法

以指、掌面为接触部位，在体表做环形而有节奏的摩擦运动，称为摩法，是推拿手法中最轻柔的一种手法。

【操作方法】

（1）掌摩法：术者手指并拢，手掌自然伸直，腕关节微伸，将手掌平放在体表上，以肘关节为支点，前臂做主动运动，带动手掌在体表施术部位做环旋摩擦运动。频率为每分钟100～120次，顺时针逆时针均可。

（2）指摩法：以食、中、无名、小指末节指面为接触部位，四指并拢，手掌自然伸直，腕关节微屈，以肘关节为支点，前臂做主动运动，带动四指指面在施术部位做环形摩擦运动，频率为每分钟100～120次，顺时针逆时针均可。

【动作要领】

（1）肩关节应放松，以前臂主动摆动为主，带动放松的腕关节做环转运动。指摩法时腕关节在放松的基础上可保持一定的紧张度，但要紧而不僵。

（2）用力要轻重得宜，速度均衡。指摩法较轻快，掌摩法稍重缓。

【注意事项】

（1）宜轻缓，不宜急重。

（2）根据病情的虚实决定手法的方向。传统认为虚证宜用顺时针方向的摩法，实证宜用逆时针方向的摩法，临床还应结合施术部位的解剖结构和病理状况选择使用不同方向的摩法。

（3）应用时，常根据病情，涂以各种性能的药膏。也可涂以葱姜汁、松节油等推拿介质，以加强摩法的作用。

（4）注意揉法和摩法的区别：揉法着力较重，操作时指掌吸定一个部位，带动皮下组织，和体表没有摩擦动作；摩法则着力较轻，操作时指掌在体表做环旋摩擦，而不带动皮下组织。临床上两者常结合使用。

（五）擦法

术者以手掌的鱼际、掌根或小鱼际着力于施术部位，做直线往返摩擦运动，使摩擦产生的热量透过体表渗透至深层，称为擦法。可分为掌擦法、鱼际擦法和小鱼际擦法。

【操作方法】

（1）掌擦法：术者以手掌掌面紧贴皮肤，腕关节平直，以肩关节为支点，上臂做主动运动，使手掌掌面在体表做直线往返的摩擦运动。频率为每分钟100～120次，多用于胸胁及腹部。

（2）鱼际擦法：术者以鱼际着力贴于体表，腕关节平直，以肩关节为支点，上臂做主动运动，使鱼际在体表做直线往返的摩擦运动。频率为每分钟100～120次，多用于胸腹、腰背和四肢部。

（3）小鱼际擦法：术者以小鱼际着力贴于体表，立掌，腕关节平直，以肩关节为支点，上臂做主动运动，使小鱼际在体表做直线往返的摩擦运动。频率为每分钟100～120次，多用于肩背、腰臀及下肢部。

【动作要领】

（1）运行路线宜直、长。不论是上下或左右摩擦，都要直线往返，不可歪斜，而且往返距离要拉长且连续，不能间歇停顿。

（2）手掌应与受术者体表接触平实，向下的压力要保持均匀，以摩擦时不使皮肤起皱为度，动作频率也应均匀。

【注意事项】

（1）术者在操作时呼吸要自然，不能屏气。

（2）产生温热刺激，掌擦法的热效应较温和；小鱼际擦法产生的热量较高；鱼际擦法产生的热量中等。临床使用擦法以患者自觉透热为度。

（3）操作时，可在施术部位涂些润滑剂，既可保护皮肤，又有利于热量渗透到体内。

（4）需直接在体表操作，应注意室内保暖。

（5）操作后，一般不宜在该施术部位再使用其他手法，避免皮肤损伤。

（六）推法

用指、掌或其他部位着力于人体一定部位或穴位上，做单方向直线或弧线的移动，称为推法。可分为平推法、直推法、旋推法、分推法、合推法等。

【操作方法】

（1）平推法：根据着力部位的不同，有拇指平推法、掌平推法和肘平推法三种。用拇指面着力紧贴体表，按经络循行或肌纤维平行方向做单方向沉缓推动。在推进过程中，可在重点治疗部位或穴位上做按揉动作。

（2）直推法：术者用拇指桡侧面或食、中两指罗纹面着力于一定部位或穴位上，做单方向的直线推动。

（3）旋推法：术者用拇指罗纹面在穴位上做螺旋形推动，频率为每分钟200～240次。

（4）分推法：术者用双手拇指罗纹面或掌面紧贴在体表上，自中心部位分别向左右两侧单方向推开，频率为每分钟120次。

（5）合推法：术者用双手拇指罗纹面或掌面紧贴体表，自穴位两旁推向穴位中间。

【动作要领】

（1）平推法是推法中着力较大的一种，推的时候需用一定的压力，用力要平稳，推进速度要缓慢，要沿直线做单方向运动。

（2）直推法以肘关节的伸屈带动腕、掌、指，做单方向的直线运动，所用压力较平推法为轻，动作要求轻快连续，以推后皮肤不发红为佳。

（3）旋推法要求肘、腕关节放松，仅靠拇指作小幅度的环旋运动，不带动皮下组织运动，类似指摩法。

（4）分推法操作时，要求两手用力均匀，动作柔和协调一致，向两旁分推时既可做直线推动，也可沿弧形推动。

（5）合推法的操作要领同分推法，只不过方向相反。

【注意事项】

（1）推法是单方向的直线或弧线运动，忌往返擦动。

（2）操作时应贴紧体表，用力平稳，均匀适中，推动的速度不宜过快。

（3）在体表操作时，可在施术部位涂滑石粉或葱姜汁等推拿介质。

（七）抹法

以拇指罗纹面贴紧皮肤，沿上下、左右或弧形路径往返推动，称为抹法。分为指抹法和掌抹法两种。

【操作方法】

（1）指抹法：术者用单手或双手拇指罗纹面着力于体表，其余四指扶持助力，拇指略用力，缓慢地做上下、左右或直线或弧线的往返移动。

（2）掌抹法：术者用单手或双手掌面着力于体表，腕关节放松，前臂与上臂协调用力，带动手掌掌面在体表做上下、左右或直线或弧线的往返移动。

【动作要领】

（1）操作时，拇指罗纹面或手掌掌面应贴紧体表。

（2）用力要均匀，动作要和缓，在施术区域内来回抹动的距离应尽量拉长。

【注意事项】

（1）刺激较表浅，操作时不宜带动皮下深部组织。

（2）易与推法相混淆。推法是单向、直线的运动，而抹法可上可下，或直线往来，或曲线运转，应用较灵活。

（3）在头面部使用时，有较固定的操作程序。

（八）扫散法

用拇指桡侧和食、中、无名、小指指端在患者颞部沿少阳经自前向后，做来回推擦运动，称为扫散法。

【操作方法】

术者一手扶患者头部，一手拇指桡侧面及其余四指指端，同时贴于头颞侧部，稍用力向耳后沿少阳经循行路线做快速来回抹动。频率为每分钟 250 次左右。

【动作要领】

（1）术者应沉肩、垂肘、肘关节屈曲 90°～120°，腕关节放松。

（2）以肘关节为支点，前臂做主动摆动，带动腕关节摆动，使着力手指在颞侧来回推擦。

【注意事项】

（1）扫散法操作时，手指着力部位稍用力紧贴头皮，向前推擦时用力稍重，回返时用力稍轻。

（2）扫散时，扶持手应固定好患者头部，避免晃动，产生不适。

（3）扫散法应自前向后循经操作，每次推擦的距离不应太长。

（九）搓法

用双手掌面夹住躯干或肢体一定部位，相对用力交替或往返快速搓动，称为搓法。

【操作方法】

（1）肩及上肢部搓法：患者取坐位，肩臂放松，自然下垂，术者站于其侧，上身略前倾，双手掌分别夹其肩前后部，相对用力快速搓揉，同时自上而下沿上肢移动至腕部，往返 3～5 遍。

（2）胁肋部搓法：患者坐位，两臂略外展，术者站其身后，以两掌分别夹其两胁肋，自腋下搓向腰部两侧数遍。

（3）下肢搓法：患者取仰卧位，屈膝约 60°，术者站于床侧，以双手掌夹其大腿两侧，自上而下搓揉至小腿部。

【动作要领】

（1）操作者应双掌对称用力，患者肢体宜放松。

（2）搓动要快，上下移动要慢。

【注意事项】

（1）用力不可过重。

（2）搓法是一种辅助手法，常用于肩及上肢部，多在推拿治疗结束时使用。

（十）抖法

以双手或单手握住患肢远端，做小幅度的上下或左右的连续抖动，称为抖法。

【操作方法】

术者用手握住上肢或下肢的远端（腕部或踝部），将被抖动的肢体抬高一定的角度（上肢在坐位下外展约 60°，下肢在仰卧位下抬离床面约 30°），在稍用力牵引状态下，做小幅度的、连续的上下抖动，使患者肢体的软组织产生颤动并传达到肢体近端。

【动作要领】

（1）患者被抖动肢体要自然伸直放松，术者呼吸自然，不可屏气。

（2）抖动的幅度要小，频率要快。

【注意事项】

（1）因下肢较重，抖动下肢的幅度可比上肢大些，频率低些。

（2）抖法常用作结束手法，上肢抖法较为常用。

（十一）按法

用手指或手掌面着力于体表特定的穴位或部位上，逐渐用力下压，称为按法。

【操作方法】

（1）指按法：拇指伸直，用拇指指端或罗纹面按压体表经络穴位上，其余四指张开，扶持在旁相应位置上以助力，单手指力不足时可用另一手拇指重叠按压其上，使拇指指面用力向下按压。

（2）掌按法：用掌根、鱼际或全掌着力按压体表，单手力量不足时，可用双手掌重叠按压。

【动作要领】

（1）按压方向要垂直，用力要由轻到重，稳而持续，使刺激充分透达到机体组织的深部，然后逐渐减轻压力，遵循从轻到重再到轻的原则。

（2）按法如需较大刺激时，可略前倾身体，借助躯干的力量增加刺激。

【注意事项】

（1）切忌用迅猛的爆发力，以免产生不良反应。

（2）用力应有节律变化。注意和较长时间持续用力的压法区别。按法在临床上常和揉法结合使用，形成复合手法按揉法。

（十二）压法

用拇指面、掌面或肘关节鹰嘴突起部着力于体表特定的穴位或部位上，持续用力下按，称为压法。

【操作方法】

术者用拇指罗纹面、手掌或屈肘以肘部前臂上段垂直向下按压体表，按压时也可在体表上逐渐滑动。肘部前臂上段按压又称为肘压法。

【动作要领】

按法和压法两者动作相似，故常混称为"按压法"。若严格区分，按法偏动，压法偏静；按法持续时间短，压法持续时间长；按法压力小、刺激轻，压法压力大、刺激强。

【注意事项】

（1）在背腰部使用时，注意控制用力大小，避免产生不良反应。

（2）肘压法的刺激较强，多用于体格健壮者的腰臀部肌肉丰厚处。

（十三）点法

以指端或关节突起部点压一定的穴位或部位，称为点法，临床上可分为指点法和肘点法。

【操作方法】

（1）指点法：术者手握空拳，拇指伸直并靠近食指中节，以拇指端着力或拇指屈曲，以拇指指间关节背侧着力或以中指指端着力，食指末节叠压于中指背侧助力，由轻而重，平稳施力，按压一定的穴位或部位。

（2）肘点法：术者屈肘，以尺骨鹰嘴突起部着力，身体略前倾，用身体上半身的重量通过肩关节、上臂传递至肘部，持续点压。

【动作要领】

点法是由按法衍化而来，要领基本相同，只不过接触面积较小，刺激较强。

【注意事项】

（1）点法接触面较小，刺激强度大，刺激时间短，多用于止痛，又称"指针"。点按后应用揉法可舒缓气血，避免局部软组织损伤。

（2）年老体弱、久病虚衰者慎用点法。

（3）肘点法和肘压法的施力部位不同，前者用尖锐的尺骨鹰嘴突起部着力，后者以肘部平钝的前臂上段着力。

（十四）捏法

用拇指和其他手指对称用力，挤压施术部位，称为捏法。用以脊柱的捏法称为"捏脊"，多用于小儿推拿。

【操作方法】

用拇指与食、中指指面或拇指与其余四指指面夹住施术部位，相对用力挤压，随即放松，重复上述动作并循序移动。

【动作要领】

拇指与其余手指用力要对称，均匀柔和，动作连贯，富有节奏。

【注意事项】

（1）以手指掌面着力，不可用指端着力。

（2）捏法对指力要求较高，尤其是拇指与其他四指的对合力，可采用相应功法练习以提高指力。

（十五）拿法

用拇指与其他四指相对用力，提捏或夹持肢体或肌肤，称为拿法。

【操作方法】

术者腕关节放松，以拇指与食、中指或其余手指的罗纹面相对用力夹紧治疗部位，将肌肤提起，并做轻重交替而连续的揉捏动作。

【动作要领】

（1）腕关节放松，手指伸直，以平坦的指腹着力挟住治疗部位，与拇指相对手指掌指关节屈曲，做类似剪刀式相对用力提捏皮肤及皮下软组织。

（2）用力缓慢柔和而均匀，由轻到重，再由重到轻，揉捏动作连贯。

【注意事项】

（1）操作时，应避免手指的指间关节屈曲，形成指端夹持肌肤或指甲抠掐的动作。

（2）操作时，应根据临床需要尽可能多地捏拿皮下软组织，避免手指在体表滑移。

（3）操作后，可用轻柔的揉摩法以舒缓气血。

（十六）捻法

用拇指和食指指面相对夹住施术部位，做对称的揉捏捻动，称为捻法。

【操作方法】

术者用拇指的罗纹面及食指桡侧面相对用力，夹住治疗部位，拇指与食指稍用力作较快速的揉捏捻动，如捻线状。捻法为辅助手法，多用于指、趾关节部。

【动作要领】

（1）动作要连贯灵活，柔和有力。

（2）速度稍快，在施术部位上的移动速度宜慢。

（十七）拨法

以拇指指腹深按于施术部位，做与筋腱、肌肉等组织走行相垂直地来回拨动，称为拨法，又称"弹拨法"。

【操作方法】

拇指伸直，以拇指指端或罗纹面着力，其余四指置于相应的位置以助力，拇指深按至患者局部有酸胀感后,再做与肌纤维或筋腱走行方向垂直地来回拨动。单手指力不足时,可双手拇指叠加操作。

【动作要领】

(1)操作时,拇指不能和体表皮肤有相对摩擦移动,应带动皮下肌纤维或筋腱韧带一起拨动。

(2)用力宜由轻渐重,以患者能忍受为度。

【注意事项】

(1)常用在压痛点上操作。

(2)刺激较强,操作后宜用轻柔的揉摩法以舒缓气血。

(十八)拍法

用虚掌在体表有节律地拍打,称为拍法。

【操作方法】

术者五指并拢,掌指关节微屈,掌心凹陷呈虚掌,有节奏地拍打治疗部位。击打频率为每分钟100~120次。

【动作要领】

(1)操作时,肩关节宜松沉,腕关节放松,击打要轻快而平稳,手掌着实后即抬起,动作富有节律,拍打次数以皮肤出现微红充血为度。

(2)可单手或双手操作。

【注意事项】

(1)手掌落在体表上应平实,不能在体表有拖抽的动作。

(2)结核、严重的骨质疏松、骨肿瘤、冠心病患者禁用拍法。

(十九)击法

用掌根、掌侧小鱼际、拳背、指尖或桑枝棒等有节奏地击打治疗部位,称为击法。

【操作方法】

(1)掌根击法:手指自然伸展,腕关节略背伸,以掌根部击打体表。

(2)侧击法:手指自然伸直,腕关节略背伸,以双手手掌小鱼际部交替击打体表。

(3)拳击法:术者手握拳,腕关节平直,以拳背平击体表,一般每次击打3~5下。

(4)指尖击法:以手的五指指端合拢轻快敲击治疗部位。

(5)棒击法:用特制的桑枝棒前段约1/2部着力,击打体表。

【动作要领】

(1)击法用劲要快速而短暂,垂直叩击体表,频率均匀有节奏。

(2)掌根击法以掌根为着力点,运用前臂的力量击打,手臂挥动的幅度可较大,每次击打3~5下。

(3)侧击法可单手或双手合掌操作,以肘关节为支点,前臂主动运动,击打时手掌小鱼际应与肌纤维方向垂直,动作轻快有节奏。

(4)拳击法以肘关节为支点,运用肘关节的屈伸和前臂的力量击打,着力宜平稳。

(5)指尖击法操作时,腕关节放松,运用腕关节的小幅度屈伸,以指端轻击体表,频率快如雨点落下。

(6)棒击法以手握桑枝棒下段的1/3,前臂做主动运动,使桑枝棒前段有节奏地击打施术部位。

【注意事项】

（1）击法操作时，应注意击打的反弹感，一触施术部位即弹起，不可在体表停顿或拖抽。

（2）严格掌握各种击法的适应部位和病证，忌暴力击打。

（3）拳击法主要用于大椎、腰骶部；掌击法可用于百会、环跳；指尖击法常用于头部；桑枝棒击法击打时要用棒体平击，不用棒尖。除腰骶部外，其他部位应用顺棒（棒体纵轴与肌纤维方向平行）击打。

（二十）弹法

用中指指腹紧压食指背侧，用力快速弹出，连续弹击某一部位或穴位，称为弹法。

【操作方法】

将食指屈曲，以中指罗纹面紧压食指背侧，然后迅速弹出，击打患处，频率为每分钟120～160次。本法常作为头面部操作的辅助手法使用。

【动作要领】

操作要均匀连续，刺激强度以不引起疼痛为度。

（二十一）振法

用手指或手掌按压在人体一定的穴位和部位上，做连续不断的快速振动，称为振法。

【操作方法】

（1）指振法：术者垂腕，用手指端置于治疗部位上，手指伸直，肘微屈，前臂和手部静止性用力，使手臂发出的振颤通过手指传递到机体，使振动部位有舒适温热感。

（2）掌振法：术者腕关节略背伸，手指自然伸直，以手掌面轻按患者体表，肘微屈，前臂和手部静止性用力，使手臂发出的振颤通过手掌传递到机体，使振动部位有舒适温热感。

【动作要领】

（1）振法操作时，肩部及上肢要求放松，肘微屈。

（2）静止性用力是将手臂与前臂肌肉绷紧，但不做自主运动。

（3）注意力应高度集中于指尖和手掌部，做到均匀自然呼吸。

（4）振颤动作应持续不断，频率为每分钟300～400次。

【注意事项】

（1）振法操作过程中除静止性用力的手部与前臂外，身体其他部位应尽量放松，不可屏气。

（2）操作过程中不可向下按压太重。

（3）振法需经过较长时间的练习。练习少林内功可有效提高振法的质量。

（二十二）掐法

用指甲缘重按穴位而不损伤治疗部位皮肤的方法，称为掐法。

【操作方法】

用拇指或食指指端甲缘重按穴位，而不损伤治疗部位皮肤。

【动作要领】

（1）要垂直向下用力，力量逐渐加大，不可抠动，以免损伤治疗部位的皮肤。

（2）掐后可在治疗部位上用拇指罗纹面轻揉以缓解疼痛。

四、实用自我推拿保健

（一）自我推拿的保健作用与要求

自我推拿保健调护法是指在中医基础理论的指导下，运用推拿的一些基本手法，在体

表一定部位或穴位进行主动推拿,或配合一定的肢体活动,以调整经络,激发营卫气血的运行,平衡阴阳,达到增强体质、防病治病、保健强身、延年益寿的目的。

1. 作用

(1)平衡阴阳:阴阳和谐是人体健康的关键,阴阳失调是疾病的内在根本,疾病的病理变化不外乎阴阳的偏盛偏衰。自我推拿通过疏通经络、协调气血而外柔四肢百骸,内养五脏六腑,调节阴阳的偏盛偏衰,使机体内外调和、阴平阳秘,保持其正常生理功能而身体健康。

(2)疏通经络:经络功能正常,气血运行通畅,脏腑体表得以沟通;若经络不畅,气血运行受阻,则会影响人体正常功能活动,导致疾病的发生。通过推拿手法刺激全身各部的经络、穴位,对身体的一些重要组织、器官的功能进行调整,疏通经络,畅达气血,促进机体新陈代谢,从而达到提高机体的自然抗病能力,起到健身防病的作用。

(3)增强体质:通过推拿可激发人体正气,促进气血运行和化生,提高机体免疫功能。推拿对脏腑有双向调节作用,可调整内脏功能紊乱,可以调畅人体气机,减轻或缓解肉体和精神的疲劳而心情愉悦;能改善局部血液循环和营养供应而达到美容减肥等效果,从而达到增强体质而健康无病的目的。

2. 要求

(1)自我推拿或家庭推拿宜在明确诊断的基础上进行,若有病患应及时就诊,以免延误病情。

(2)推拿时保持环境温湿度适宜,防止外感。给予舒适体位,于推拿部位暴露的皮肤施以适量皮肤润滑剂,如按摩膏等。

(3)推拿手法应协调柔和,用力适中,先轻后重,由浅入深。每次以20～30分钟为宜,因人而异,以舒适愉快为佳。自我推拿应持之以恒、循序渐进方显持久效果。

(4)孕妇腹部、腰骶部及有些穴位如合谷、三阴交等一般慎用推拿手法。如剧烈运动、过饱或饥饿、酒醉、极度疲劳、情绪不稳或在妇女经期等情况下不宜实施推拿。病情严重者、外伤及传染病禁忌推拿。

(5)实用推拿自我保健调护法简便易行、安全有效,适用于各种年龄层次的人进行养生保健、防病强身。

（二）实用推拿自我保健调护手法

1. 全身自我推拿保健法 成人在自身体表部位或穴位进行推拿手法操作,以舒缓疲劳、愉悦心情,并达到强身健体、防病治病、延年益寿的目的,也是保健养生调护的常用方法。具体操作依自身状况而灵活掌握,可以结合五脏循经进行,亦可形成从头到脚连续的动作完成全身自我推拿,施之有法,行之有效。

叩齿→净口→摩面→熨目→点睛明→擦迎香→按太阳→鸣天鼓→梳头→拿颈项→捏肩→甩手→揉胸→摩腹→捶背→搓腰→点环跳→擦大腿→抓小腿→摩涌泉

2. 宽胸法 肺的生理功能正常可使人体呼吸、营养、水液代谢保持良好的状态,反之则出现呼吸不利、胸闷、咳喘,甚至水肿等病证。因此,采用此保健推拿法对肺系疾患起防治作用。

(1)揉胸部:以一手中指罗纹面沿锁骨下、肋间隙,由内向外,由上而下,用力按揉,可感觉酸胀为宜。

(2)拿胸膺:先用右手从腋下捏拿左侧胸大肌约9次,再换左手如法操作。然后双手十指交叉抱持于后枕部,双肘相平,尽力向后扩展,同时吸气,向前内收肘呼气,一呼一吸,操作 9 次。一呼一吸,一提一拿,慢慢由里向外松之。

(3)拍胸:用右手虚掌置于右乳上方,适当用力拍击并渐横向左侧移动,来回 9 次,以热为度。

(4)擦胸:以两手掌交叉紧贴胸部体表,横向用力往返擦动 36 次,以热为度。

(5)推膻中:双手手掌相叠,置于两乳中间的膻中穴,上下推擦 36 次。

(6)揉中府:两手掌交叉抱于胸前,用两手中指指端置于两侧的中府穴,稍用力作顺时针、逆时针方向的揉动,各 36 次。

(7)勾天突:用食指指尖置于天突穴处,向下勾点,揉动 1 分钟。

(8)疏肺经:坐位或立位,右掌先置左乳上,环摩至热后,以掌沿着肩前、上臂内侧前上方、前臂桡侧至腕、拇、食指背侧(肺经的循行路线),做往返推擦 36 次,然后换左手操作右侧。

3.健脾法 脾的生理功能健运则饮食精微不断吸收,化生气血,营养充足,口唇红润光泽;反之则形体消瘦,肌肉痿软,口淡无味或异味,口唇淡白无光泽。采用此保健推拿法可对脾胃疾患起防治作用。

(1)摩中脘:用左手或右手手掌置于中脘部,先逆时针,从小到大摩脘腹 36 圈,然后再顺时针,从大到小摩 36 圈。

(2)揉天枢:坐位或仰卧位,用双手的食、中指同时按揉天枢穴,顺、逆时针各 36 次。

(3)按脘腹:左手或右手并拢四指放置于中脘穴上,采用顺腹式呼吸,吸气时稍用力下按,呼气时作轻柔的环形揉动,如此操作 36 次。

(4)分阴阳:两手相对,全掌置于剑突下,稍稍用力从内向外沿肋弓向胁肋处分推,并逐渐向小腹移动,操作 9 次。

(5)摩脐:一手掌心贴脐部,另一手按手背,顺时针方向旋转摩动 3 分钟~5 分钟。

(6)按足三里:双手拇指或食、中指置于足三里穴位上,稍用力作按揉,使局部有酸胀感,约 3 分钟。

(7)点血海:取坐位,两手分别置于大腿部,拇指点按于血海穴,再作顺、逆时针方向的揉动各 36 次。

(8)捏合谷:右手拇、食指相对捏、拿左侧合谷穴 1 分钟,然后换左手操作右侧。

4.安神法 心的生理功能正常,则可见人精神振奋,思维敏捷,动作灵活,脉搏和缓有力,舌质淡红润泽;反之则见精神萎靡,反应迟钝以及脉涩不畅,节律不整,舌质紫暗或苍白等。经常采用此保健推拿法可对心系疾病有防治作用。

(1)摩胸:右掌按置两乳正中,指尖斜向前下方,先从左乳下环行推摩心区复原,再以掌根在前,沿右乳下环行推摩,如此连续呈"∞"(横 8 字)形,操作 36 次。

(2)拍头顶:用手掌心有节律地拍击头顶,初做时,拍击力量宜轻,若无不适反应,力量可适当加重,每次拍击 10 次左右。

(3)拿心经:右手拇指置于左侧腋下,其余四指置上臂内上侧,边做拿捏,边做按揉,沿上臂内侧渐次向下操作到腕部神门穴,如此往返操作 9 次,再换左手操作右侧。

(4)揉神门:坐位,用右手食、中指相叠,食指按压在左手的神门穴,按揉 1 分钟,换手操作。

（5）挤内关：坐位，用右手拇指按压在左手的内关穴位上，其余四指在腕背侧起到辅助作用，稍用力用拇指指端向上、下挤按内关穴9次。再换左手如法操作右侧。

（6）鸣天鼓：双手掌分按于两耳上，掌根向前，五指向后，以食、中、环指叩击枕部3次，双手掌骤离耳部1次，如此重复9次。

（7）搅沧海：舌在口腔上、下牙龈外周从左向右，从右向左各转9次，产生津液分3口缓缓咽下。

5. 疏肝法 肝的生理功能正常则筋强力壮，爪甲坚韧，眼睛明亮；否则筋软弛缩，视物不清。经常施行本法进行保健推拿，对于肝胆病变有很好的防治作用。

（1）揉膻中：坐位，用左手，四指并拢置于膻中穴，稍用力作顺时针、逆时针方向的揉动各36次。

（2）擦胁肋：坐位，两手五指并拢置于胸前乳头，左手在上，右手在下，从胸前横向沿肋骨方向擦动并逐渐下移至浮肋，然后换右手在上，左手在下操作，以胁肋部有透热感为度。

（3）擦少腹：坐或卧位，双手掌分置于两胁肋下，同时用力斜向少腹推擦至耻骨，往返36次。

（4）点章门：用两手的中指指尖分别置于两侧的章门穴上，稍用力点按，约1分钟，以酸胀为度。

（5）揉期门：坐或卧位，用左手的掌根置于右侧的期门穴位上，用力沿顺时针、逆时针方向，各揉动36次，然后换右手操作左侧，动作相同。

（6）掐太冲：坐位，用两手拇指的指尖置于两侧太冲穴上，稍用力按掐，以酸麻为度，约1分钟，换用拇指的罗纹面轻揉该穴位。

6. 固肾法 肾为"先天之本"，是人体生命的动力源泉。主要功能是贮藏人体精气，主管人体生殖与发育，并可调节人体水液代谢，肾的纳气功能对人体呼吸亦有重要意义。选用本法推拿保健可对肾系疾病有防治作用。

（1）摩关元：用左或右掌以关元穴为圆心，作逆时针和顺时针方向摩动各36次，然后随呼吸向内向下按压关元3分钟。

（2）擦少腹：双手掌分置两胁肋下，同时用力斜向少腹部推擦至耻骨，往返操作以透热为度。

（3）擦腰骶：身体微前倾，屈肘，两手掌尽量置于两侧腰背部，以全掌或小鱼际着力，向下至骶尾骶部快速来回擦动，以透热为度。

（4）摩肾府：两手掌紧贴肾腧穴，双手同时按由外向里的方向作环形转动按摩，共转动36次（此为顺转，为补法；反之为泻。肾腧穴宜补不宜泻，转动时要注意顺逆），如有肾虚、腰痛诸病者，可以增加转动次数。

（5）揉命门：以两手的食、中两指点按在命门穴上，稍用力作环形的揉动，顺逆各36次。

（6）搓涌泉：盘膝而坐，双手掌对搓至发热后，沿足三阴经并过内踝关节至足大趾根，往返摩擦至透热为止，然后左右手分别搓涌泉穴至局部发热。搓揉时要不缓不急，略有节奏感。

（7）缩二阴：处于安静状态下，全身放松，用顺腹式呼吸法（即吸气时腹部隆起，呼气时腹部收缩），并在呼气时稍用力收缩前后二阴，吸气时放松，重复36次。

第三节 穴位按压法

穴位按压法，是指在中医理论指导下，运用手指、手掌、指间关节、肘等部位按压刺激穴位，以激发经络之气，调整阴阳，从而达到预防治疗疾病的方法。穴位按压法源自于针刺疗法，两者刺激的穴位和经脉相同，针刺法以各种针具刺激穴位，穴位按压法则是以各种手法刺激穴位。穴位按压法操作简便、经济安全、适应证广、疗效理想，是中医护理中最常用的方法之一。

一、穴位按压法的适应证

穴位按压法具有缓解紧张、舒筋止痛、活血化瘀、疏通经络等作用，适用范围广泛，可用于内、妇、外、儿、伤科等多种病证的护理。尤其适用于疼痛性疾病、软组织损伤、情绪紧张、脏腑功能失调等病证的护理和康复。

1. 伤科病证 肌筋膜炎、腰痛、颈椎病、肩周炎、慢性肌肉劳损、踝关节扭伤和膝关节扭伤等。

2. 内科病证 感冒、头痛、眩晕、失眠、咳嗽、哮喘、胃痛、泄泻、便秘、阳痿、高血压、冠心病、中风后遗症、慢性疲劳综合征、抑郁症等。

3. 外科病证 乳腺增生、术后胃肠功能紊乱、放化疗反应等。

4. 妇科病证 月经不调、痛经、更年期综合征等。

5. 五官科病证 近视、耳鸣、鼻炎等。

二、穴位按压常用手法及穴位

大部分推拿手法均可用于穴位按压法中，尤其是以手指、手掌等部位作用于穴位的推拿手法。持久、有力、均匀、柔和、渗透，也是穴位按压手法的基本要求。一般而言，持久而有渗透力的压力宜缓慢施加于穴位，每穴持续按压大约 3 分钟。按压穴位的力度取决于患者的体型及穴位所在的部位。不同患者及不同部位所需的按压力度不同，按压局部可出现酸、麻、重、胀、痛等感觉。如果疼痛明显，则应减少按压力度，以更轻柔的手法代替。小腿部、面部以及外阴部穴位较为敏感，一般按压力度较轻。背部、臀部、肩部等肌肉丰厚部位可采用较大力度、更为深透的按压力度。

常用的穴位按压手法有一指禅推法、揉法、摩法、擦法、抹法、按法、压法、点法、拿法、拨法、掐法等。这些手法的具体操作方法、动作要领及注意事项见本书第三章第一节"推拿法"部分。

穴位按压的常用穴位及按压手法详见本书第二章第二节"经络腧穴"部分表2-3。

三、穴位按压禁忌证

1. 某些外科疾病如急性腹膜炎、肠穿孔、急性阑尾炎、骨折等。

2. 各种急慢性传染病如伤寒、流行性脑脊髓膜炎、乙脑、肝炎、结核、梅毒、淋病、艾滋病等。

3. 急性中毒如食物中毒、煤气中毒、药物中毒、酒精中毒、毒蛇咬伤等。

4. 各种严重出血性疾病如脑出血、胃出血、子宫出血、便血、尿血、外伤出血等。

5. 各种严重的、危及生命的疾病，如急性心肌梗死、严重肾衰竭、心力衰竭等。

四、穴位按压注意事项

1. 穴位按压前，操作室要保持适宜的温度和空气流通。

2. 根据受术者的病情、体质、年龄、性别及操作部位等情况，选择适当的治疗体位，务使受术者感到舒适。

3. 穴位按压时动作应缓慢、有节奏，以使身体不同组织及内脏对刺激产生适宜的反应。切忌生硬、暴力按压方式。

4. 患者在过于饥饿、疲劳、精神过度紧张时，不宜立即进行穴位按压。避免饭后立即进行穴位按压，一般在餐后一小时左右再进行穴位按压为宜。

5. 妇女怀孕 3 个月以内者，小腹部的腧穴不宜穴位按压。若怀孕 3 个月以上者，其腹部、腰骶部腧穴也不宜穴位按压。至于三阴交、合谷、昆仑、至阴等一些通经活血的腧穴，在怀孕期禁穴位按压。如妇女行经期，若非为了调经，亦不应穴位按压。

6. 皮肤有感染、溃疡、瘢痕或肿瘤的部位，不宜穴位按压。

7. 淋巴结部位，如腹股沟、耳后、颌下、乳腺外上侧靠近腋窝部等只能轻用摩法，而不能按压。

第四节　灸　　法

灸法是指用艾绒或药物为主要灸材，点燃后悬置或放置在穴位或病变部位，进行烧灼、温熨，借灸火的热力以及药物的作用，达到治病、防病和保健目的的一种外治方法。

灸法具有温经通络、祛风解表、温中散寒、温肾健脾、回阳固脱、益气升阳、消瘀散结、防病保健等作用。

用于施灸的原料以艾绒最为常用。将干燥的艾叶经过反复捣碎，去除杂质，留取纯净细软的部分，即为艾绒。艾叶气味芳香、辛温味苦，易于燃烧，火力温和，主灸百病。

一、灸法的适应范围

灸法的适应证广泛，以虚证、寒证和阴证为主。如治疗寒凝血滞，经络痹阻引起的风寒湿痹、痛经、经闭、腹痛等证；外感风寒表证及中焦虚寒呕吐、泄泻等；脾肾阳虚之久泄、遗尿、遗精、阳痿、早泄；阳气虚脱而出现的大汗淋漓、四肢厥冷、脉微欲绝的虚脱证；中气不足，气虚下陷之内脏脱垂、阴挺、脱肛等；外科疾患，如疮疡初起，疔肿未化脓者，瘰病及疮疡溃久不愈等。

二、灸法的禁忌证

1. 无论外感或阴虚内热证，凡脉象数疾者禁灸；高热、抽搐或极度衰竭、形瘦骨弱者，亦不宜灸治。凡属阴虚阳亢、邪实内闭及热毒炽盛等病证，应慎用灸法。

2. 心尖搏动处、大血管处、妊娠期妇女下腹部以及腰骶部，睾丸、乳头、阴部不可灸。颜面部不宜着肤灸。关节活动处不能瘢痕灸。

三、灸法的种类

灸法的种类很多，根据用物不同，临床常用的灸法见图 3-5。

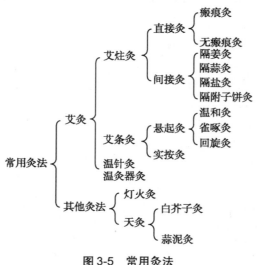

图 3-5　常用灸法

四、常用灸法操作

（一）艾炷灸

艾炷灸是把艾绒搓捏成规格大小不同的圆锥形艾炷，置于施灸部位，点燃灼烧而治病的方法。艾炷大小可根据患者病情及施灸部位而定，小者如麦粒大，中者如半截枣核大，大者如半截橄榄大。每燃烧一个艾炷，称为一壮。施灸时，艾炷灸可分为直接灸和间接灸。

1. **直接灸**　又称为"着肤灸"和"明灸"。即选择大小合适的艾炷，直接放在所选部位的皮肤上施灸的方法。根据灸后皮肤是否留有瘢痕，又分为瘢痕灸和无瘢痕灸两种。因瘢痕灸给患者带来的痛苦较大，目前临床已很少使用，在此仅介绍无瘢痕灸。

无瘢痕灸，又称为非化脓灸，即灸后不留有瘢痕的治疗方法。临床常用于治疗风寒痹痛以及虚寒性的腹痛、泄泻和痛经等。治疗时在所选部位的皮肤上涂少量凡士林，再放置艾炷点燃，当艾炷燃剩 2/5 左右，患者感觉疼痛时，用镊子将燃剩的艾炷夹去，置于污物盘内，换炷再灸。一般连续灸 3～7 壮，以患者局部皮肤充血、红晕，但以不起疱为度。

2. **间接灸**　又称隔物灸，即在艾炷与施灸部位的皮肤之间，隔垫上某种物品而施灸的一种方法。一般常用的有隔姜灸、隔蒜灸、隔盐灸和隔附子饼灸等。

（1）隔姜灸：是以生姜为间隔物而施灸的一种方法。临床常用于治疗虚寒性病证，如腹痛、泄泻、呕吐及痛经等。将生姜切成直径为 2～3cm，厚约 0.2～0.3cm 的薄片，中间以针刺上数孔。在所选部位的皮肤上涂少许凡士林，放上姜片，再将艾炷置于姜片上，点燃施灸。待艾炷燃尽后，除去灰烬，换炷再灸。一般灸 5～10 壮，以局部皮肤红晕，但以不起疱为度。

（2）隔蒜灸：是以大蒜片为间隔物而施灸的一种治疗方法。临床主要用于治疗肺结核及疮疡初期等病证。将大蒜头切成 0.2～0.3cm 的薄片，中间以针穿刺数孔。在所选部位的皮肤上涂少许凡士林，放上大蒜片，再将艾炷置于蒜片上，点燃施灸。待艾炷燃尽后，除去灰烬，换炷再灸。一般灸5～7壮，以局部皮肤红晕，但以不起疱为度。

（3）隔盐灸：是以盐为间隔物而施灸的一种治疗方法。常用于急性寒性腹痛、吐泻、痢疾以及中风脱证等证。一般多选用神阙穴。先用精盐将肚脐填平，在盐上放一中间刺数孔的姜片，以防食盐受热爆起而引起烫伤，再将艾炷置于姜片之上，点燃施灸。燃尽后，除去灰烬，易炷再灸，壮数不拘，直至病情缓解。

（4）隔附子饼灸：是以附子片或附子饼为间隔物而施灸的一种治疗方法。常用于治疗因命门火衰引起的阳痿、早泄、疮疡久溃不愈等症。将附子研成细末，用黄酒调合，制成直径为3cm，厚约0.8cm的附子饼，中间用粗针刺数孔，上置艾炷，放于施灸部位上，点燃施灸。燃尽后，除去灰烬，易炷再灸，一般灸5～7壮。

（二）艾条灸

艾条灸是指用桑皮纸将纯净的艾绒（或加入中药）卷成圆柱形艾条，将其一端点燃，对准腧穴或患处施灸的一种方法。按照施灸时操作手法的不同，可分为悬起灸和实按灸。

1. 悬起灸　按其操作方法又可分为温和灸、雀啄灸、回旋灸。用物包括：治疗盘内置艾条、打火机、镊子、清洁弯盘。

（1）温和灸：备齐用物，根据病情选取穴位，协助患者取合理舒适体位，暴露治疗部位，点燃艾条一端，一手持艾条与施灸部位皮肤保持2～3cm的距离进行持续熏灸，以患者局部皮肤有温热感而无灼痛感为宜。一般每个部位灸10～15分钟，直至局部皮肤红晕为度。临床常用于治疗慢性虚寒性疾病，如腹痛、痛经等。

（2）雀啄灸：备齐用物，根据病情选取穴位，协助患者取合理舒适体位，暴露治疗部位，点燃艾条一端，一手持艾条与施灸部位皮肤保持2～5cm距离，像鸟雀啄食般一上一下不停移动，进行反复熏灸，一般每个部位灸5分钟左右。此法温热感较强烈，常用于治疗急性病证。

（3）回旋灸：备齐用物，根据病情选取穴位，协助患者取合理舒适体位，暴露治疗部位，点燃艾条一端，在距离施灸部位皮肤约3cm处，左右来回或旋转移动，进行反复熏灸，一般每个部位可灸20～30分钟。临床常用于治疗急性病证。

以上三种方法，可单独使用，亦可混合使用。

2. 实按灸　施灸时，先在施灸腧穴或患处垫上布或纸数层。然后将艾条的一端点燃后按到施术部位上，使热力透达深部。若艾火熄灭，再点再按。适用于风寒湿痹和虚寒证。

（三）天灸

又称药物灸、发疱灸。即将一些具有刺激性的药物，涂敷于穴位或患处，敷后皮肤可起疱，或仅使局部充血潮红。常用的有蒜泥灸和白芥子灸等。

1. 蒜泥灸　将大蒜捣烂如泥，取3～5g贴敷于穴位上，敷灸1～3小时，以局部皮肤发痒发红起疱为度。如敷涌泉穴可治疗咯血，敷合谷穴可治疗扁桃体炎等。

2. 白芥子灸　将适量白芥子研成细末，用水调和成糊状，贴敷于腧穴或患处，敷以油纸，胶布固定。一般可用于治疗关节痹痛，或配合其他药物治疗哮喘等证。

（四）灸法注意事项

1. 施灸前应向患者做好解释，并协助患者摆好体位，避免患者因疲劳而移动体位，造成烫伤。

2. 应遵循施灸的先后顺序。一般先灸阳经，后灸阴经；先灸上部，后灸下部。先灸艾炷小者，后灸艾炷大者；壮数少的部位先灸，壮数多的后灸。

3. 操作者可用自己的手来测知温度，以便及时调整距离，防止烫伤。

4. 及时除去灰烬，防止烫伤皮肤。污物盘内可盛少许水，将燃剩的艾灰放入，以防复燃。

5. 施灸后如局部皮肤出现潮红或有灼热感，属正常现象，无需处理。如灸后局部起疱，小者可自行吸收，较大的水疱可用无菌注射器抽出液体，用无菌纱布覆盖，防止感染。

第五节　拔　罐　法

拔罐法是指以罐为工具，借助抽吸或燃烧热力，排除罐内空气，使之形成负压，将罐吸附于施治部位的体表或腧穴上，使局部皮肤充血、淤血，以达到防治疾病目的的一种方法，亦称"吸筒法"。因古时多用牛角作为拔罐工具，故又称"角法"。

一、拔罐法的适应范围

拔罐法具有通经活络、祛风散寒、消肿止痛、吸毒排脓等功效。临床常用于治疗外感风寒的头痛，风寒湿痹导致的关节疼痛、腰背酸痛、虚寒性咳喘以及毒蛇咬伤的排毒等。

二、拔罐法的禁忌证

1. 骨骼凹凸不平、毛发较多部位不宜拔罐。

2. 治疗局部皮肤有溃疡、水肿以及有大血管分布处一般不宜拔罐。

3. 孕妇腹部和腰骶部不宜拔罐。

4. 高热、抽搐及凝血机制障碍患者不宜拔罐。

5. 严重心脏病、心力衰竭、重度水肿不宜拔罐。

6. 精神紧张、疲劳、饮酒后，以及过饥、过饱、烦渴时不宜拔罐。

三、罐　的　种　类

目前临床使用的罐具主要有竹罐、陶罐、玻璃罐及负压吸引罐等，其中以玻璃罐最为常用。

1. **竹罐**　是用直径为 3～5cm 的竹子，截成 6～10cm 不同长度，一端留节作底，另一端作罐口，并用砂纸磨光而成。其优点为取材容易，制作简单，轻巧价廉，不易损坏，适于水（药）煮。缺点是易爆裂、漏气。用后可煮沸消毒。

2. **陶罐**　是用陶土烧制而成，吸附力强，但质地较重，易摔碎损坏。用后可煮沸消毒或用消毒剂浸泡消毒。

3. **玻璃罐**　是临床较为常用的拔罐器具，用玻璃制成，形如球状，有大、中、小三型。其优点是质地透明，使用时可直接观察局部皮肤的变化情况，便于掌握留罐时间。缺点是传热较快而易烫伤，易破碎。用后煮沸或用消毒剂浸泡消毒。

4. **负压吸引罐**　用透明塑料制成，顶部设置活塞，便于抽气。使用方便安全且不易破碎。用后可用消毒液浸泡消毒。

四、罐的吸附方法

罐的吸附方法是指采用一定的方法排除罐内空气，使之形成负压，吸附于拔罐局部的方法。目前常用的有火吸法、水吸法和抽气吸法三种。

1. **火吸法** 是指利用燃烧时火的热力排除罐内空气,形成负压,将罐吸附于治疗部位皮肤上。临床常用闪火法。

操作者一手持大小适宜的罐具,另一手用止血钳夹紧 95% 的乙醇棉球,点燃后尽快伸入罐内,在罐壁中段绕 1～2 圈后立即退出,同时迅速将罐扣在所拔部位皮肤上。此种点火方法比较安全,也是临床最常用的点火方法。需要注意的是点燃的乙醇棉球应尽快伸入罐内中部,不要在罐口停留,以免将罐口烧热,引起烫伤。

2. **水吸法** 又称煮罐法,是指利用高温的水排除罐内空气,使之形成负压,并将罐吸附于局部皮肤的一种方法。可以用水,亦可以用中药汤剂煮罐,临床多用竹罐。将大小适宜的竹罐投入沸水或药液中煮 5～10 分钟,用长镊子夹住罐底,使罐口朝下,甩去罐内余水,立即用湿冷毛巾紧扪罐口,再迅速将罐扣在应拔部位上。

3. **抽气吸法** 是指将负压吸引罐扣于局部皮肤上,将抽气筒连接罐顶部抽气活塞,抽出罐内空气,使之形成负压,待吸牢后,将抽气筒取下,关闭气门,即能吸住。

五、起 罐 方 法

待拔罐局部皮肤出现明显瘀斑或留罐时间已到,即可起罐。起罐时操作者一手握住罐体,另一手的拇指或手指按压罐口皮肤,待空气进入罐内,即可取下。不可强行上提或旋转提拔,以免引起疼痛或损伤皮肤。

六、火罐操作法

(一)用物准备

需准备玻璃罐(根据所拔部位,选择大、中、小罐具及数量)、95% 乙醇棉球或纸片、打火机、止血钳、弯盘;如为走罐,则需另备凡士林或按摩乳。

(二)操作步骤

1. 备齐用物,携至患者床前,解释操作时注意事项,再次核对医嘱。
2. 根据病情,协助患者取合理舒适体位,暴露拔罐部位,注意保暖。
3. 选择大小合适的罐具,检查罐口边缘是否光滑。
4. 用闪火法将罐吸附于局部皮肤上,留罐 10～15 分钟。
5. 留罐过程中,注意观察局部皮肤颜色变化及火罐吸附情况。
6. 起罐,擦去污渍,协助患者穿衣,取舒适体位。
7. 整理用物,洗手,记录。

七、拔罐法的临床应用

(一)留罐

留罐是指待罐吸牢后,将罐留置 5～15 分钟,待局部皮肤充血,皮下出现瘀血时即可起罐。如果罐体较大,吸附力较强时,可适当缩短留罐时间,以免局部皮肤起疱。此法较为常用,一般疾病均可使用,可单罐留罐,亦可多罐同时留罐。

(二)走罐

走罐是指先在罐口或预拔部位涂一些润滑油或凡士林,再将罐拔住,用手握住罐体,进行上下或左右往返推移,直至所拔部位皮肤出现红润、充血或瘀血时,将罐起下。一般适用于面积较大、肌肉丰厚部位，如背部、腰臀部以及大腿部等。常选用罐口口径较大，且罐口较圆滑的玻璃罐。可用于治疗急性热病、瘫痪麻木、风湿痹证、肌肉萎缩等病证。

（三）闪罐

闪罐是指将罐拔住后立即起下，反复多次地拔住、起下，直至局部皮肤出现潮红、充血或瘀血为止。多适用于局部麻木、疼痛等证。

八、拔罐法的注意事项

1. 拔罐时要选择肌肉丰厚的部位和舒适合理的体位。

2. 根据所拔部位选择大小适宜的罐，注意检查罐口是否圆滑、有无裂缝。

3. 拔罐时动作要稳、准、快。

4. 拔罐过程中注意询问患者的感觉，观察局部皮肤情况。当患者感觉所拔部位发热、发紧、发酸、疼痛、灼热时，应取下重拔。

5. 留罐时应帮助患者盖好衣被以保暖。

6. 拔火罐或水罐时要避免灼伤或烫伤皮肤。若烫伤或留罐时间过长而皮肤出现小水疱时，可外敷无菌纱布加以保护，防止擦破感染；水疱较大时应经消毒后用无菌注射器将渗液抽出，再用无菌纱布覆盖以防感染。

7. 注意有无晕罐先兆。当患者出现头晕、恶心、面色苍白等晕罐反应时，应立即停止拔罐，将罐具全部起下。使患者平卧，注意保暖，轻者仰卧片刻，给饮温开水或糖水后，即可恢复正常。重者可通知医生并对症处理。

第六节　刮　痧　法

刮痧法，是用边缘钝滑的器具，在人体一定部位的皮肤上反复刮动，使局部皮下出现痧斑或痧痕，以达到防治疾病目的的一种方法。通过刮痧，脏腑秽浊之气经腠理通达于外，使周身气血迅速得到畅通，从而达到治疗目的。

一、刮痧法的适应范围

刮痧法适用于外感湿邪所致的高热、头痛、恶心、呕吐及外感暑湿所致的中暑、腹痛、腹泻等证。

二、刮痧法的禁忌证

1. 凡危重病证，如急性传染病、严重心脏病等禁止刮痧。

2. 有出血倾向的疾病，如血小板减少症、凝血功能障碍等禁用刮痧。

3. 各种皮肤溃疡、疮疡、烫伤，或外伤骨折处及皮肤不明病因的包块等禁止直接在病灶部位刮拭。

4. 年老久病、过于消瘦者不宜刮痧。

5. 妊娠妇女的腹部及腰骶部、及身体的一些穴位禁刮，如三阴交、合谷、肩井、昆仑等。囟门未闭合的小儿头部禁用刮痧。

6. 过饥、过饱、过度疲劳或过度紧张者禁用刮痧。

三、刮痧工具

刮痧板是目前最常用的刮痧工具,临床使用最多的是水牛角刮痧板,亦可选择硬币或边缘光滑而无破损的瓷匙。

四、常用刮痧部位

1. **头部** 常取眉心、太阳穴部位。
2. **颈项部** 取颈部、项部两侧。
3. **胸部** 各肋间隙、胸骨中线。乳头禁止刮痧。
4. **肩背部** 两肩部、背部脊柱两侧为最常用的刮痧部位。
5. **上下肢** 上臂内侧、肘窝、下肢大腿内侧及腘窝。

五、刮痧法的操作

(一)用物准备

治疗盘,刮具,治疗碗内放润滑剂(可用清水、香油或活血剂)、治疗巾或纸巾。

(二)操作步骤

1. 备齐用物,携至患者床旁,向患者做好解释,取得合作。
2. 根据病证帮助患者取舒适体位,并协助其暴露刮痧部位。一般可选用仰卧位、俯卧位、仰靠等姿势,以患者舒适为宜。
3. 检查刮具边缘,确定光滑无缺损。
4. 手持刮具,蘸润滑剂,在选定部位施刮。刮具与刮拭方向皮肤保持 45°～90°。颈部、脊柱旁从上至下,胸背部从内向外,单一方向刮拭皮肤,不可来回刮拭。用力应均匀,力度适中,禁用暴力。刮痧过程中,应保持刮具边缘湿润。一般刮至局部皮下出现红色或紫红色痧痕为度。
5. 刮痧的条数应视具体情况而定。一般每次刮 8～10 条,每条刮 6～15cm,每条刮 20 次左右。
6. 刮痧结束,擦干油或水渍,协助患者穿好衣裤,整理床单。

六、刮痧法的注意事项

1. 保持室内空气新鲜、流通,避免直接吹风。
2. 刮痧用具一定要注意清洁,用后清洗并用 75% 的酒精消毒。最好专人专板,固定使用。
3. 刮痧时用力应均匀,力度适中,以患者能耐受为宜。每次每个部位刮拭不超过 10 分钟为宜,或以出痧为度,对不出痧或出痧少者不可强求出痧。
4. 操作中注意观察患者局部皮肤颜色变化情况,随时询问其感觉。如患者出现疼痛异常、冷汗不止、胸闷烦躁等,应停止刮痧。
5. 嘱患者刮治期间,注意休息,保持心情愉快;饮食清淡易消化,禁食生冷油腻之品;出痧后避免受凉。
6. 两次刮痧间一般间隔 3～6 天,以皮肤痧退为准,3～5 次为一疗程。

(马良宵)

第七节　热　熨　法

热熨法是将加热后的药物装入布袋,在人体局部或腧穴来回移动或回旋运转,利用温热及药物的共同作用,以达到治疗目的的一种方法。常用的热熨法包括药熨法、葱熨法、盐熨法等。

一、热熨法的目的

利用温热及药物的共同作用,以达到温经通络、散寒止痛、行气活血、祛瘀消肿等功效。

二、热熨法的禁忌证

各种实热证或神昏患者禁用;腹部疼痛或包块性质不明者,孕妇腹部及腰骶部、身体大血管处、皮肤有破损处及局部无知觉处忌用。

三、热　熨　方　法

(一)药熨法

药熨法是将中药用白酒或食醋搅拌后加热,装入布袋中,在患者患处或穴位来回移动滚熨的一种方法。

1. **适应证**　脾胃虚寒引起的胃脘疼痛、腹冷泄泻;风湿痹证引起的关节冷痛、麻木、酸胀等。

2. **用物准备**　治疗盘、药物、白酒或醋、治疗碗、双层纱布袋 2 个、棉签、凡士林,另备大毛巾、炒锅、电磁炉、竹铲或竹筷。

3. **操作步骤**

(1)操作者衣帽整洁,洗手、戴口罩;根据医嘱,将药物倒入锅中,加入适量白酒或食醋,搅拌均匀后,用文火炒至 60～70℃,装入双层布袋中,用大毛巾包裹后,保温备用。

(2)备齐用物,携至床旁,再次核对;解释治疗目的、方法,以取得患者的配合;根据病情协助患者取舒适、合理的体位,暴露药熨部位,注意保暖,必要时帷帘遮挡患者。

(3)局部皮肤涂少许凡士林后,将药熨袋放在患处或相应穴位处,用力来回推熨,力量要均匀。开始时用力要轻,速度可稍快,随着药袋温度的降低,用力可逐渐增大,同时速度减慢。药袋温度过低时,及时更换药袋,以保持温度,加强效果;药熨过程中应随时注意观察局部皮肤情况,询问患者局部有无灼痛感,防止烫伤。

(4)药熨时间一般为 15～30 分钟,每天 1 次～2 次。

(5)药熨后清洁局部皮肤,协助患者穿好衣服,取舒适卧位。

(6)整理用物,洗手,记录。

4. **注意事项**

(1)加热药物的过程中要注意安全,中途加入白酒时要将炒锅离开热源,以免发生危险。

(2)药熨前向患者做好解释,嘱患者排空小便。

(3)冬季注意保暖,室内温度要适宜,以免感受风寒。

(4)热熨过程中要随时观察皮肤变化,预防烫伤。药熨袋内温度应保持在 50～60℃,一般不超过 70℃,年老、婴幼儿不宜超过 50℃。

（5）操作过程中应保持药袋温度，保证及时更换或加热。如患者感到不适，应停止操作。

（二）葱熨法

葱熨法是将新鲜大葱白 200～250g（切成 2～3cm 长）加入白酒 30ml 炒热，装入布袋中，在患者腹部热熨，达到升清降浊之功效的一种治疗方法。癃闭者可用葱熨袋从脐周右侧向左侧进行上下滚熨，右升左降，以达到排出腹内腹水、积气，通利大小便的作用；痿证、瘫痪者直接滚熨患处。每次葱熨时间一般为 20 分钟，每日 2 次。

（三）盐熨法

盐熨法是将颗粒大小均匀的大青盐或海盐 500～1000g 炒热，装入纱布袋中，待温度适宜时，在患处或特定部位来回运转的一种方法。慢性虚寒性胃痛、腹泻患者可在胃脘部或腹部滚熨；痹证、痿证、瘫痪、筋骨疼痛患者直接熨患处；癃闭者熨神阙或小腹；耳鸣头晕者可将盐熨袋枕于头下；肾阳不足者熨足心。每次熨 20～30 分钟，每日 2 次。

第八节　熏　洗　法

熏洗法是用中药煎煮后，先用蒸汽熏蒸，待温后再用药液淋洗、浸浴全身或局部患处的一种外治方法。

一、熏洗法的目的

利用中药的热力和加热后产生的蒸汽渗透入人体皮肤、深层组织，以达到开泄腠理、清热解毒、消肿止痛、杀虫止痒、温经通络、活血化瘀、疏风散寒、祛风除湿、协调脏腑功能的目的。

二、熏洗法的适应证

熏洗法的适应范围很广，涉及内、外、妇、儿、骨伤、五官、皮肤科的多种疾病，如风寒感冒、疮疡、痈疽、肛周脓肿、外阴瘙痒、筋骨疼痛、风寒痹证、麦粒肿、湿疹、皮肤瘙痒、手足癣等。

三、熏洗法的禁忌证

发热、昏迷、局部水肿、精神病患者、恶性肿瘤、黄疸、有出血倾向、气血两亏、严重心脏病、哮喘发作时禁熏洗，孕妇及妇女月经期间禁止坐浴、全身药浴。

四、熏洗法的用物准备

1. **眼部熏洗法**　治疗盘，治疗碗（内盛煎好的中药滤液），水温计，纱布，镊子。
2. **四肢熏洗法**　面盆或木桶，药液，水温计，浴巾或中单，卵圆钳，小毛巾。
3. **坐浴法**　治疗盘，小毛巾，药液，水温计，坐浴盆，坐浴椅，有孔木盖。
4. **全身药浴法**　浴缸或大浴盆，药液，热水，水温计，坐架，罩单，浴巾，软毛巾，衣裤，拖鞋。

五、熏洗法的操作步骤

1. 操作者衣帽整洁，洗手、戴口罩；根据医嘱，将药液配制好备用。

2. 备齐用物，携至床旁，再次核对；解释治疗目的、方法，以取得患者的配合；根据病情协助患者取舒适、合理的体位，并暴露熏洗部位，必要时帷帘遮挡患者，根据患者的具体情况调节病室的温度。

3. 不同部位的熏洗方法

（1）眼部熏洗法：将煎好的药液倒入治疗碗中，碗口围一纱布，中间露一小孔，患者取端坐姿势，将患眼对准小孔先熏蒸，待药液温度降至 40℃ 时，用镊子夹取消毒纱布蘸药液频频淋洗患眼。时间约 15～30 分钟。

（2）四肢熏洗法：药液趁热倒入盆内，将患肢架于盆上，用浴巾或布单围盖住患肢及盆，使药液蒸汽熏蒸患肢。待药液温度降至 38～41℃ 时，将患肢浸泡于药液中，时间约 10～20 分钟。

（3）坐浴法：将药液倒入坐浴盆内，置盆于坐浴椅上，盖上有孔木盖。协助患者将裤脱至膝盖，露出臀部，坐在木盖上熏蒸，待药液温度降至 40℃ 时，移去木盖，臀部坐入盆中泡洗，时间约 20～30 分钟。

（4）全身药浴法：将药液倒入浴缸或浴盆内，调整浴缸内的药液温度至 50℃，放好坐架以保证安全。协助患者脱掉衣服，坐在浴盆坐架上，用罩单围住全身，仅露出头面，使药液蒸气熏蒸全身。待药液温度降至 38～41℃ 时，将全身浸泡于药液中，用软毛巾协助患者拭洗，活动四肢关节。时间约 20～40 分钟。

4. 熏洗过程中，密切观察患者的反应，若感不适，应立即停止，给予对症处理。

5. 熏洗结束，清洁局部皮肤。协助患者穿好衣服，取舒适卧位。

6. 整理用物，洗手，记录。

六、注 意 事 项

1. 冬季注意保暖，防止受凉。

2. 熏洗的药液温度不宜过高，一般为 50～70℃，淋洗的药液温度一般为 40℃，以防烫伤。

3. 熏洗一般每日 1 次，每次 20～30 分钟，视病情也可每日 2 次。

4. 患者不宜空腹熏洗，进餐前后半个小时内不宜熏洗。年老体质虚弱者不可单独熏洗，且熏洗的时间不宜过长，以防虚脱。

5. 在伤口部位进行熏洗时，严格执行无菌操作。

（杨晓玮）

第四章
一般调护方法

调护，即调理、养护。广义的调护，是指运用中医理论和方法来预防疾病，促进健康。狭义的调护，是指中医护理的具体方法。中医一般调护包括起居调护、饮食调护、情志调护和运动调护等。

第一节　起居调护

起居是指人们在日常生活中的基本生存活动，包括生活方式、生活习惯、劳作风格等。起居调护是指顺应自然变化的规律，合理安排日常生活、作息时间等。生活起居与健康有着密切的关系，要保持身体健康，延年益寿，应懂得顺应自然变化的规律，适应四时气候变化，做到饮食有节，起居有常，生活规律；若饮食不节，起居无常，就会多病早衰。

一、顺应四时，调养形神

（一）"顺应四时、调养形神"的意义和基本原则

世间万物变化的根本原因，是四时阴阳的变化。春夏为阳气当令，阳主生发，阴主长养，万物应以生、长；秋冬为阴气所主，阳主肃杀，阴主闭藏，万物趋于收、藏。《黄帝内经·素问》认为，人体的生命机能与天地自然之气相通应，生命本于自然阴阳变化。四时调养从根本上说，就是根据自然界阴阳的盛衰，来调节人体阴阳的盈虚，使人体的阴阳变化适应自然界阴阳变化的规律。

《素问·四气调神大论》曰"春夏养阳，秋冬养阴"，这是根据自然界和人体阴阳消长、气机升降、五脏盛衰的不同时间、特点、状态而提出的调摄原则。春夏时节，万物从冬藏中复苏、生发，以至于繁荣茂盛，这种生机的由弱而强，是天地间春夏阳气的象征。人类在这一阶段的生命活动须适应自然界阴阳的变化以养阳。秋冬之令，万物渐趋结实、肃杀而至闭藏，是阴气主政，人体也以阴气为主导，宜适应自然变化以潜藏阳气，滋养阴精。背离这一阴阳变化的至理，就有可能影响人体整个阴阳的平衡，导致各种疾病的出现。所以，四时养生必须遵循"春夏养阳，秋冬养阴"的基本原则。

（二）四时起居调护

1. 春季起居调护　春季，经过隆冬的秘藏，阳气已由弱而旺，自然界阳气当令，主万物的生发，自然界呈现蓬勃向上、生机盎然的景象。人们应顺应春时生发之气，调摄作息。

（1）调护原则：应顺应自然界阳气生发的积极趋势，与天地万物蓬勃向上的趋势一致，扶助机体阳气，调畅肝胆气机，规避春季各种致病因素，保持人体少阳之气的旺盛，并为夏季的养"长"打下充实的基础。

（2）日常活动调养：春季各种起居活动均要考虑到舒展、宣泄通达。应稍迟些睡觉，在保证基本睡眠的前提下尽可能早起，进行一些室外活动，衣服保持宽松舒适，披散头发，尽量舒缓身体，在没有任何压抑束缚的情况下，促进阳气的生发。白天尽可能抽时间进行活动以舒缓机体的疲惫，晚上适当进行有益身心的娱乐活动以缓解一天的劳累。基本要求是：根据个人不同体质及个人喜好，选择不同的活动，以舒缓、畅达为要。尽量进行强度不大而舒缓的活动，使机体尽可能处于调达舒畅的状态。但不可过于疲惫，亦不宜久坐不动、久视不移、久睡不起，以免阻碍肌肉筋骨的舒缓，使经络气血瘀积，有碍于肝胆之气的调畅。尽量少守舍，可选择空气清新的户外适宜场所，如公园、草地等地进行户外活动，多接触大自然，以呼吸自然界的清晰空气，舒缓筋骨，使春天阳气生发。

（3）"春捂"以养阳气："春捂"指春季尽可能迟地卸减冬装，"捂"住身体的热气，以保证阳气生发的体内环境。春季阳气刚升而未盛，寒气将去而未衰，乍暖乍寒，机体很难适应这种变幻莫测的气候。寒温冷热不时，过早地脱去棉衣，寒气则乘虚而入，初生的阳气尚不足以与春寒抗衡，抵御能力减弱，极易感受各种疾病。"春捂"得宜，阳气旺则正气盛，"虚邪贼风"便无缘侵袭人体。春季着装既要宽松、柔软保暖，还应注意随气候变化而增减，切忌减衣太快。此外，由于寒多自下而上，传统养生主张春时衣着宜下厚上薄，青年女性尤为注意，不可过早换裙装。

（4）"虚邪贼风，避之有时"：认识各种致病因素以适时趋避。春季，晴时阳光普照、温暖宜人，阴时阴雨绵绵、寒气袭人，乍寒乍暖的气候易引起疾病，如流行性感冒、腮腺炎等呼吸道传染病，神经性皮炎、荨麻疹等皮肤病及胃肠道疾病等。因此，春季应尤其注意天气变化对人体的影响，在瞬息转变的时候，避开"虚邪贼风"的侵袭。

2. 夏季起居调护　夏季阳气旺盛，天阳下济，地热上蒸，天地阴阳之气上下交合，万物繁华茂盛。

（1）调护原则：应根据自然界阳气极度旺盛的特点，与天地间万物生长的趋势一致，顺盛阳以养阳，护阳气以养"长"，养心气以辅阳，既要盛夏防暑邪，长夏防湿邪，同时又要注意保护人体阳气，不离"春夏养阳"的总规律，为秋季的养"收"打下基础。

（2）日常活动调养：夏季人们应顺应自然界养长之势，宜入夜晚睡，清晨早起，以适应日出早而落日晚的规律。白天时间长，夜卧早起，午间适当小眠，以恢复体力。夏日炎热，腠理开泄，易受风寒湿邪侵袭，不可过于避热趋凉，或饮冷无度，致使中气内虚，暑热与风寒之邪乘虚而入。因此夏季穿衣不可太薄，尤其腹、背部更要注意保暖。因为人的背部是督脉所在，主管着人体一身的阳气，背部受寒易阻碍全身阳气的运行，而脐部属于任脉，调节阴经的气血。脐部和背部受寒不仅会影响到脾胃，使人体出现腹痛、腹泻等症状，更可引起痛经、月经紊乱等疾病。同时夏季睡眠时不宜夜晚露宿，空调房间不宜室内外温差过大。纳凉时勿在房檐下、过道里，应远离门窗缝隙，以防贼风入内。汗孔张开，不宜立即用冷水冲凉，或入冷水游泳，或冒雨贪凉，以防寒湿入侵。过热时，提倡温水浴，或用温湿毛巾擦抹，使机体腠理毛孔不致骤然闭拒，气不得泄，而致邪闭于内。夏季日照时间长，阳光充足，人体养护也要尽可能地进行户外活动，多接触阳光，使汗液排泄，排除体内毒素。夏季活动要注意：最好选择清晨或傍晚较凉爽时进行，场地宜选择公园、庭院等空气清新处，以散步、慢跑等强度较低的项目为宜，活动量要适度。

（3）防病避邪：暑热过度可使人头昏、胸闷、恶心、口渴、甚至昏迷。因此，安排劳动或体育锻炼时，要避开烈日炽热之时，并注意加强防护。夏季还要防湿邪侵袭。长夏是湿邪最盛之时，湿邪与热邪相缠绕，极易损伤人体脾胃之阳气，使体内的水液不能正常代谢。暑湿伤人后引起的疾病，病程很长，不易恢复，所以在居住环境上要切忌潮湿，更不要久卧湿地。同时应注意预防一些常见病证，如夏季感冒（也称"热伤风"）、中暑（俗称发痧）、细菌性痢疾、急性胃肠炎（也称"六月泻"）、日光性皮炎、食物中毒等。

3. 秋季起居调护　秋季，自然界阳气渐降，阴气渐长，是由阳盛转变为阴盛的过渡时期。人体的阴阳盛衰也与天地阳消阴长相应，由阳盛的气机开泄，转为阴长的气机收敛，随"夏长"到"秋收"而相应改变。

（1）调护原则：应遵循"秋冬养阴"的基本规律，养阴、养收、养肺、防秋燥；应当适应自然界阴气渐生而旺的规律，把保养体内的阴气作为首要任务，为冬藏打基础。

（2）日常活动调养：秋季的起居作息要适应秋燥之气和收敛之性，应早睡以顺应阴精的收藏，早起以顺应阳气的舒张。日常活动不可过度劳累，不可泄汗过多，以防阳气和阴液受损伤。秋季养生锻炼分为三个层次：一是以静养为主的气功锻炼法，强调呼吸内守、形神内敛；二是轻度运动养生法，如太极拳、太极剑、散步等，以舒展肌肉筋骨为目的，不要求大汗淋漓、消耗体力；三是对形体肥胖而需要减肥者，可以考虑运动量大一点的项目。

（3）"秋冻"以辅阳气：四季养生的一个原则是"春捂秋冻"，春捂以助阳气的升发，秋冻则是辅佐阳气的敛藏。"秋冻"含有积极意义，是古今养生都十分强调的秋天养生方法。秋虽凉还不至于寒，人们还能耐受，有意识地进行防寒锻炼，逐渐增强体质和避免因穿衣过多产生身热汗出而致阴津伤耗、阳气外泄，以顺应秋天阴精内蓄、阳气内守的需要。当然"秋冻"还要因人、因天气变化而异，如老人、小孩，由于抵抗力弱，在进入深秋时就要注意保暖，适时增加衣服。

（4）避虚邪贼风以防病：秋季气候变化较大，热、燥、寒气皆有，起居若不慎，便容易患病。故应慎起居，避虚邪，防秋病于未发之前。主要应注意以下病证的预防：支气管哮喘，多半在秋季气候由热转凉时发作；便秘，因秋天气候干燥，燥伤津液，肠道干涩而引起；秋季腹泻，是典型的季节病，要注意婴幼儿腹部保暖，因秋季气候渐凉，婴幼儿腹部容易受寒。

4. 冬季起居调护　冬季，自然界阳气潜藏于内，阴气当令，主万物闭藏。人体阳气也顺应天地阴阳升降的规律而秘藏于内。

（1）调护原则：应顺应自然界冬气闭藏的特点，与天地间万物潜藏能量的趋势一致，滋养人体阴精，蓄养机体生机，保养阳气，防寒保暖，以保护肾气为根本，为春天的生发奠定基础。

（2）日常活动调养：冬令时节，由于风寒气冷，寒邪最易伤人体之阳气，故日常活动的重要原则就是防寒护阳。人们在寒冷的冬天应早睡、晚起，起床的时间最好在日出之后。因为冬令夜愈深则寒气愈重，早睡可以使人体阳气免受阴寒的侵扰；待日出再起床，则能避开夜间的寒气。以自然界的阳气主张机体的阳气，是人们防寒保暖的基本措施。冬季要特别注意头部、颈部、背部和两足的保暖，年老体弱者尤应注意。背部是人体的阳中之阳，风寒等邪气极易通过背部侵入而引发呼吸系统疾病和心脑血管疾病。"寒从脚起"，冬季要注重两足的保暖，两足温暖者不易受寒感冒，而足部受寒，势必影响内脏，可引致腹痛、腹泻等疾病。

（3）冬季防病保健：严寒季节，寒气最易伤人，可诱发多种疾病。当过度的寒冷刺激时，对高血压、心脏病、脑血管病和其他循环系统疾病都有诱发作用；寒冷可使人体裸露部位的皮肤粗糙或皲裂、老化，耳、手指等常发生冻疮；冬天若让头部突然遭受冷空气，或长时间受到冷风的侵袭，易发生面神经麻痹症。这些疾病的预防主要是防寒保暖。

二、起居有常，劳逸适度

（一）起居有常

起居有常要求人们做到：按时作息，力戒贪睡；适当锻炼，筋骨强健；一日三餐，定时定量；荤素粗细，搭配合理；劳逸结合，动静有度。《素问•上古天真论》曰："饮食有节，起居有常，不妄作劳，故能形与神俱，而尽终其天年，度百岁乃去。"起居有常是调养神气的重要法则。人们若能起居有常，合理作息，就能保养神气，使人体精力充沛，生命力旺盛。反之，若起居无常，天长日久则神气衰败，就会出现精神萎靡，生命力衰退。

（二）劳逸适度

劳包括神劳、形（体）劳和房劳。神劳很重要的一个方面是嗜欲，嗜欲是因为喜好太过而致偏爱成癖，欲望太过，必伤心神。中医通过断嗜源、寡嗜欲等节精神以养生；关于体劳，《彭祖摄生养性论》云："不欲甚劳，不欲甚逸。"人体日常的运动，不宜过于劳累，要循序渐进，过劳于人不利；也不宜过于清闲安逸，静而少动甚至不动易导致精气郁滞，筋伤肉痿，从而缩短寿命。过多睡卧伤人元气，过多地坐着不动伤人肌力；性欲虽为人之天性，不可放纵而应有所节制。古人云："房中之事，能生人，能煞人，譬如水火，知用之者，可以养生，不能用之者，立可死矣。"

三、睡　眠　有　节

睡眠有节，是指根据自然界与人体阴阳变化的规律，采用合理的睡眠方法和调护措施，以保证睡眠质量，消除疲劳，恢复精力和体力，从而达到防病强身，益寿延年的目的。祖国医学历来重视睡眠科学，认为"眠食两者为养生之要务"。人的一生中有三分之一的时间在睡眠中度过，这既是生理的需要，也是健康的保证和恢复精神的必要途径。

中医学认为天体的运行、阴阳的变化促成了昼夜的交替，昼为阳，夜为阴。人体应与昼夜阴阳消长的规律相适应。当阳气衰、阴气盛的时候就该闭目安眠，而当阴气尽、阳气盛时就该起床。

（一）睡眠环境宜忌

1. 睡前宜忌

（1）睡前神宜定。忌七情过极，读书思虑，大喜大怒则神不守舍，读书思虑则神动而躁，致气机紊乱，阳不入阴。睡前亦不可剧烈运动，以免影响入睡。睡前应减慢呼吸节奏，可以适当静坐、散步、看慢节奏的电视、听低缓的音乐等，使身体逐渐入静，静则生阴，阴盛则寐。

（2）睡前宜暖足。其要点有二：一是睡前用温热水浸足，使血液下行，改善脑部充血状态，以利入眠；二是按摩足涌泉穴，该穴是足少阴肾经要穴，长期按摩以利睡眠。现代医学研究证明，经常按摩刺激脚部，能调节自主神经和内分泌功能，促进血液循环，有助于消除疲劳，改善睡眠，防治心脑血管疾病。

（3）睡前饮食宜少食多餐，不宜过饱，也不宜过少。《彭祖摄生养性论》曰："饱食偃卧则气伤。"饱食即卧，则脾胃不运，食滞胸脘，化湿成痰，大伤阳气。饥饿状态入睡则饥肠辘辘，难以入眠。浓茶、咖啡能兴奋中枢神经，使人难以入睡，不宜多饮。睡前不宜大量饮水，饮水过多则排尿次数增多，特别是老年人，夜尿增多则起夜多，影响夜间休息。睡眠不佳者就寝前可饮用牛奶或酸奶，也可食用养心阴的食物，如冰糖百合莲子羹、百合莲子汤等，将有良好的催眠效果。饮食后宜休息半小时左右再就寝。

2. 睡中禁忌

（1）寝卧忌当风，对炉火。睡眠时头对门窗或大开门窗，风易入脑户引起面瘫、偏瘫。卧时头对炉火、暖气，易使火攻上焦，造成咽干目赤鼻衄，甚则头痛。

（2）卧忌言语哼唱。古人云"肺为五脏华盖，好似钟磬，凡人卧下肺即收敛"，如果卧下言语，则肺震动而使五脏俱不得宁，影响睡眠质量。

（二）睡眠时间和姿势

1. 睡眠时间　子午觉是古人睡眠养生法之一，即每天于子时（23～1点）、午时（11～13点）入睡。中医认为，子午之时，阴阳交接，极盛极衰，体内气血阴阳极不平衡，必欲静卧，以候气复。根据天地阴阳之气在一天中消长变化的规律，每天晚上的子时是阴气最盛、阳气最弱、阴阳之气交接之时，故此时是睡眠的最佳时期，此时最能养阴，而子时也是经脉运行到肝、胆的时间，养肝的时间应该熟睡。现代研究也发现，夜间0～4点，机体各器官功能降至最低；中午11～下午1点，是人体交感神经最疲劳的时间，因此睡子午觉更符合人的生理规律，可以起到事半功倍的作用。午休时间不宜过长，以30分钟～1小时为佳。

每人每天睡眠时间因不同年龄、性别、体质、性格、环境因素等而不同，通常应为8小时，而年龄越小，睡眠时间越长，次数也越多。

2. 睡眠姿势　有仰卧、俯卧、侧卧三种。侧卧者似卧龙，任督相通，阴阳和顺，中医养生专家认为侧卧是首选的睡姿。俯卧位，伏床而卧，背朝上腹朝下，虽四肢有力经气畅达，但五脏受压，阴阳不和，难于安眠。仰卧位，虽四肢舒展放松，但阴阳倒逆，阴脉在上、阳脉在下，督脉被压，尽管阴脉畅达，但阳气无法激荡，一觉睡熟，阳气尽为阴浊所陷，经气未能畅达四肢末梢。

3. 睡眠方位　睡眠的方位与健康紧密相关，中国古代养生家根据天人相应、五行相生理论，对寝卧方向提出过几种不同的主张。有的主张按四时阴阳定东西，认为春夏属阳，头宜朝东卧；秋冬属阴，头宜朝西卧，以符合"春夏养阳，秋冬养阴"的原则；有的主张一年四季都应寝卧东向，认为头为诸阳之会，人体之最上方，气血升发所向，而东方震位主春，能够升发万物之气，故头向东卧，可保证升清降浊，头脑清楚。而大多数养生家认为要避免北首而卧，认为北方属水，阴中之阴位，主冬主寒，恐北首而卧阴寒之气直伤人体元阳，损害元神之府。

四、二便调畅

（一）大便通畅

古代医家对保持大便通畅非常重视。汉代王充在《论衡》中载有"欲得长生，肠中常清，欲得不死，肠中无滓"，提示人们保持大便通畅可延年益寿。如果大便秘结不畅，粪便在肠内停留时间延长，水分和有毒物质就会被大量重吸收，可引起多种疾病，如痔疮、肛裂、肠癌等。

要培养良好的排便习惯：养成定时作息、定时进餐、按时排便的好习惯；排便要做到顺其自然，做到有便不强忍、大便不强挣。

注意饮食调节：饮食宜多样化，以五谷杂粮为主食，适当多用蔬菜和水果，此外要多饮水。

（二）小便通利

古人云："要长生，小便清；要长活，小便洁。"保持小便清洁、通利，是保证身体健康的重要方面。小便通利与肺、脾、肾、膀胱等脏腑的功能有关，而水液代谢的状态反映了机体脏腑功能的正常与否，特别是肾气是否健旺，因为肾是新陈代谢的原动力，调节着水液代谢的各个环节，中医理论中"肾主水"。

饮食要注意少食、素食、食久后饮、渴而才饮等。此外，有小便要及时排出，强忍不解、努力强排都会对身体健康造成损害。

（郝玉芳 周 芬）

第二节 中医饮食调护

合理饮食是人体生命活动的需要，是健康长寿的保障。饮食调护得当，可增进健康、防病治病；调护失宜，则伤身害病、衰老损寿。中医倡导以食养生，以食疗病。

一、食物的性味

中医认为"药食同源"，食物同药物一样，具有寒、热、温、凉之四性（古称四气），酸、苦、甘、辛、咸之五味。选择不同性味的食物进行配膳，使寒热相宜，五味调和，在充饥和营养的同时，亦可起到保健和治疗的作用。

（一）四气
寒凉性食物具有清热、泻火、解毒、滋阴等功效，用于热证，如西瓜、萝卜、绿豆、莲子等。

温热性食物具有温中、助阳、散寒等作用，用于寒证，如羊肉、鲤鱼、核桃、荔枝等。

有些食物没有明显的寒热之偏性，其性较平和，称之为平性，具有补益、和中的功效，如猪肉、山药、花生、鸡蛋等。

（二）五味
辛味食物具有发散、行气、活血的功效，用于外感表证、气血瘀滞等证，如生姜、大蒜、白酒等；

苦味食物具有清热、泻下、燥湿的功效，用于火热证、实热便秘、湿热证等，如杏仁、苦瓜等；

酸味食物具有收敛、固涩、开胃、生津的功效，用于虚汗、久泻、滑精、遗尿等证，如刺梨、山楂等；

甘味食物具有补益和中、缓急止痛的功效，用于虚证、脾胃不和、疼痛等，如蜂蜜、大枣等；

咸味食物具有软坚、泻下的功效，用于便秘、瘰疬、癥瘕等证，如海藻、海带等。

有些食物气味不明显，称之为"淡味"，能利水渗湿，归于甘味，如冬瓜；还有些食物具有涩味，常与酸味并存，附于酸味上，如柿子。

总之，每种食物都具有性和味，不能孤立地看待，两者必须综合起来分析应用。

二、饮食调护的基本原则

（一）平衡阴阳，扶正祛邪
阴阳学说是概括人体生理、病理的基础理论。正常情况下人体阴阳处于平衡状态，一旦出现阴阳偏盛或偏衰的变化，则会表现不同程度的病证。

疾病的发生、发展主要涉及人体的正气和致病的邪气，其变化的过程就是正邪交争、各有盛衰的过程。因此,协调阴阳是施膳的重要原则,即有余者损之,不足者补之。饮食调护的目的就是祛除邪气,扶助正气,以达到正胜邪却,阴阳平衡,恢复健康。

(二)全面膳食,谨和五味

《黄帝内经》提出的"五谷为养,五果为助,五畜为益,五菜为充,气味合而服之,以补精益气",概述了膳食的结构与内容,即以谷类、动物类食物补益人体,以蔬菜、水果类食物辅助补充,如此食物多样,荤素搭配,避免五味偏嗜,促进全面营养。

五味对不同的脏腑有相对的倾向性,如酸先入肝,苦先入心,甘先入脾,辛先入肺,咸先入肾,这种倾向性主要表现在食物对不同脏腑的作用上。如果五味偏嗜太过,久之会引起相应脏气的偏盛偏衰,导致五脏的功能活动失调。如过食甜腻之品,则会壅塞滞气、助湿生痰而伤脾碍胃。故五味调和能滋养五脏,补益五脏之气,强壮身体。

----- 知识链接4-1 -----

以类补类

这是中医备受争议的食养方法。如"以脏补脏"之血肉有情之品,能产生"同气相求"的药效,其补脏的作用远在草本植物之上,因此在食疗中广泛应用。明代著名医家李时珍有:"以胃治胃,以心归心,以血导血,以骨入骨,以髓补髓,以皮治皮。"如"以形养形",核桃似人之大脑,有益肾健脑之功。"猪肾煮核桃"的药膳,补肾益脑治疗肾虚,适用于脑转耳鸣、腰酸、遗精等症。

(三)审因用膳,辨证选食

审因用膳指针对影响健康的因素,可因人、因地、因时、因证、因病不同而分别施膳。

饮食调护应根据人的年龄、性别、体质、个性、心理、职业等方面的差异,分别予以不同的调摄。如老年期,五脏逐渐虚衰,老年人又厌于药而喜于食,可适当食补肺、脾、肾,促进新陈代谢,祛病延年。

由于四时气候的变化对人体的生理、病理有很大影响,因此应当在不同的季节合理选择调配不同的饮食以增进健康。如冬季天寒地冻,万物伏藏,可食补肾温阳的当归生姜羊肉汤。

不同地域,人之适应性有异而形成差别体质,易发不同病证,宜选择性进食。如中国的地理环境,东南地区气温偏高,湿气重,宜食清淡、渗湿之物;西北地区气温偏低,燥气盛,宜食温热、生津、润燥之品。

辨证选食配膳时,应根据病证的阴阳、表里、虚实、寒热而分别选择不同的饮食,如阳虚当给予甘温益气之品,如桂圆、山药、大枣等。

(四)合理搭配,趋利避害

安身之本,必资于饮食,但食物之间或食疗药膳应当合理搭配,使人全面吸收营养,满足生命需要。合理的饮食搭配宜荤素结合,粗细均衡,寒温适度,顾护脾胃,改变不良饮食习惯与嗜好,避免食用不利于人体健康及加重或恶化病情的食物。

如患病期间所忌食物:①生冷:冷饮、冷食、生的蔬菜和水果等。为寒证、虚证、脾胃虚寒或平时易感风寒者所忌;②黏滑:糯米、大麦、小麦等所制的米面食品等,如粽子、元宵。为脾虚纳呆或外感初起患者所忌,尤其在暑湿季节;③油腻:肥肉、煎炸或乳制品等。脾虚或痰湿者所忌;④辛辣:热证或阴虚内热者均忌辛辣食物,如生姜、葱、大蒜、花椒、辣椒、酒等；⑤腥膻：水产品、羊肉、狗肉等。为哮喘、斑疹疮疡患者所忌；⑥发物：指能引起旧病复发、新病加重的食物，如鱼、虾、蟹、豆芽、茼蒿、韭菜、鸡头等。哮喘、皮肤病、过敏体质者忌食腥膻、辛辣之品及一些特殊食物如香菜。

三、辨 体 施 膳

体质是指人体秉承先天（父母）遗传、受后天多种因素影响，所形成的与自然、社会环境相适应的功能和形态上相对稳定的固有特性。体质决定对某种致病因素或疾病的易感性及病变过程的倾向性。因人施养，如辨体施膳，可根据体质的不同进行饮食调护。

（一）平和质（A 型）

特征：阴阳气血调和，见体态适中、面色红润、精力充沛等表现。

饮食调护：体质平和是健康之源，此类人"养生之道，莫先于食"，原则是膳食平衡。保持饮食有节，饥饱适度；进食规律，细嚼慢咽；食后保健，摩腹散步，以调养气血，协理阴阳，即"有粗有细不甜不咸，三四五顿七八分饱"。

（二）气虚质（B 型）

特征：元气不足，见疲乏神倦、气短懒言、自汗等表现。

饮食调护：益气健脾，培补元气。多食养气补益之物，如粳米、小米、山药、马铃薯、扁豆、胡萝卜、香菇、豆腐、鸡肉、鸡蛋、牛肉、菜花等。亦可选用补益药膳缓缓调补，如人参莲肉汤、黄芪汽锅鸡等补养佳品。

（三）阳虚质（C 型）

特征：阳气不足，见形体白胖、畏寒怕冷、手足不温等表现。

饮食调护：温补脾肾以祛寒补阳，宜多食甘温、壮阳之品，如羊肉、带鱼、虾、栗子、韭菜、洋葱等。忌性寒生冷之物。夏勿贪凉，冬宜温补，如当归生姜羊肉汤。

（四）阴虚质（D 型）

特征：阴液亏少，见体形瘦长、口燥咽干、手足心热、面色潮红等表现。

饮食调护：滋阴养体，阴虚体质者关键在滋养肝肾之阴。宜食芝麻、糯米、蜂蜜、海参、牡蛎、蛤蜊、银耳、甘蔗、鸭肉、牛奶等甘凉清润、生津养阴之物。阴虚火旺之人忌温热辛辣香燥之品。

（五）痰湿质（E 型）

特征：痰湿凝聚，见形体肥胖、胸闷痰多、口黏苔腻等表现。

饮食调护：宜健脾利湿、化痰祛湿的食物，如薏米、红小豆、扁豆、花生、鲤鱼、鲫鱼、萝卜、山药、竹笋、荸荠、海蜇等，亦可选茯苓饼、杏仁霜等食疗方。忌暴饮暴食，少食肥甘厚味、酸涩苦寒之物，酒勿过饮。

（六）湿热质（F 型）

特征：湿热内蕴，面垢油光、口苦口干、舌红苔黄腻等表现。

饮食调护：宜清化湿热、分消走泄。多选用芳香的蔬菜如香菜、藿香等以利清除湿气，或薏苡仁、莲子、茯苓、冬瓜、红小豆、蚕豆、鸭肉、鲫鱼、鲤鱼、海带、苦瓜、黄瓜、西瓜、白菜、芹菜、卷心菜、胡萝卜、绿豆芽等有利湿作用的食物。少食甘酸滋腻之品及温热菜蔬水果如辣椒、蒜、荔枝、芒果。不可过食酒、奶油、动物内脏等。

（七）血瘀质（G 型）

特征：血行不畅，瘀血内阻，见肤色晦黯、口唇暗淡、舌黯有瘀点或瘀斑等表现。

饮食调护：可常服桃仁、油菜、黑大豆、陈皮、木耳、玫瑰等具有缓和的行气、活血祛瘀作用的食物。淡酒可少量常饮以行气血、助药势。食疗方选用山楂粥、花生粥等。忌寒凉、温燥、油腻、酸涩之物如柿子、石榴、蛋黄等。

（八）气郁质（H 型）

特征：气机郁滞，长期情志不畅所致，见忧郁脆弱、神情郁闷、胸胁胀满疼痛，常伴善太息、喉间异物感、乳房胀痛等表现。

饮食调护：多食具有行气解郁功效的食物，如橙子、萝卜、洋葱、菊花、玫瑰、茴香菜、刀豆等，以疏肝理气、调畅气机、调节情绪。气郁质者应少食收敛酸涩之物，如乌梅、南瓜、泡菜、草莓、李子、柠檬等，以免阻滞气机。

（九）特禀质（I 型）

特征：先天禀赋不足或遗传，以生理缺陷、过敏反应等为主要特征。

饮食调护：特禀质者应根据个体的实际情况选择保健食谱。如过敏体质者避免食用各种致敏之物，减少发作机会。如饮食过敏所致的哮喘病，饮食宜清淡，忌食生冷、辛辣、肥甘油腻及各种发物，如酒、鱼、虾、蟹、辣椒、肥肉，以免引动伏痰宿疾。

----- 知识链接 4-2 ---

彭祖

中国上古有一个志于养生的寿者，他善于烹调雉鸡羹，精通药物补养和导引之术。尧帝时他进献此羹，尧帝遂把彭城封与他，世称"彭祖"；舜帝时他师从尹寿子，隐居武夷山；商王曾向他请教长生之术。他不慕名利，摄养为生。彭祖成为健康长寿的象征。

四、四季饮食养生

春、夏、秋、冬四时季节的交替，昼夜长短的不同体现了一年中时间的变化，气候的变化表现为春温、夏热、秋凉、冬寒的更迭，物候的变化表现为世间万物春生、夏长、秋收、冬藏的变动，而这些皆反映四时阴阳的盛衰。因此四时养生，即调节人体阴阳的盈虚，以适应自然界阴阳变化的规律。因时调摄，如因时施膳，指在不同的季节合理选择调配不同的饮食，增强体质，促进健康。

（一）春季

春三月，包含了立春、雨水、惊蛰、春分、清明、谷雨六个节气。

春季风和日暖，阳气升发，宜食清温平淡之物，如小麦、鸡肝、鸭血、菠菜、香蕉等，少食生冷、粘腻之品。食疗方可选韭菜炒鸡蛋、醋泡黄豆、芹菜粥等。

中医论四时阴阳以东方之气应春气时，五味之酸味、五色之青色、五脏之肝脏，皆应于春。因此春季养生应注重养阳气，调肝脏，适当选用青色、酸味的食物以助春生之气。但肝旺则伤脾，宜"省酸增甘"以养脾。

（二）夏季

夏三月，包括立夏、小满、芒种、夏至、小暑、大暑六个节气。

夏季酷热难耐，宜清淡消暑、解渴生津之品，如西瓜、冬瓜、绿豆汤、乌梅小豆汤、荷叶粥等，忌寒凉、厚味之物。饮食温养为宜，讲究卫生，防止病从口入。

中医论四时阴阳以南方之气应夏气时，五味之苦味、五色之赤色、五脏之心脏，皆应于夏。因此夏季养生亦应注重养阳气，调心脏，适当选用赤色、苦味的食物以助夏长之气，如苦瓜、莲子、番茄。

中医亦有长夏之论，乃四时之外的另一个季节概念，常指夏秋之交的一段时间。湿气是其主气，易伤脾阳，当食健脾利湿之物，如薏苡仁、扁豆、山药等。

（三）秋季

秋三月，包括立秋、处暑、白露、秋分、寒露、霜降六个节气。

秋季炎暑渐消，气候干燥，饮食应以滋阴润肺为主，如芝麻、蜂蜜、菠萝、乳品、甘蔗、藕、糯米等。少食葱、姜、辣椒等辛辣之物。进补时也应注意在平补的基础上再合以生津养液之品，如秋梨膏、银耳冰糖羹等。

肺应秋气，其味辛，其色白，因此秋季养生应注重养阴气，润肺燥，适当选用白色、辛味的食物以顾护秋季收敛之气。但肺气过盛则伤肝，宜少辛多酸以保肝。

（四）冬季

冬三月，包含立冬、小雪、大雪、冬至、小寒、大寒六个节气。

冬季万物凋零，朔风凛冽，宜滋阴潜阳作用的食物，如谷类、羊肉、鸡蛋、黑木耳、牛肉、黑芝麻、鳗鱼等，去寒就温，以保护阳气。冬季以养精、藏精为主，此时进补可扶正固本，有助于体内阳气生发，增强抵抗力，能有效地预防开春的时行瘟病。食疗方如栗子鸡、八宝粥、葱烧海参等。

肾应冬气，其味咸，其色黑，因此冬季养生应注重养肾阴，温肾阳，适当选用黑色、咸味的食物以顾护冬季收藏之气。但水能克火，饮食之味宜减咸增苦以养心。

总之，四季饮食养生当遵循阴阳的变化规律，理解"春夏养阳，秋冬养阴"的基本原则。中医认为一日亦分四季，朝则为春，日中为夏，日入为秋，夜半为冬。故每日皆当摄生调护，针对不同时辰保养相对脏腑，顺天应时，和谐养生之道。

（陈　岩）

第三节　情志调护

所谓情志，指人的七种情绪，即喜、怒、忧、思、悲、恐、惊，简称七情。七情属于人的精神情志活动，与人体脏腑功能活动有密切的关系。在正常情况下，七情不会使人致病，只有突然强烈或长期持久的情志刺激，超过人体的正常生理活动范围，使人体气机紊乱，脏腑、阴阳、气血失调，导致疾病的发生。七情不仅可以引起多种疾病的发生，而且对疾病发展也有重要影响。因此，作为护理工作者，应设法消除患者的紧张、恐惧、愤怒、忧虑等不良情志的刺激，帮助患者调节情志以保持良好精神状态，促进健康。

一、中医"养心"思想

中国医家在长期的探索和实践中形成了系统的"养心"思想，包括清静养神、养心贵在养德、情欲适度、内守精神等，体现了养生中"和"的内涵，以及恬淡虚无、真气从之、精神内守、病安从来的思想。

（一）清静养神

老子庄子的清静养神思想反映了道家积精全神的观点：顺应事物自然之理，主张思想清静，戒除杂念，少私寡欲。中医养生学认为，精气神是人体三宝。神聚则气聚，神散则气消,若葆惜精气而不知存神,犹如断其根基。心神宜静,动而不妄,用而不过;若杂念过多,则伤神。

(二)养性修德

中国古代学者意识到道德与一个人的心理状态和寿命有密切关系。良好的道德修养可维持脏腑阴阳平衡,修身积德,阴阳气和,能度百岁而动作不衰。此外,良好的道德修养能使人保持开朗、乐观的心境。

(三)怡养性情

中医养生学认为,"精神内守"是"养心"的核心,是指对人的精神意识、思维活动及心理状态进行自我控制、自我调节,使机体与环境保持平衡协调而不紊乱。主张人要保持适度的欲望,并以思想、理性和意志力控制人的过度欲望,如节制过度的财欲、名利欲、性欲等。

(四)四气调神

"天人合一"、"天人感应"是中国古代哲学思想。从养生角度看,人的情志活动必须顺应四时气候的变化,以适应自然界生长和收藏的规律,达到养生防病的目的。春天和肝属木,春天是木旺的时候,要求精神要豁达调畅,赏心怡情;夏天与心属火,天气的炎热使人容易激动、发火。此时应保持情志愉快,使体内阳气向外宣泄;秋天阴气始盛,阳气始衰,此时为不使阳气外泄,避免秋天肃杀之气的伤害,情志应是收敛的,应神气内敛,志意安宁;冬天阳气潜藏,阴气盛极,精神志意宜内守,保持心神安宁。

二、不良情志的调护方法

情志变化可以直接影响人体的生理功能。《素问·汤液醪醴论》曰:"精神不进,志意不治,故病不愈。"历代名医一再提倡:"善医者,必先医其心,而后医其身。"因此,加强情志护理,对疾病的康复及维持健康都有重要的意义。情志护理的方法有多种,可根据个体的实际情况选择合适的方法,以便取得最佳效果。

(一)以情胜情法

又叫情志制约法,指以一种情志抑制另一种情志,以淡化或消除不良情绪,保持良好精神状态的一种方法。《素问·阴阳应象大论》指出:"怒伤肝,悲胜怒"、"喜伤心,恐胜喜"、"思伤脾,怒胜思"、"忧伤肺,喜胜忧"、"恐伤肾,思胜恐"。以情胜情法是根据情志及五脏间存在的阴阳五行生克原理,用相互制约、相互克制的情志来转移和干扰原来对机体有害的情志,借以达到协调情志的目的。此为祖国医学独特的心理治疗与康复方法。著名医家张子和指出:"悲可以制怒,以怆恻苦楚之言感之;喜可以治悲,以谑浪戏狎之言娱之;恐可以治喜,以恐惧死亡之言怖之;怒可以制思,以污辱欺罔之事触之;思可以治恐,以虑彼志此之言夺之。凡此五者,必诡诈谲怪,无所不至,然后可以动人耳目,易人听视。"

在使用以情胜情法时,要在患者有所预感时,再进行正式的情志治疗,不要在患者毫无思想准备之时突然地进行,并且还要掌握患者对情志刺激的敏感程度,以便选择适当方法,避免太过或不及。

1. 喜胜悲法 指火制约金法,即用各种幽默、逗人的语言,或使人兴奋的语言,让患者尽快高兴起来,以克制其原有悲忧过度所致情绪障碍及相关的躯体疾病。对于由于神伤而表现得抑郁、低沉的种种病证,皆可使用。

----- **知识链接 4-3** ---

在《医苑典故趣拾》中有一病例：清代有位巡按大人，郁郁寡欢，成天愁眉苦脸。家人特请名医诊治，当名医问完其病由后，按脉许久，竟诊断为"月经不调"。巡按大人听罢，嗤之以鼻，大笑不止，连连说道："我堂堂男子焉能'月经不调'，真是荒唐到了极点。"从此，每回忆及此事，就大笑一番，乐而不止。

名医朱丹溪曾遇一青年秀才，婚后不久突然亡妻，故终日哭泣悲伤，终成疾病。求尽名医，用尽名药，久治无效。朱丹溪为其诊脉后说："你有喜脉，看样子恐怕已有数月了。"秀才捧腹大笑，并说："什么名医，男女都不分，庸医也！"此后，每想起此事，就会自然发笑，亦常将此事作为奇谈笑料告诉别人，与众人同乐。秀才食欲增加，心情开朗，病态消除。

以上两例为运用喜胜悲法的典型例证。常用的方法有两种：其一，可以以开玩笑或不庄重的语言刺激患者，使患者兴奋起来，以消除因过度悲伤忧愁所致疾病；其二，若患者是因意念未遂、所求不得、郁郁寡欢，积久成疾者，则应顺其意，使患者情志舒畅而促使病愈。

2. **悲胜怒法** 即金制约木法，即用各种语言或方法使患者产生悲哀的情绪，以克制其原有愤怒过度所致情绪障碍及相关的躯体疾病。护理人员可创设不同情境，或以悲伤凄苦的动情语言感化患者，唤起他悲痛的情感；或用威吓的语言震慑患者，使其恐惧，继而转悲，悲则气消，胸中郁怒之气得以排解。

3. **怒胜思法** 指木制约土法，即用各种方法使患者发怒，以克制其原有思虑过度所致情绪障碍及相关的躯体疾病。适用于长期思虑不解、气结成疾或情绪异常低沉的病证。

----- **知识链接 4-4** ---

《续名医类案》载："一富家妇人，因思虑过甚，二年余不寐。张子和看后曰：'两手脉俱缓，此脾受之也，脾主思故也。'乃与其丈夫怒而激之也，多取其财，饮酒数日，不处一法而去，其人大怒，汗出，是夜困眠，如此者，八九日不寤，自是而食进，脉得其平。"

《四川医林人物载》里亦记载一例郁病怒激的病例：青龙桥有位姓王的儒生，得了一种怪病，喜欢独居暗室，不能接近灯光，偶尔出来则病情加重，遍寻名医而屡治不验。一天名医李健昂经过此地，家人忙请他来诊视。李氏诊毕，并不处方，却索取王生昔日之文，乱其句读，高声朗诵。王叱问："读者谁人"，李则声音更高。王气愤至极，忘记了畏明的习惯，跑出来夺过文章，就灯而坐，并指责李氏："你不解句读，为何在此高声嘶闹？"儒生一怒之后，郁闷得泄，病也就好了。

以上两例，说明思之甚可以使人的行为和活动调节发生障碍，致正气不行而气结，或阴阳不调，阳亢不与阴交而不寐，当怒而激之时，逆上之气冲开了结聚之气，兴奋之阳因汗而泄，致阴阳平调而愈。

4. **思胜恐法** 指土制约水法，即采用让患者思考问题的方法，以克制其原有惊恐过度所致情绪障碍及相关的躯体疾病。

----- **知识链接 4-5** ---

《晋书·乐广传》记载："尝有亲客，久阔不复来，广（乐广）问其故。答曰：'前在坐，蒙赐

酒。方欲酒，见杯中有蛇，意甚恶之，既饮而疾。'于时河南听事壁上有角弓，漆画作蛇，广意杯中蛇即角影也。复置酒于前处，谓客曰：'酒中复有所见不？'答曰：'所见如初。'广乃告其所以，客豁然意解，沉疴顿愈。"

"杯弓蛇影"这一成语所讲的历史事实，说明由恐惧引起的疾病，可以用"深思"的方法来解除其恐惧紧张的心理状态，从而使疾病消除，恢复健康。

5. 恐胜喜法 指水制约火法，即用各种方法使患者产生惊恐，以克制其原有的因喜乐过极所致情绪障碍及相关躯体疾病。适用于神情兴奋、狂躁的病证。

----- **知识链接 4-6** ---

《儒门事亲》里载：有一位庄医师治以喜乐之极而病者，庄切其脉，为之失声，佯曰："吾取药去，数日更不来。"于是患者便渐渐由怀疑不安而产生恐惧，又由恐惧产生悲哀，认为医生不再来是因自己患了重病。病者悲泣，辞其亲友曰："吾不久矣！"庄知其将愈，慰之。

《泂溪医书》里亦记载一例喜病恐胜之病例：某人新考上状元，告假返乡，途中突然病倒，请来一位医生诊视。医生看后说："你的病治不好了，七天内就要死，快赶路吧，抓紧点时间可以回到家中。"新状元垂头丧气，日夜兼程赶回家中，七天后安然无恙。其仆人进来说："那位医生有一封信，要我到家后交给您。"只见信中讲到："公自及第后，大喜伤心，非药力所能愈，故假以死恐之，所以治病也，今无妨矣。"

（二）移情易性法

又称转移法，即通过一定的方法和措施转移或改变人的情绪和注意力，以解脱不良情绪的方法。有些人患某种疾病后，往往将注意力集中在疾病上，担心病情恶化，担心预后不佳，担心因病影响工作、劳动、学习和生活，整天胡思乱想，陷入苦闷、烦恼和忧愁之中，甚至紧张、恐惧。在这种情况下，应分散患者对疾病的注意力，使其思想焦点从疾病转移于他处；或改变周围环境，使患者避免与不良刺激接触。移情易性的具体方法很多，应根据不同人的心理特点、环境等，采取不同的措施，灵活运用。主要方法如下：

1. 琴棋书画移情法 《北史·崔光传》曰："取乐琴书，颐养神性。"《理瀹骈文》曰："七情致病者，看书解闷，听曲消愁，有胜于服药者矣。"故在烦闷不安、情绪不佳时可根据各自的兴趣爱好，从事自己喜欢的活动，如书法、绘画、音乐等，用这些方法排解愁绪、寄托情怀、舒畅气机、怡养心神。欧阳修《送杨置序》中记载了他"尝有幽忧之疾"，后来"受宫音数引，久而久之，不知疾之在体也"。

2. 运动移情法 在情绪激动时或与别人争吵时，最好的方法是转移一下注意力，参加适当的活动，如打球、散步、打太极拳等；或参加适当的体力劳动，用形体的紧张去消除精神上的紧张。旅游亦可以驱除烦恼，有利于身心恢复健康。当思虑过度，心情不快时，应到郊外游玩，领略大自然的风光，让山清水秀的环境调节消极情绪。

（三）说理开导法

说理开导法是指通过运用正确、巧妙的语言，对人进行劝说开导，端正人对事物的看法，认识自己的行为所造成的危害，解除不必要的忧愁顾虑，提高战胜疾病的信心，积极配合治疗，使机体早日康复。

运用时要针对不同人的精神状态和个性特征，做到有的放矢、动之以情、晓之以理、喻之以例、明之以法,解除患者的思想负担,提高其自信心,以逐渐改善患者的精神状态和躯体状况。

《黄帝内经》曰:"告之以其败,语之以其善,导之以其所便,开之以其所苦。"此为说理开导法的起源。其含义是:第一,"告之以其败",是向患者指出疾病的性质、原因、危害、病情的轻重,引起患者对疾病的注意,使患者认真对待疾病,既不轻视忽略,也不畏惧恐慌。第二,"语之以其善",指告知患者只要与医务人员配合,及时治疗,是可以恢复健康的,以增强患者战胜疾病的信心。第三,"导之以其所便",告诉患者调养和治疗的具体措施。第四,"开之以其所苦",指帮助患者解除消极的心理状态,克服内心不良情绪。

历代著名医家在临床诊疗中,善于运用疏导的方法治疗疾病。《四有斋丛说》载:邝子元求官不顺,郁闷积病,一老僧分析其疾病的原因是"妄想太多",要想病好,就要消除"妄想",按老僧建议"静坐月余,心疾如矢。"

(四)节制法

节制法指调节情绪,节制感情,防止七情过激,从而达到心理平衡的方法。

中医养生学认为:七情内伤是造成发病的重要原因,七情过用必成灾,人必须注意精神修养,节制自己的感情,维持心理平衡。《黄帝内经》指出"智者养生",要"和喜怒"。《医学心悟》归纳了"保生四要","戒嗔怒"即为一要。

愉悦的心情在一定程度上来说对人体是有益的,但如果是突然的狂喜,就会喜则气缓,即心气涣散。心主血脉,心气虚则不能行血,血运无力导致血液瘀滞于心脉,出现心悸、心痛、中风,甚至死亡。

清代医学家喻昌《寓意草》里载:"昔有新贵人,马上扬扬得意,未及回寓,一笑而逝。"《岳书传》中牛皋因打败了完颜兀术,兴奋过度,大笑三声,气不得续,当即倒地身亡。《儒林外史》里载范进少时多次进京赶考,屡考屡败,到五十多岁终于中举,由于过度高兴,突然颠狂。这些均是喜伤心的病例。

适度的生气有利于气机的宣泄和情志的调畅。但若暴怒,"怒则气上",暴怒伤肝,则会导致肝气不疏,上犯头目,出现头胀头痛,面红目赤,肝区疼痛;或者气极反静,不言不语,重者会因气厥而四肢抽搐,甚至昏厥死亡。

人在遇到烦心事的时候适当地忧愁担心无可厚非,但是忧虑太过,表现为终日忧心忡忡,郁郁寡欢,轻者愁眉苦脸、闷闷不乐、少言少语、意志消沉、独坐叹息,重者难以入眠、精神萎靡或紧张、心中烦躁,就会因气机紊乱而导致脏腑功能失调,出现心悸、胃痛、食欲减退、失眠等种种不适。

每个人在遇到问题时都要思考,但若思虑过度也会导致多种病证。中医认为"思则气结","脾在志为思",故过度思虑最易伤脾气,脾胃运化失职,就会造成食欲减低、胃脘胀满、腹胀腹痛等。

从以上我们可以认识到七情过激对身体有很大的伤害,故需要注意有意识地控制自己的情绪,做到大喜临门,不过分激动;悲伤时,适可而止。只要善于避免嗔怒、忧郁、悲伤等不愉快的消极情绪,使心理处于怡然自得的乐观状态,可大大提高机体免疫能力。如能提高大脑及整个神经系统的功能,使各个器官系统的功能协调一致,不仅可避免焦虑、失眠、头痛、神经衰弱等轻度的心理疾病,也会减少精神分裂症等严重心理疾病的发生。

（郝玉芳　周　芬）

第四节　运 动 调 护

运动调护是指通过运动的方式达到维护健康、增强体质、延缓衰老的目的。运动调护方式众多,中国传统健身术为其中之一。中国传统健身术内容十分丰富,如太极拳、太极剑、八段锦、五禽戏、易筋经等。因其种类不同,锻炼方式及要求也各有特色。本节重点介绍太极拳、八段锦、五禽戏的作用和注意事项,以及运动调护的一般要求和注意事项。

一、中国传统健身术

（一）太极拳

太极拳是中华民族宝贵的民族遗产,以其姿势优美,动作柔和,男女老幼皆宜,且不受时间和季节限制的特点,加上既能锻炼身体,又能防治疾病的作用,而深受中国人民喜爱。

1. 作用

（1）调节呼吸功能,增加肺活量:练太极拳时要求气沉丹田,呼吸匀、细、深、长、缓,保持腹实胸宽的状态,这可起到保持肺组织弹性、改进胸廓活动度、增加肺活量、提高肺的通气和换气功能的作用。

（2）调节心血管系统功能,增强血管的弹性:太极拳动作包括各肌肉、关节的活动,其动作舒展,且要求有意识地使呼吸与动作呼应,以保证静脉血液回流,加强血液及淋巴的循环,以及增强血管弹性。

（3）调节神经系统功能:由于练太极拳时,要求精神贯注,"意守丹田",不存杂念,即要"心静用意"。这样人的意念始终集中在动作上,故使大脑专注于指挥全身各器官系统功能的变化和协调动作,提高了神经系统自我意念控制能力,从而达到改善神经系统功能的作用,有利于大脑充分休息,消除机体疲劳。

（4）畅通经络,培补正气:坚持练习太极拳,达到一定程度便可通任、督、带、冲诸脉,增加丹田之气,使人精气充足、神旺体健。还可补益肾精、强壮筋骨、抵御疾病,能防止早衰、延缓衰老,并可预防脊柱老年性退行性病变,使人延年益寿。

2. 动作要领

（1）虚领顶劲:头颈似向上提升,头向上顶,项部保持正直,松竖而不僵硬,这样利于保持身体重心的稳定。

（2）含胸拔背、沉肩垂肘:指胸、背、肩、肘的姿势,胸要含不能挺,背要松沉直竖,躯干正直,前后均要平正,不凹不凸。两肩平齐,肩不能耸而沉,不可一高一底;肘要松垂,肘关节微屈,手臂伸缩运转时,轻灵沉着而不漂浮。

（3）手眼相应,以腰为轴,移步似猫行,虚实分清:指打拳时必须上下呼应,融为一体,要求动作出于意,发于腰,动于手,眼随手转,两下肢弓步和虚步分清而交替,练到腿上有劲,轻移慢放没有声音。

（4）用意识导引动作，用意不用力：用意念引出肢体动作来，随意用力，劲虽使得很大，外表却看不出来，即随着意而暗用劲的意思。

（5）意气相合，气沉丹田：就是用意与呼吸相配合，呼吸要用腹式呼吸，一吸一呼正好与动作一开一合相配。

（6）动中求静，动静结合：即肢体动而脑子静，思想要集中于打拳，所谓形动于外，心静于内。

（7）动作连贯均匀，连绵不断：指每一招一式的动作快慢均匀，而各式之间又是连绵不断。

（二）八段锦

八段锦，即八段动作，古人认为这八段动作美如画锦，故称"八段锦"。它起源于北宋（960—1127），距今已有800多年的历史，是作用较好的一套健身操。全套动作简单，简单易学，运动量适中，适合各类人群练习，尤其是老年人和慢性病患者。

八段锦功法分坐式和立式两种。立式八段锦风格上一般分为南派和北派，南派以柔为主，北派以刚为主。从文献和动作上考察，不论是南派还是北派，都同出一源。现比较流行的是南派立式八段锦。

1. 作用　八段锦能改善神经体液调节功能和加强血液循环，对腹腔脏器有柔和的按摩作用，对神经系统、心血管系统、消化系统、呼吸系统、免疫系统及运动器官都有良好的调节作用，有助于促进身心健康，达到延缓衰老、延年益寿的功效，是一种较好的体育运动。八段锦除了具有强身益寿的作用外，对于头痛、眩晕、肩周炎、腰腿痛、消化不良、神经衰弱诸症也有防治功效。

2. 动作要领　练习八段锦应精神安定，意守丹田，头似顶悬，闭口，舌抵上腭，双目平视，全身放松，呼吸自然。

（1）呼吸均匀、自然：八段锦同样要配合呼吸，呼吸自然、平稳，做到呼吸深、长、匀、静。同时呼吸、意念与每个动作的要领相配合，利用意识引导练功。

（2）意守丹田：八段锦的运动要求"用意引导动作"。意到身随，动作不僵不拘。要心情舒坦，精神安定，意识与动作配合融会一体。姿势自如，强调"意守丹田"，意练重于体练。

（3）刚柔相济：在练习八段锦时要求全身肌肉、神经均放松，身体重心放稳。然后根据动作要领，轻缓、用力地进行。练功时始终注意松中有紧，松力时要轻松自然，用力时要均匀，稳定而且含蓄在内。

八段锦包括八节连贯的健身法，具体内容如下：双手托天理三焦；左右开弓似射雕；调理脾胃需单举；五劳七伤往后瞧；摇头摆尾去心火；背后七颠百病消；攒拳怒目增力气；两手攀足固肾腰。

（三）五禽戏

五禽戏是指模仿虎、鹿、熊、猿、鹤五种动物的动作，组编而成的一套锻炼身体的方法。两千多年前的名医华佗在总结前人的基础上，创编了五禽戏。坚持练习五禽戏具有防病治病、强壮筋骨、延年益寿的功效，因其行之有效，而备受后世推崇。

1. 作用

（1）调心作用：五禽戏要求练功者在练功前和习练每一戏时都要进行心理调节，以缓解精神紧张的状况，提高情绪的稳定性，保持心理健康。

（2）调身作用：五禽戏每一戏都各具特色，连起来又浑然一体。经常练习可起到调气血、益脏腑、通经络、活筋骨、利关节的作用。

（3）调息作用：五禽戏可以疏通经络，调畅气血，使肺主呼吸，肾主纳气的功能得到加强，气通则血通，气足则神旺，气的功能改善，则整个人体的经络血脉畅通，从而达到促进身体健康的作用。

2. 动作要领

（1）全身放松：练功时，首先要全身放松，情绪要轻松乐观。乐观轻松的情绪可使气血通畅，精神振奋；全身放松可使动作不至过分僵硬、紧张。

（2）呼吸自然均匀：呼吸要平静自然，使用腹式呼吸，均匀和缓。吸气时，口要合闭，舌尖轻抵上腭。做到"吸气用鼻，呼气用嘴"。

（3）专注意守：要排除杂念，精神专注，根据各戏意守要求，将意志集中于意守部位，以保证意、气相随。

（4）动作自然：五禽戏动作各有不同，如熊之沉缓、猿之轻灵、虎之刚健，鹿之温驯、鹤之活泼等。练功时，应根据其动作特点而进行，动作宜自然舒展，不要拘紧。

二、运动调护的一般要求和注意事项

（一）动静结合

运动调护时，要动静结合，动静适宜。运动时，一切顺乎自然，进行自然调息、调心，神形兼顾，内外俱练，动于外而静于内，动主练而静主养神。这样，在锻炼过程中内练精神、外练形体，使内外和谐，体现"由动入静、静中有动、以静制动、动静结合"的思想。

（二）持之以恒

锻炼身体非一朝一夕之事，要坚持不懈，每天应坚持进行一定时间和一定强度的锻炼，方能达到运动养生的目的。

（三）运动适度，循序渐进

运动调护，应该根据个体差异掌握合适的运动量，并应循序渐进，逐渐增加运动量和动作的复杂程度。一般来说，以每次锻炼后不感觉到过度疲劳为宜；也有人以脉搏及心跳频率作为运动量的指标。对于正常成年人的运动量，以每分钟心率增加至 140 次为宜；而对于老年人的运动量，以每分钟心率增加至 120 次为宜。若运动后食欲减退、头昏头痛、自觉劳累汗多、精神倦怠，说明运动量过大，超过了机体耐受的限度，会使身体因过劳而受损。

（四）因时制宜

一般而言，早晨运动较好，因为早晨的空气较新鲜，室外运动有助于将体内积聚的二氧化碳排出，吸入更多的氧气，增加机体的新陈代谢。午睡前后或临睡前不可剧烈运动，以免引起神经系统的兴奋，影响睡眠。另外，进食前后也不宜剧烈运动，因进食前机体处于饥饿状态，易发生低血糖症；而饭后剧烈运动，不仅影响消化，还可引起胃下垂、慢性胃肠炎等疾病。

（五）因人制宜

体育项目的选择，既要符合自己的兴趣爱好，又要结合自身特点。老年人由于肌肉力量减退、神经系统反应较慢、协调能力差，宜选择动作缓慢柔和、肌肉协调放松、全身能得到锻炼的运动，如步行、太极拳、慢跑等。年轻力壮、身体素质较好的人，可选择运动量较大的锻炼项目，如长跑、打篮球等。此外，每个人工作性质不同，所选择的运动项目亦应有差别，如教师、营业员等行业，工作需要长时间站立，易发生下肢静脉曲张，可选择仰卧抬腿类运动；经常伏案工作者，可选择一些扩胸、伸腰、仰头的运动项目等。

（苏春香）

第五章
实用中医自我调护

　　人体是一个有机的整体，任何局部病变均与其所属的内在脏腑的病变密切相关，所以局部功能障碍必然会影响到整体功能。每个人根据个人的实际情况，有针对性地进行某个特定部位的自我调护，有益于人体整体的生理功能。

第一节　口　腔　调　护

　　口腔是人体"开放门户"之一，"病从口入"是人尽皆知的道理。做好口腔卫生保健，不仅可以预防口腔和牙齿的疾病，而且可以有效地防治多种全身性疾病。

一、固齿保健法

　　我国古代养生家提出"百物养生，莫先口齿"的主张，养成良好的卫生习惯，重视固齿保健术，是养生保健的一项重要任务。

（一）口宜勤漱

　　《礼记》谓："鸡初鸣，咸盥漱。"《千金要方》亦说："食毕当漱口数过，令人牙齿不败，口香。"漱口能清除口中的浊气和食物残渣，清洁口齿。一日三餐之后，或平时甜食后皆需漱口。漱口用水种类很多，如水漱、茶漱、津漱、盐水漱、食醋漱、中药泡水漱等。

（二）早晚刷牙

　　刷牙的作用是清洁口腔，按摩齿龈，促进血液循环，增进抗病能力。刷牙的次数，要根据需要和现实条件。提倡"早晚刷牙，饭后漱口"，睡前刷牙比早晨刷牙更为重要。另外，要特别注意使用正确的刷牙方法，即顺牙缝方向竖刷，先里后外，力量适度。横刷和用力过大，不易清洁牙间污物，又可能损伤牙周组织，导致牙龈萎缩。

（三）齿宜常叩

　　晋代葛洪《抱朴子》一书指出："清晨叩齿三百过者，永不动摇。"自古以来，很多长寿者，都重视和受益于叩齿保健，尤其清晨叩齿意义更大。叩齿的具体方论是：排除杂念、思想放松，口唇轻闭，然后上下牙齿相互轻轻叩击，先叩臼齿 50 下，次叩门牙 50 下，再错牙叩大齿部位 50 下。每日早晚各一次。

（四）搓唇按摩

　　将口唇闭合，用右手四指并拢，轻轻在口唇外沿顺时针方向和逆时针方向揉搓，直至局部微热发红为止。其作用是促进口腔和牙龈的血液循环，健齿固齿，防治牙齿疾病，且有颜面美容保健作用。

（五）正确咀嚼

咀嚼食物应双侧，或两侧交替使用牙齿，不宜只习惯于单侧牙齿咀嚼。使用单侧牙齿的弊端有三：一是使用的一侧，因负担过重而易造成牙本质过敏或牙髓炎；二是不使用的一侧易发生牙龈失用性萎缩而致牙病；三是往往引起面容不端正。

（六）饮食保健

口腔、牙齿患病与营养不平衡有一定关系，因此营养要合理。维生素 A、D、C 族，以及钙、磷、蛋白质等，是牙齿发育不可缺少的营养成分。应适当食用一些含维生素 C 丰富的新鲜蔬菜、水果，含上述维生素及钙、磷、蛋白质丰富的食品，如动物的肝、肾、蛋黄及牛奶等。妊娠期、哺乳期的妇女，及婴幼儿童尤应注意适当补充这类食品，保证牙釉质的发育。

（七）纠正不良习惯

不良习惯也是导致牙病的一个原因。儿童应自幼养成不吮手指不咬铅笔写字的卫生习惯。饭后不宜用牙签或火柴棒等物剔牙，这种方法极易损伤齿龈组织，继而造成感染、溃烂等。

长期吸烟者，牙面易有黑褐色烟斑沉着，有利于结石沉积，局部菌斑刺激也可使牙周病加重。烟草中含有多种有害物质，烟雾中化学成分可直接刺激牙周组织或进入血液循环，造成牙周组织的慢性损害。

（八）防药物损齿

牙齿有病应及时治疗，但应避免一些不利于牙齿的药物，尤其在妊娠期、哺乳期的妇女和婴幼儿童不宜服用四环素类药物，如四环素、土霉素等。否则，易使乳牙发黄，且造成永久性黄牙，或引起牙釉质发育不全，易发生龋齿。

二、唾液保健法

唾液俗称口水，为津液所化。中医认为，它是一种与生命密切相关的天然补品，所以古人给予"金津玉液"、"甘露"、"华池之水"等美称。漱津咽唾，古称"胎食"，是古代非常倡导的一种强身方法。

（一）唾液的保健作用

《素问·宣明五气篇》说"脾为涎，肾为唾"，唾液由脾肾所主。脾肾乃先天、后天之本，与健康长寿密切相关。因此，唾液在摄生保健中具有特殊价值。

1. 帮助消化　唾液中的淀粉酶使食物中的淀粉分解为麦芽糖，进而分解为葡萄糖使食物得到初步消化。

2. 清洁口腔和保护消化道　唾液清洁口腔、保护牙齿，还有中和胃酸、修补胃黏膜等作用。

3. 解毒作用　唾液与食物充分混合，通过口腔里的化学变化能使致癌物质毒性失灵，被誉为"天然的防癌剂"，故有"细嚼慢咽，益寿延年"之谚。

4. 延缓衰老作用　《养性延命录》指出："食玉泉者，令人延年，除百病。"这些功效已被历代养生家和气功家的长期实践所证实。此外，唾液还有防病治病、促使伤口愈合等作用。唾液中包含了血浆中的各类成分，含有多种酶、维生素、矿物质、有机酸和激素等，经常保持唾液分泌旺盛，直接参与机体的新陈代谢过程，从而改善毛发、肌肉、筋骨、血液、脏腑的功能，增强免疫功能，预防疾病，达到祛病延年的目的。

（二）漱津咽唾法

漱津咽唾的方法很多，常用的有两种。

1. **常食法**　坐、卧、站姿势均可，平心静气，以舌舔上。或将舌伸到上颌牙齿外侧，上下搅动，然后伸向里侧，再上下左右搅动，古人称其为"赤龙搅天池"，待到唾液满口时，再分3次把津液咽下，并以意念送到丹田。或者与叩齿配合进行，先叩齿36次，后漱津咽唾。每次三度九咽，时间以早晚为好。若有时间，亦可多做几次。

2. **配合气功服食法**　以静功为宜，具体功法可根据自己的爱好选择。具体做法是：排除杂念，意守丹田，舌抵上腭，双目微闭，松静自然，调息入静，吸气时，舌抵上齿外缘，不断舔动以促进唾液分泌；呼气时，舌尖放下，气从丹田上引，口微开，徐徐吐气，待到唾液满口时，分三次缓缓咽下。每日早晚可各练半小时。上述二法，简而易行，只要长期坚持练功，就可收到气足神旺，容颜不枯，耳目聪明，保健延寿的效果。

第二节　颜面调护

颜面调护，又可称美容保健。面部是脏腑气血上注之处，血液循环比较丰富。中医还将面部不同部位分属五脏。即左颊属肝，右颊属肺，头额属心，下颏属肾，鼻属脾。面部与脏腑经络的关系非常密切，尤以心与颜面最为攸关。同样，面部的变化可反映出脏腑经络气血的盛衰和病变。颜面部位暴露在人体上部，六淫之邪侵犯人体，颜面首当其冲。颜面是反映机体健康状况的一个窗口，故凡养生者，皆重视颜面调护。

一、科学洗面

面部是五脏精气外荣之处，经常洗面能疏通气血，有促进五脏精气外荣的作用。但洗面用水的水质、水温、次数都应符合人体生理特点。

洗面宜用软水，软水含矿物质较少，对皮肤有软化作用。

对于水温，宜因人而异。非油性皮肤和混合肤质的人，最好用高于30℃但低于体温的水洗脸。这种温水不仅可以轻松洗去面部浮尘，还可使毛孔张开，利于皮肤的深层清洁。注意水温不宜过热，超过人体正常体温时，面部血管壁的活力就会减弱，皮肤容易变得松弛无力、发干，出现皱纹。油性肤质不宜使用冷水，冷水能使毛孔收缩，无法洗净堆积于面部的大量皮脂、尘埃及化妆品残留物等，不但不能达到美容的效果，反而引发痤疮或加重痤疮之类的皮肤问题。此外，还可冷温水交替洗面，既可清洁面部皮肤，也可使皮肤浅表血管扩张、收缩，加强皮肤血液循环，使皮肤细腻净嫩。

对于洗脸次数，每天应至少早、晚两次用洁面皂或洁面乳清洗面部。洗脸时的手势以中指和无名指从脸的中央往外、从下往上画圆圈式地轻柔移动。洗脸时，先用温水将洁面用品揉出泡沫，敷于面部，轻柔按摩1分钟。彻底冲净泡沫，最后用冷水洗脸。冷水可以增强血液循环，提高皮肤弹性。

二、按摩美容

历代养生家强调"面宜多擦"。古人是非常重视用按摩的方法来美容的。

美容按摩可分两类：一类是直接在面部进行的，即直接按摩美容法；另一类是通过按摩远离面部的经络而达美容效果的，即间接按摩美容。按摩方法很多，现仅介绍一种传统按摩保健美容法。

彭祖浴面法(《千金翼方》)：清晨起床用左右手摩擦耳朵，然后轻轻牵拉耳朵；再用手指摩擦头皮,梳理头发;最后把双手摩热,以热手擦面,从上向下 14 次。此法可使颜面气血流通,面有光泽,头发不白,且可预防头病。

三、饮 食 美 容

为了预防颜面皮肤早衰,应注意饮食营养平衡,适当增加对皮肤有益的保健食品。从中医角度讲,要进行饮食美容,须遵循饮食养生原则和宜忌。中医古籍中记载有很多美容作用的食品,如芝麻、蜂蜜、香菇、人乳、牛乳、羊乳、海参、南瓜子、莲藕、冬瓜、樱桃、小麦等。现代科学研究证实,这些食品营养极为丰富,含有多种维生素、酶、矿物质,多种氨基酸等,不仅可使面色嫩白、红润光泽,而且还能延年益寿。此外,还可进行食疗药膳美容保健。美容粥:糯米、燕窝(干品)适量煮粥,有润肺补脾,益颜美容之效。胡萝卜、粳米适量煮粥,有健胃补脾,润肤美容作用。薏苡仁、百合适量煮粥,可清热润燥,治疗面部扁平疣、痤疮、雀斑等。

四、药 物 美 容

药物美容,就是运用美容方药使皮肤细腻洁白,滋养肌肤,去皱防皱,并祛除面部的皮肤疾患。具有美容作用的方药很多,可分为内服美容方药和外用美容品两类。

(一)内服美容方药

本方法又可分为两类。一类是通过内服中药,起到调整脏腑、气血、经络的功能,达到润肤、增白、除皱减皱、驻颜美容的目的;另一类是通过活血祛瘀、祛风散寒、清热解毒、消肿散结等法,治疗各种影响颜面美容的疾病。例如,隋炀帝后宫面白散(《医心方》):橘皮30g、冬瓜仁50g、桃花40g,捣细为末即可,每次2g,每日3次。有燥湿化痰,活血益颜的功效。

还可适当饮用药酒,例如枸杞子酒(《延年方》),可补益肝肾、驻颜美容。桃花美容酒(《图经本草》),可润泽颜面,使人面如桃花。根据历代研究和实践,认为下述药物有润泽皮肤,增加皮肤弹性的作用,如白芷、枸杞子、杏仁、桃仁、黑芝麻、桃花等。

(二)外用美容品

外用美容品涂敷于面部或洗面,通过皮肤局部吸收,达到疏通经络、滋润皮肤、除去污秽、增白除皱、防御外邪侵袭的目的。玉容西施散(《东医宝鉴》):绿豆粉60g,白芷、白芨、白蔹、白僵蚕、白附子、天花粉各30g,甘松、山奈、茅香各15g,零陵香、防风、藁本各6g,肥皂荚二锭。诸药研为细末,每次洗面用之,其作用是祛风润肤、通络香肌、令面色如玉。

五、情 志 美 容

中医认为,"面由心生"。红润亮丽的容颜、蓬勃的朝气和优雅的风度来自健康的心理。老子在《道德经》指出,天下无形的东西比有形的东西更重要。情绪的好坏不仅会影响人体的生理功能,而且还会直接影响到人的肤色,要善于释放心理压力,在日常生活中要保持乐观的情绪、豁达的胸怀,避免情志过极。

第三节　头 发 调 护

中国人美发的标准是:发黑而有光泽,发粗而密集。故未老发早灰白、发枯焦稀疏、脱发等均属病态。头发除了是健康的标志外，还有保护头部和大脑的作用，同时健康的头发又有特殊的美容作用，使人显得精神饱满，容光焕发。

中医认为"肾主骨，其华在发"、"发为血之余"。人的肾精、气血充足，就会有健康而秀美的头发。头发与五脏的关系十分密切，头发的荣枯能直接反映出五脏气血的盛衰。而头发的变化又能反映出人的情志、生理和病理的变化。七情过极，亦可引起头发的变化，一般而言，头发由黑变灰、变白的过程，即是机体精气由盛转衰的过程。因此历代养生家都很重视美发保健，把头发的保养方法看作是健康长寿的重要措施之一。

一、梳理、按摩

古代养生家主张"发宜多梳"，《诸病源候论》说："千过梳头，头不白。"常梳头能疏通气血，散风明目，荣发固发，促进睡眠，对养生保健有重要意义。中医认为，"头为诸阳之会"，有许多经穴，血管神经十分丰富，梳子在头皮上来回划摩，可刺激头皮神经末梢和经穴，并通过神经和经络的传导，作用于大脑皮层，调节经络系统和神经系统功能，改善头部神经紧张状态，促进局部血液循环。梳发时间，一般可在清晨、午休、晚睡前，或其他空余时间皆可，但以早晨最佳，早晨是人的阳气升发之时，早晨梳头有助人体阳气升发。梳头的正确做法应是：由前向后，再由后向前；由左向右，再由右向左，如此循环往复，梳头数十次或数百次，最后把头发整理，把头发梳到平滑光整为止。

梳头时还可以结合手指按摩，即双手十指自然分开，用指腹或指端从额前发际向后发际，做环状揉动，然后再由两侧向头顶揉动按摩，用力均匀一致，如此反复做 36 次，至头皮微热为度。梳理和按摩两项，可以分开做，亦可一起做。

二、合 理 洗 发

《老老恒言》说："养生家言发宜多栉，不宜多洗。当风而沐，恐患头风。"洗发过勤会洗去对头发有保护作用的皮脂，缩短头发的正常寿命，严重的还可招致毛发癣菌感染。一般而言，干性头发宜适当减少洗发次数；油性头发可适当增加洗发次数。洗发水温不宜太凉或太热，37～38℃为佳。水温太低，去污效果差；水温过高，损伤头发，使其变得松脆易断。对于洗发剂的选择，干性和中性头发用偏于中性的香皂或洗发护发精；油性头发可用普通肥皂、硫磺皂，或偏于碱性的洗发剂。婴幼儿皮肤娇嫩，老年人皮肤干燥，可用脂性香皂或洗发液洗发。洗发结束后不要用毛巾使劲地搓干或拧干，应让头发自然晾干。也尽量不用热电吹风吹头发，若使用，吹风温度要尽量低，吹得时间尽量短。因头发在潮湿的情况下，其强度明显降低，容易被拉断。洗头后，不能湿气未干就卧床，否则易生湿热，损伤头发。

三、饮 食 健 发

日常饮食多样化，合理搭配，保持体内酸碱平衡，对健发、美发，防止头发早衰有重要作用。可适量食用含蛋白质、碘、钙及维生素 A、B、E 等较丰富的天然食物，如鲜奶、鱼、蛋类、豆类、绿色蔬菜、瓜果、粗粮等。芝麻、大枣、冬瓜、桃仁、杏仁、松子仁、蘑菇、山药、黄豆、百合、龙眼肉、草莓、花生等都是健发美发的营养食品，可根据情况适当选用。现举一款美容粥，可供食用。仙人粥（《遵生八笺》）：何首乌、粳米适量，熬粥，经常食服，有补肝肾、益气血、乌发驻颜之效。

四、药 物 美 发

药物美发是以中医理论为指导,运用中药进行美发保健的方法。药物美发既有美发保健作用,又有健发治疗作用。美发药品可分为外用和内服两类。

(一)外用类药

根据不同情况选用相应的中药洗浴头发,直接作用于皮肤组织和头发,以达到健发目的。外用药物有润发、洁发、香发、茂发、乌发,防治脱发等作用。古代医学和养生家在这方面有很多记载,现仅举几例。

1. 香发散(《慈禧太后医方选议》) 零陵香 30g,辛夷 15g,玫瑰花 15g,檀香 18g,川大黄 12g,甘草 12g,丹皮 12g,山奈 9g,丁香 9g,细辛 9g,苏合香油 9g,白芷 9g。研药为细末,用苏合香油搅匀,晾干。药面掺发上,篦去。本方有洁发香发作用,久用发落重生,至老不白。

2. 令发不落方(《慈禧光绪医方选议》) 榧子 3 个,胡桃 2 个,侧柏叶 30g,共捣烂,浸泡雪水内,用浸液洗发。本方有止发落、令发黑润之效,尤其对血热发落有良效。

(二)内服药

内服药主要通过调整机体整体功能,促进气血运行,而起到健发作用。具有健发作用的中药很多,如胡麻、油菜籽、核桃、黑大豆等。内服也有很多剂型,如汤剂、膏剂、酒剂、丸剂等。

瓜子散(《千金翼方》):瓜子、白芷、当归、川芎、炙甘草各 60g,研药为散,饭后服 1g 左右,日 3 次,酒浆汤饮,经常服用有活血补血、美发荣肤的作用,可防衰抗老,预防头发早白。

第四节 眼 睛 调 护

眼睛的功能与脏腑经络的关系非常密切,它是人体精气神的综合反映。《灵枢》指出"五脏六腑之精气,皆上注于目",因此,眼睛调护既要重视局部,又须重视整体与局部的关系。历代养生家都把养目健目作为养生中的一项重要内容,并积累了不少行之有效的方法和措施,兹简述如下:

一、运 目 保 健

运目,即指眼珠运转,以锻炼其功能,可采取多种方法进行。

(一)运睛

此法有增强眼珠光泽和灵敏性的作用,能祛除内障外翳,纠正近视和远视。具体做法:早晨醒后,先闭目,眼球从右向左,从左向右,各旋转 10 次;然后睁目坐定,用眼睛依次看左右,左上角、右上角、左下角、右下角,反复 4~5 次;晚上睡觉前,先睁目运睛,后闭目运睛各 10 次左右。

(二)远眺

用眼睛眺望远处景物,以调节眼球功能,避免眼球变形而导致视力减退。例如,在清晨,休息或夜间,有选择地望远山、树木、草原、蓝天、白云、明月、星空等。

二、按 摩 健 目

（一）熨目

《圣济总录》说："摩手熨目"，其做法是：双手掌面摩擦至热，在睁目时，两手掌分别按在两目上，使其热气煦熨两目珠，稍冷再摩再熨，如此反复 3～5 遍，每天可做数次，有温通阳气，明目提神作用。

（二）捏眦

即闭气后用手捏按两目之四角，直至微感闷气时即可换气结束，连续做 3～5 遍，每日可做多次。

（三）点按穴位

用食指指腹或大拇指背第一关节的曲骨，点按丝竹空、鱼腰，或攒竹、四白、太阳穴等，手法由轻到重，以有明显的酸胀感为准，然后再轻揉抚摩几次。此法有健目明目、治疗目疾的作用。

三、闭 目 养 神

历代养生家都主张"目不久视"、"目不妄视"，说明养目和养神是密切相关的。在日常生活或工作、学习中，看书、写作、看电视等时间不宜过久，当视力出现疲劳时，可排除杂念，全身自然放松，闭目静坐 5～10 分钟；或每天定时做几次闭目静养。此法有消除视力疲劳、调节情志的作用，也是医治目疾有效的辅助方法。

四、饮 食 健 目

一般而言，多吃蔬菜、水果、胡萝卜、动物的肝脏，或适当用些鱼肝油，对视力有一定保护作用，切忌贪食膏粱厚味及辛辣大热之品。同时，还可配合食疗方法，以养肝明目。

五、药 物 健 目

中医认为视疲劳与脾、肝、肾、气、血关系密切，故中药养目主要从健脾、养肝、益肾、补气血入手。中药健目分外用和内服两类，可根据不同情况，选择食用。如明目枕，用荞麦皮、绿豆皮、黑豆皮、决明子、菊花做成枕芯，有疏风散热、清肝明目之功。

根据需要选服中成药，如视物易疲劳、双目干涩、属于肝肾阴亏，可选用补益肝肾的六味地黄丸、杞菊地黄丸、石斛夜光丸等；视物易疲劳、平日体弱无力，属于气血不足，可选用气血双补的八珍丸；视物易疲劳、素体虚弱、纳食不香，属于脾气虚弱，可选用补中益气丸。

第五节　耳 部 调 护

中医学认为，耳为肾之窍。耳的功能与五脏皆有关系，而与肾的关系尤为密切。耳的听觉能力能够反映出心、肾、脑等脏腑的功能。

一、耳 勿 极 听

极听耗伤精气，损害听力。《淮南子》谓："五声哗耳，使耳不聪。"在有噪音环境中工作和学习应做好必要的保护性措施，如控制噪声源；在噪声大的环境有意识地张开口，以利进入耳道的声波能较快扩散开来,减轻对耳膜、内耳鼓膜的过大压力,做好个人防护。

二、按摩健耳

按摩健耳功法可分为以下几步:①按摩耳根:用两手食指按摩两耳根前后各 15 次;②按摩耳廓:以两手按摩耳轮,一上一下按摩 15 次;③摇拉两耳:以两手拇食二指摇拉两耳廓各 15 次,但拉时不要太用力;④弹击两耳:以两手中指弹击两耳 15 次;⑤鸣天鼓:以两手掌捂住两耳孔,五指置于脑后,用两手中间的三指轻轻叩击后脑部 24 次,然后两手掌连续开合 10 次。此法使耳道鼓气,以使耳膜震动,称之为"鸣天鼓"。

耳部按摩可促进耳部气血流通,调动体内正气,以增强机体对疾病的抵抗力,保持生理功能相对平衡;可润泽外耳肤色,抗耳膜老化,预防冻耳,防治耳病;活跃肾脏元气,强壮身体,抗衰老,利健康,助长寿。

三、梳 耳 法

一般采用不太硬细刷梳耳部。

1. 刷擦耳背 可将耳廓前折,刷擦耳背 20～30 次,直至耳背皮肤微红、发热为止。如无细刷,可用手部鱼际处刷擦。

2. 揉耳窝 两手食指指腹同时按揉两侧耳廓上耳甲艇(耳轮脚上面的凹窝)10～20 次,再按揉耳甲腔(耳轮脚下面的凹窝)10～20 次。然后用细刷对上述两个部位刷擦至有发热感觉为止。

3. 刷擦耳轮 用细刷从耳轮上端向下分别刷擦两侧耳垂 20～30 次,然后紧握两耳向上、向下分别用力提拉耳轮各 3～5 次。如无细刷可用手指指腹代替。

梳耳法在临床上可应用于防治耳部冻疮:先取茄片或茄根水煎洗,洗后采用梳理法,直至耳部有明显热感为止。

四、药 枕 保 健

古人用药枕作为聪耳保健手段,现举两个药枕方如下:

菊花枕:选用菊花干品 1000g,川芎 400g,丹皮、白芷各 200g,装入枕套内,使药香缓慢挥发,一般每个药枕可连续使用半年左右。现代医学研究证实,本药枕内成分含有多种挥发油,具有清肝明目、降压、清热凉血、活血化瘀等功效。常用菊花枕的人,会感到神清气爽,精神饱满。

磁石枕和柏木枕:古代道家养生倡导用磁石枕和柏木枕。磁石枕是将磁石镶嵌在木枕上制成的,经常使用有聪耳明目之效。柏木枕用柏木板制成,四壁留有 120 个小孔,内装当归、川芎、防风、白芷、丹皮、菊花等多种药物,外套布套,药味缓慢散出。药枕的养生原理是依靠草本植物特有的芳香气味和磁石的磁场作用,达到闻香疗病的效果。

第六节 鼻 部 调 护

《内经》指出"肺气通于鼻"。鼻是呼吸道的门户,是防止致病微生物、灰尘等侵入的第一道防线。鼻腔内有鼻毛,又有黏液,故鼻内常有很多细菌、污垢,有时会成为播散细菌的疫源。因此,为了有效防止呼吸道疾病,鼻部调护非常重要。

一、浴 鼻 训 练

浴鼻训练，就是用冷水浴鼻。一年四季提倡冷水洗鼻，尤其是早晨洗脸时，用冷水清洗几次鼻腔，可改善鼻黏膜的血液循环，增强鼻对天气变化的适应能力，可预防感冒及其他呼吸道疾患。

在污染较为严重的环境中工作的人、鼻部干燥较为严重者或鼻部手术后的人可以到医院进行鼻部冲洗，可有效缓解鼻部不适，在家里也可以用清水或淡盐水进行鼻部清洗。具体方法如下：将鼻孔浸在盐水中，随吸气将水吸入鼻腔，让其充分与鼻黏膜接触，稍停一会儿，再将水呼出，反复 1～3 分钟。注意防止水呛入气管。鼻部干燥可滴几滴植物油在鼻腔中，以保持鼻部的滋润。

二、鼻 部 按 摩

鼻部按摩分拉鼻、擦鼻、刮鼻、摩鼻尖和"印堂"按摩，这些按摩手法均可增强鼻部的血液流通，使鼻的外部皮肤润泽、光亮，还能起到养肺、预防感冒、防治各种鼻炎的功效。

拉鼻：用拇指和食指夹住鼻根两侧，用力向下拉，连拉 16 次。

擦鼻：用两手鱼际相互摩擦至热后，按鼻两侧，顺鼻根至迎香穴，上下往返摩擦 24 次。

刮鼻：用手指刮鼻梁，从上向下 36 次。

摩鼻尖：分别用两手手指摩擦鼻尖各 36 次。

"印堂"按摩：即用中指和食指、无名指的指腹点按"印堂"穴 16 次，也可用两手中指，一左一右交替按摩"印堂"穴位。通过按摩，可增强鼻黏膜上皮细胞的增生能力，并能刺激嗅觉细胞，使嗅觉灵敏。

三、药 物 健 鼻

平常鼻腔内要尽量保持适当湿度，若过于干燥易使鼻膜破裂而出血。在气候干燥的情况下，可配合药物保健，如在鼻内滴一些复方薄荷油，或适量服用维生素 A、D 等，以保护鼻黏膜。此外，还可服用中药，如：

润鼻汤：天冬 9g，黑芝麻 15g，沙参 9g，麦冬 9g，黄精 9g，玉竹 9g，生地 9g，川贝母 9g。本方有润肺养脾之效，加减服用，可起滋润护鼻之功。

健鼻汤：苍耳子 27g，蝉衣 6g，防风 9g，白蒺藜 9g，玉竹 9g，炙甘草 4.5g，苡仁 12g，百合 9g。本方以祛风健鼻为主，润肺健脾，使肺气和，脾气充，对易伤风流涕之人，有良好的保健预防作用。

四、纠正不良习惯

在鼻部养护时，应注意以下几个方面：

第一，擤鼻涕是鼻炎患者最频繁的举动，不正确的擤鼻涕方法会使鼻膜黏液充满鼻窦，使得鼻窦变成病菌滋生的温床。故应养成正确擤鼻涕的习惯，即交替将左右鼻翼压向鼻中隔，不要用手捏紧双侧鼻孔擤鼻涕，以免增加鼻、咽部压力，使鼻涕倒流进入耳内。

第二，不可挖鼻孔、拔鼻毛或剪鼻毛。鼻部处于医学上的"危险三角区"内，如果炎症控制不好，有可能侵入颅内，危及生命，所以最好戒除挖鼻孔的坏习惯。

第三，不可吞咽鼻涕。吞咽鼻涕容易刺激咽喉和肠胃。鼻涕中含有尘土、细菌等微小的有害物质和过敏原，咽下时会对咽喉部黏膜造成刺激，引起咳嗽，长期如此会引发慢性咽喉炎，吞咽到胃肠中的细菌和病毒也会对胃肠黏膜产生刺激，引起疾病。

第七节 颈 椎 调 护

有研究表明，近年来颈椎病的发病率呈上升趋势，且有低龄化倾向。人们对颈部保养方法不当，使颈部长期处于不良姿势，极易导致颈椎周围组织形成慢性劳损而发生纤维组织炎或逐步退变。

一、保持正确的坐姿

经常伏案工作的人颈椎病发病率较高。其主要原因是坐立姿势不正确。因此，端正坐姿是预防颈椎病非常重要的措施之一。

正确的坐姿为：保持自然舒服的端坐位，上身挺直，收腹，下颌微收，两下肢并拢，头部略微前倾，头、颈、肩、胸保持正常生理曲线为准。同时，还要注意桌与椅的距离适中。

注意纠正一些生活中的不良习惯，如：看电视时最好不要倚着沙发，或半躺半卧靠在床头；打麻将时间不可过长，要经常变换身体姿势等。

二、加强颈部功能锻炼

长时间近距离看物，尤其是处于低头状态者，既影响颈椎，又易引起视力疲劳。对长时间伏案工作者，每工作 0.5～1 小时，就要进行适当活动。每当伏案过久后，应抬头向远方眺望半分钟左右。可根据颈椎运动功能特点进行颈部锻炼，如前屈和后伸、左侧屈和右侧屈、左侧旋转和右侧旋转、左侧环转和右侧环转，也可进行耸肩、双臂划圈等局部运动。

平常还可练习"凤凰"颈部保健操。具体做法：闭上眼睛，以自己的下巴为笔，身体不动，在空中写出繁体字"鳳凰"两个字，连续写 10 遍，每天练 3 次。可在休息、等车等时间段内，随时练习，皆有良好效果。这个练习可带动颈部各个环节的活动，但动作幅度不宜过大，动作柔和有序，有预防和辅助治疗颈椎病之效。

三、合 理 用 枕

颈椎病的早期表现为颈部脊柱生理弯曲的异常改变，如变小、变直或后凸。因此，预防颈部脊柱生理弯曲的异常改变是预防该病的关键。可以通过合理用枕进行预防，枕头的选择要符合颈椎生理曲度、质地柔软、透气性好。形状最好为圆柱形，直径大约 20cm。卧床休息时，枕头应放在头颈下，这样可使颈后部的肌肉松弛，保持颈椎正常生理曲度。枕头中央应略凹进，应呈中间低两端高的形状，颈部应充分接触枕头并保持略后仰，不要悬空。这样既可对头部起到相对固定作用，又减少在睡眠中头颈部的异常活动，还可以对颈部起到保暖作用。枕头不可以过高或过低、过软或过硬。此外，要注意睡眠姿势，睡觉时不可俯卧，习惯侧卧位者，应使枕头与肩同高。

此外，可使用药枕，对顽固性失眠、颈椎病、高血压、神经性头痛、紧张性头痛、偏头痛、头晕、焦虑症、抑郁症等疾病起到一定的防治作用。药枕配方如下：川芎、吴茱萸、川乌、草乌、当归、没药、细辛、威灵仙、甘草、冰片、樟脑、薄荷。将方中前 9 味药共研细末，用醋在微火上炒至有焦味时加入冰片、樟脑及薄荷粉拌匀。然后用晾干的绸布包药末做成枕芯，夜间枕,白天用塑料袋封装。

四、自 我 按 摩

　　自我按摩:选腕骨、外关、肩中、风池等穴位进行按摩,同时缓缓转动颈部,每次 10～15 分钟,每日 2 次。

　　拿颈项:将手掌握在后颈部,以四指和掌根用力捏起后颈 6～9 次,每日 3 次,经常练习,对颈椎保健很有好处。

第八节　手 足 调 护

　　手足是上肢和下肢阴经和阳经交接的部位。机体的气血阴阳的盛衰,与手足的功能状态有密切关系。历代养生家都非常重视手足的卫生保健。

一、手 的 调 护

　　在日常生活中,手最易被污染。不注意手的卫生保健,可以导致很多疾病,下面介绍几种护手方法。

(一)甩动双手

　　双手轻握拳,由前而后,甩动上肢,先向左侧甩动,再向右侧甩动,然后两肢垂于身体两侧甩动,各 24 次。有舒展筋骨关节、流通经络气血、强健上肢的作用,可预防肩、肘、腕关节疾病,还可调节气血,防治高血压。

(二)手部按摩

　　将手部按摩和上臂按摩结合在一起做。具体做法:双手合掌互相摩擦至热,一手五指掌面放在另一手五指背面,从指端至手腕来往摩擦,以局部有热感为度,双手交替。按摩时间可安排在晚上睡前和早晨醒后,本法可以促进肌肤的血液循环,增进新陈代谢及营养的吸收,使肌肉强健,可柔润健手,防治冻疮。

(三)药物润手

　　采用药物方法,保护手部皮肤,使其滋润滑嫩、洁白红润。以下举二方为例:

　　千金手膏方(《千金翼方》):桃仁 20g,杏仁 10g(去皮尖),橘核 20g,赤芍 20g,辛夷仁、川芎、当归各 30g,大枣 60g,牛脑、羊脑、狗脑各 60g。诸药加工制成膏,洗手后,涂在手上擦匀,忌火炙手。本品有光润皮肤、护手防皱之效。

　　太平手膏方(《太平圣惠方》):瓜蒌瓤 60g,杏仁 30g,蜂蜜适量。制作成膏,每夜睡前涂手。本品防止手部皲裂,使皮肤白净柔嫩,富有弹性。

二、足 的 调 护

　　俗话说:"树枯根先竭,人老脚先衰"、"种树护根,养人护脚。"脚对人体健康具有重要意义,足部不适是人体早衰和发生病变的一个征象。足部反射区保健疗法早已被列为替代医学并被广泛应用于临床。

(一)足部宜保暖

　　一般健康人脚部的正常温度应该是:脚尖约为 22℃ 左右,脚掌的温度约为 28℃ 左右。人的双脚温度为 28～33℃ 时,感觉最舒服。若降到 22℃ 以下时,则易患感冒等疾病。中医学认为："诸病从寒起，寒从足下生。"所以，天气寒冷时要保持足部适当的温度。鞋袜宜保暖、宽大、柔软和舒服，鞋子要防水、透气性能好，并要及时更换。脚部保暖对于预防感冒、鼻炎、哮喘、心绞痛等有一定的益处，保持双足的适当温度是预防疾病的一种重要方法。

（二）足宜勤泡洗

中医养生学认为："足是人之底，一夜一次洗。"民间流传着四季洗脚的歌谣："春天洗脚，升阳固脱；夏天洗脚，暑湿可祛；秋天洗脚，肺润肠濡；冬天洗脚，丹田温灼。睡前洗脚，睡眠香甜；远行洗脚，解除疲劳。"足宜勤泡洗，经常用温水洗脚，能刺激足部穴位，增强血液运行，调整脏腑，疏通经络，安神定志，从而达到强身健体、祛病除邪的目的。

除温水泡脚外，还可以用药浴的方法。

1. 取夏枯草 30g，钩藤、菊花各 20g，桑叶 15g，煎水浴足，每日 1～2 次，每次 10～15 分钟，适用于高血压患者。

2. 取透骨草、寻骨风、老鹳草各 30g，黄蒿 20g，乳香、没药、桃仁、独活各 10g，水煎趁热洗足，每日 2 次，适用于下肢关节炎。

3. 取苏木 30g，桃仁、红花、土鳖虫、血竭、乳香各 10g，自然铜 20g，趁热浸浴患足，适用于足部损伤。

4. 取丁香 15g，苦参、大黄、明矾、地肤子各 30g，黄柏、地榆各 20g 水煎取汁，待药液温后洗足，每次 10～15 分钟，每日 5～6 次，每日 1 剂，可用于脚癣。

（三）足宜常按摩

足部按摩简便易行，是一种常用的自我保健和防病治病方法。足部按摩主要是通过按摩穴位和刺激脚部反射区，起到舒筋活络、改善血液循环、协调脏腑功能、平衡阴阳、解除疲劳的作用，还可防治很多局部和全身性疾病。常用的方法有：

1. **摩涌泉法**　"涌泉穴"是"足少阴肾经"中一个重要穴位，也是肾脏在脚部的"反射区"。每晚洗脚后临睡之前，一手握脚趾，另一手摩擦足底"涌泉穴"30～60 次，以热为度，两脚轮流摩擦，具有调肝、健脾、安眠、强身的作用。

2. **按摩足部**　对足部进行按摩，可用手指头、指关节，也可使用按摩棒、按摩球等按摩工具。根据身体情况用揉搓或按压等方法按摩。作为日常保健，可在每个反射区按摩 2～3 分钟，先左脚后右脚，每次按摩半小时左右。按摩的力度顺序为轻—重—轻，以能忍受为限。按摩中如发现有异常的酸、胀、刺、麻、痛的感觉，或皮肤有结节状、条索状、沙粒状等印迹出现时，说明其对应部位可能有功能性疾病，需要重点按摩。

（四）外用药物护足

秋冬季节，足部常因经脉阻滞，肌肤失养，皮肤枯燥，而出现皲裂。用散寒活血、润燥养肤的中药，外涂足部，可收到良好的防治效果。

冬月润足防裂方：猪脂油 12g，黄蜡 60g，白芷、升麻、猪牙皂荚各 3g，丁香 1.5g，麝香 0.6g。制备成膏，洗脚后涂上。本方有祛邪通络、祛风消肿、防裂防冻之效。

第九节　胸背腰腹调护

胸、背、腰、腹是人体脏腑所居的部位，其功能盛衰直接关系到内部脏腑功能活动。历代养生家都非常重视这四个部位的保养，保养得当，可促进气血运行，协调和增强全身各部的联系，提高新陈代谢的能力，达到健身防病的目的。

一、胸 部 调 护

胸部是人体重要脏腑心脏和肺脏所在的位置,胸部的气血运行及寒暖直接影响脏腑的功能,胸部调护的基本方法包括注意保暖和自我按摩。

(一)衣服护胸

中医养生学认为:"胸宜常护",《老老恒言》说:"夏虽极热时,必着葛布短半臂,以护其胸。"说明胸部的保护以保暖避寒为主,目的在于保护胸阳,年老体弱者更应注意。日常生活中,人们穿的背心、上衣,均是以保护胸背的阳气为主。

(二)胸部按摩

乳房按摩:取坐位或仰卧位,用左手掌在胸部从左上向右下推摩,右手从右上向左下推摩,双手交叉进行,推摩 30 次。然后,两只手同时揉乳房正反方向各 30 圈,再左右与上下各揉按 30 次。女性还可做抓拿乳房保健:两小臂交叉,右手扶左侧乳房,左手扶右侧乳房,然后用手指抓拿乳房,1 抓 1 放为 1 次,可连续做 30 次。胸部按摩可以振奋阳气,促进气血运行,增强心肺功能,可以防治胸闷、气喘、咳嗽、心悸等病证。

拿胸肌:两手交叉于胸前,拇指按于腋前,食指、中指按于腋下,捏拿胸大肌。具有行气活血、增强呼吸系统功能等作用。

拍胸部:用虚掌或空拳轻轻拍击胸部。可增强心肺功能和促使痰液的排出,用以防治呼吸和循环系统病证。

推胸胁:用一手的手掌平放在同侧胸部的乳头上方,斜行向下推抹,途经前胸正中两乳头之间,推向对侧的胁肋部。具有宽胸理气、止咳化痰、平喘降逆、舒肝利胆、消食散瘀等作用。

二、背 部 调 护

背为足太阳膀胱经、督脉所过之所,五脏的腧穴都汇聚于背,背的寒暖与脏腑的功能直接相关。合理的背部运动、按摩保健可提高人体的免疫力,调节血压,增强心脏功能,促进消化功能,有益于健身防病。

(一)背部宜常暖

背部保暖方法有三:①衣服护背:平时穿衣注意背部保暖,随时加减衣服,以调护其背;②晒背取暖:避风晒背,能暖背通阳,增进健康;③慎避风寒:因为背为五脏腧穴所会,尤其是天热汗出腠理开时,若被风吹,则风寒之邪易于内侵,引起疾病。夏日汗出后不可背向电扇,以免风寒之邪伤人。

(二)背宜常捶摩

历代医家和养生家都强调保护背部的重要性,而且提出了捶背、搓背、等自我调护背部的方法。

1. 自我捶背 本法可以和调五脏六腑,促进气血运行,舒筋通络,振奋阳气,强心益肾,增强人体生命活力。方法:两腿开立,全身放松,双手半握拳,自然下垂。捶打时,先转腰,两拳随腰部的转动,前后交替叩击背部及小腹。左右转腰 1 次,可连续做 30~50 次。叩击部位,先下后上,再自上而下。

2. 自我搓背 本法有防治感冒、缓解腰背酸痛和胸闷腹胀等病证的功效。方法:可在洗浴时进行。以湿毛巾搭于背后,双手拉紧毛巾两端,用力搓背,直至背部发热为止。注意用力不宜过猛,以免搓伤皮肤。

三、腰 部 调 护

腰是躯体的中点，此处活动大，负重多，为人体运动的枢纽，中国传统功夫十分强调"以腰为轴"、"主宰于腰"。把腰部活动看作生命活动之本。日常生活和工作特别容易导致其劳损，故腰部保健尤为重要。

（一）正确用腰

在搬、抬重物时，应将两足分开与肩等宽，屈膝，腹肌用力，再搬动物体。此时大腿和小腿的肌肉同时用力，分散了腰部的力量。在膝关节伸直状态下，从地上搬取重物，腰部承受的压力可增加 40%，极易损伤腰部的韧带、肌肉和椎间盘。搬物时不要弯腰，而应屈膝，要保持腰部正常直立位置时的曲度，避免力量集中在腰部。如物体太重，不可强行用力。

直立挺直的姿势对腰椎关节是最好的，弯腰时，对腰部组织的负担均有不同程度的加重，长时间弯腰可致腰肌劳损、继而发展为脊柱的劳损退变。若弯腰角度小于 20°，腰部负担较小。因此在日常生活中尽量保持背部挺直，避免长时间弯腰工作，以减轻腰部的负担。

（二）传统运动练腰

中国传统锻炼腰部的方法很多。很多传统健身术都非常强调腰部活动，如五禽戏、易筋经、八段锦、太极拳等，皆以活动腰部为主。通过松胯、转腰、俯仰等活动，达到强腰健体作用。

（三）腰宜常按摩

"腰为肾之府。"腰部保健按摩具有温补肾阳、强腰壮肾，润肠通便等作用，还可以舒筋通络，促进腰部气血循环，消除腰肌疲劳，缓解腰肌痉挛与腰部疼痛，使腰部活动灵活、健壮有力。

1. **腰部按摩** 搓手令热，以两手掌面紧贴腰部脊柱两旁，直线往返摩擦腰部两侧，1 上 1 下为 1 次，连做 108 次，使腰部有热感。每天摩擦腰部，具有行气活血、温经散寒、壮腰益肾等作用。

2. **揉按命门穴** 右手或左手握拳，以食指掌指关节突起部（拳尖）置于命门穴上，先顺时针方向压揉 9 次，再逆时针方向压揉 9 次，如此重复操做 36 次，意守命门穴。每天按揉此穴，具有温肾阳、强腰脊等作用。

3. **揉腰眼穴** 两手握拳，以食指掌指关节突起部放在两侧腰眼穴上，先顺时针方向压揉 9 次，再逆时针方向压揉 9 次，连做 36 次，意守腰眼穴。每天按揉此穴，具有活血通络、健腰益肾等作用。

4. **叩击腰骶** 两手四指握大拇指成拳，以拳背部有节奏地叩击腰部脊柱两侧到骶部，左右皆叩击 36 次。意守腰骶部，并意想腰骶部放松。每天叩击腰骶，具有活血通络、强筋健骨等作用。

四、腹 部 调 护

腹部是六腑所在部位，做好腹部的保健可加强消化系统、泌尿生殖系统的功能，防治肥胖、高血压和妇科疾病。

（一）腹部保暖

古代养生家很注意腹部的保暖。《老老恒言》说："腹为五脏之总，故腹本喜暖，老人下元虚弱，更宜加意暖之。"并主张对年老和体弱者进行"兜肚"或"肚束"保健。

1. **兜肚**　将艾叶捶软铺匀，盖上丝棉（或棉花），装入双层肚兜内，将兜系于腹部即可。

2. **肚束**　又称为"腰彩"。即为宽约七、八寸的布系于腰腹部。养生家曹慈山谓此法"前护腹，旁护腰，后护命门，取益良多"。此二法均可配以有温暖作用的药末装入其中，以加强温暖腹部的作用。

（二）腹部按摩

腹部按摩不仅起到局部治疗作用，而且对全身组织、器官功能起着调节的作用。临床实践证明，腹部按摩对冠心病、高血压、糖尿病、胃肠功能紊乱、小儿消化不良、月经不调、更年期综合征、痛经等有很好的治疗作用和辅助治疗作用，并能提高人体对疾病的抵抗力，防治风、寒、暑、湿、燥、火等外邪的侵袭。

揉腹保健养生法在我国已有几千年的历史，是一种比较适合于中老年人的自我保健方法。祖国医学指出，"脾胃为后天之本"，"六腑以通为养"，说明人体消化、吸收、排泄功能与人体健康有密切关系。揉腹可以充实五脏，通和六腑，驱外感之诸邪，清内生之百症。

揉腹不受时间及体位限制，一般以夜晚睡眠前仰卧位为佳。应该注意的是：揉腹前应排空小便；过饱时不宜马上进行；局部皮肤感染者，腹腔急性炎症者，腹部肿瘤者不宜揉腹。

自我按摩的具体做法是：先搓热双手，然后双手相重叠，置于腹部，用掌心绕脐沿逆时针方向由小到大转摩 36 圈，再逆时钟方向由大到小绕脐摩 36 圈，立、卧均可，饭后、临睡前均可进行。可健脾胃、助消化，并有安眠和防治胃肠疾病的作用。按摩手法要轻柔缓和适中，切忌马虎粗暴。整个操作需 10～15 分钟。患者饭前饭后 1 小时内和酒醉后不宜按摩治疗。

（乔　雪）

第六章

常见病证的中医调护

常见病证的中医调护属于中医临床护理范畴，主要内容涉及常见病证的基本概念、基本证型和护理措施。护理措施包含生活起居护理、给药护理、饮食护理和对症护理，重点强调中医调护方法的临床辨证应用。本章节重点介绍的常见症状包括感冒、不寐、胃痛、积滞、便秘、痛经等。

第一节 感　冒

感冒是因感受病邪，出现鼻塞、流涕、喷嚏、头痛、恶寒、发热及全身不适等为主要临床表现的一种外感病证。感冒一年四季均可发生，以冬春季为多见。在一个时期内广泛流行，症状相似者则称为"时行感冒"，多为疫疬之毒所致。

一、基 本 证 型

1. **风寒束表**　恶寒重，发热轻，无汗，头痛身疼，鼻塞流清涕，喷嚏，舌苔薄白，脉浮紧或浮缓。

2. **风热犯表**　发热，微恶风寒，头痛，鼻塞流黄涕，咽痛咽红，咳嗽，舌边尖红，舌苔薄黄，脉浮数。

3. **暑湿袭表**　见于夏季，头昏胀重，鼻塞流涕，发热或热势不扬，微恶风寒，无汗或少汗，胸闷泛恶，舌苔黄腻，脉濡数。

4. **气虚感冒**　发热恶寒，头身疼痛，咳嗽鼻塞，自汗出，倦怠无力，短气懒言，舌淡苔白，脉浮而无力。

5. **阴虚感冒**　身热微恶风寒，头痛无汗，头晕心烦，口渴咽干，手足心热，咳嗽少痰，舌红，脉细数。

二、护 理 措 施

1. 生活起居护理

（1）病室应安静、整洁，保持空气清新，阳光充足，定时开窗通风换气，做好空气消毒。开窗通风时，应给患者加衣被，避免因空气对流，复感风邪。风寒及气虚感冒者应注意防寒保暖，室温可稍高；风热及阴虚感冒者，室温可稍低，湿度应适中；暑湿感冒则应降低室内温度与湿度。

（2）感冒患者应保证充分的休息和睡眠，以尽快恢复体力，驱邪外出。病轻者要避免过重的体力劳动和剧烈的运动锻炼；病重、体虚者要卧床休息，以免增加机体消耗，降低抵抗力,加重病情。

(3)时行感冒患者应注意呼吸道隔离,室内空气要每日消毒1～2次,患者擦拭口鼻分泌物的用品不可随意丢弃,相关用具亦应每日消毒。

(4)根据气候变化随时增减衣被,以免复感外邪。

2.给药护理

(1)解表药多为辛散轻扬之品,有效成分易挥发,不宜久煎。

(2)发散风寒药应热服,稍加衣被;体实者服药后可饮适量热汤以取汗;体虚者服药后可饮热稀粥,益胃气、养津液,以助汗出。发散风热药宜温服。服药后以遍身微汗出为佳,不要汗出当风,再次受邪,避免过汗伤正。

3.饮食护理

(1)多喝水以补充津液、以助汗源。因脾胃运化功能降低,饮食应清淡、易消化,以稀饭、面条等半流质或软食为主,多食新鲜蔬菜及多汁水果。禁忌辛辣、肥腻、煎炸食物,戒酒烟。

(2)风寒感冒:饮食中佐用生姜等辛味发散之品,可助药力散寒祛邪。

(3)风热感冒:可用薄荷叶、菊花茶等以清凉解热。

(4)暑湿感冒:应避免过食生冷及甜品,可用鲜藿香、佩兰开水冲泡代茶饮。

(5)气虚感冒:宜选用温性食物,如鸡汤等。

(6)阴虚感冒:用银耳等凉性之品。

4.对症护理

(1)发热且有恶寒者,不采用凉敷或冰敷降温,避免腠理闭塞,汗不易出而留邪。高热而恶寒不明显者可用温水擦浴,亦可针刺退热。推拿护理风寒感冒取大椎、曲池、风池、合谷等穴,并可加灸;风热感冒穴选大椎、曲池、尺泽、可刺十宣放血;头身困重,可用拧挤疗法,施术部位取印堂、太阳、颈部等处。亦可配合刮痧,部位取夹脊两侧、背部胸肋处、肘窝、腘窝等。

(2)鼻塞不通可推按鼻的两侧至鼻根,指压或针刺迎香穴。

(3)头身疼痛可予按摩疗法:从印堂开始,向上沿前额发际推至头维、太阳,配合按印堂、鱼腰、太阳、百会等穴;沿膀胱经从头顶拿至风池、大椎两侧;然后按、揉大椎、曲池,配合拿肩井、合谷。连续拍击背部两侧膀胱经,以皮肤微红为度。

(4)拔罐法:适用于缓解头身痛。走罐在膀胱经,亦可留罐在大椎、肺腧等。

第二节 不 寐

不寐是经常不能获得正常睡眠的病证。轻者入睡困难或寐而不酣、时寐时醒、醒后难以再寐,重者彻夜不眠。

一、基本证型

1.心脾两虚 多梦易醒,心悸健忘,头晕目眩,肢倦神疲,面色不华,舌淡,苔薄,脉细弱。

2.阴虚火旺 心烦不寐,心悸健忘,五心烦热,腰膝酸软,头晕耳鸣,口干少津,舌红,苔少,脉细数。

3. **心虚胆怯**　夜寐多梦易惊，心悸胆怯，气短倦怠，舌淡，苔薄，脉弦细。

4. **痰热内扰**　不寐，头重目眩，心烦口苦，胸闷痰多，舌质红，苔黄腻，脉滑数。

5. **肝郁化火**　不寐多梦，烦躁易怒，目赤口苦，便秘尿黄，舌红，苔黄，脉弦数。

二、护 理 措 施

1. **生活起居护理**

（1）为患者提供有利于入睡的环境：保持卧室安静，避免嘈杂；卧具平整，舒适；室内遮光，室温冷暖适宜。

（2）指导患者作息规律，起居有节，建立良好的睡眠习惯。

（3）建议晚餐后睡觉前户外散步，放松心身。

2. **给药护理**　一般睡前约半小时服用安神药物。如果还需要服用治疗其他疾病的药物（如抗高血压药等）应该分开服用，不宜同时服用。如果同时服用其他镇静类药物主要观察不良反应如头晕、头痛等。

3. **情志护理**　通过语言疏导、情志引导等方式，解除情志不遂及各种精神刺激因素，避免过度思虑。对肝郁化火患者劝其保持心情舒畅，沟通中应态度和蔼，耐心倾听，细心解释，语言亲切。心虚胆怯患者，心理承受力差，胆怯易惊，害怕独自睡卧，在进行情志护理的同时建议其家人给以更加私密、安全的居住环境，或是给予更多帮助与照顾，以消除其胆怯心理。

4. **饮食护理**　晚餐的食量适度，不宜过饱或过饥；食物性质不宜过油腻，进食时间不宜距就寝时间过短。晚餐时或晚餐后不宜饮浓茶、烈酒、咖啡等饮料。建议睡前饮适量热牛奶。

5. **对症护理**

（1）按摩、推拿：常用的穴位有百会、内关、神门、三阴交、涌泉等。按摩的时间选择在睡前进行效果更佳，按摩手法适宜轻柔。

（2）睡觉前半小时温热水或草药水泡足或泡浴等。

（3）指导患者使用放松术，如缓慢地深呼吸，或听轻松的音乐，让心境宁静平和。

（4）使用植物芳透剂，如薰衣草精油、或是熏香等，芳香之气不仅可以愉悦心神，同时助于诱导入睡。

第三节　胃　　痛

胃痛又称胃脘痛，是指以上腹胃脘部近心窝处疼痛为主要表现的病证。寒邪、情志、饮食等因素是引起胃痛的常见原因。

一、基 本 证 型

1. **寒邪犯胃**　胃痛暴作，恶寒喜暖，脘腹得温则痛减，遇寒则痛增，口不渴，或渴喜热饮，苔薄白，脉弦紧。

2. **食滞肠胃**　胃痛，脘腹胀满，嗳腐吞酸，或吐不消化食物，吐食或矢气后痛减，或大便不爽，苔厚腻，脉滑或实。

3. **肝胃气滞**　胃脘胀闷，攻撑作痛，脘痛连胁，嗳气频繁，大便不畅，每因遇烦恼郁怒而痛作，苔薄白，脉弦。

4. **脾胃湿热**　胃脘灼热疼痛，泛酸嘈杂，心烦，口苦或粘，舌红，苔黄或腻，脉滑数。

5. **瘀阻胃络**　胃痛较剧，痛如针刺或刀割，痛有定处，拒按，或大便色黑，舌质紫暗，脉涩。

6. **胃阴亏虚**　胃痛隐作，灼热不适，嘈杂似饥，似饥而不欲食，口干，大便干燥，舌红少津，脉细数。

7. **脾胃虚寒**　胃痛隐隐，绵绵不休，空腹为甚，得食则缓，喜热喜按，泛吐清水，神倦乏力，手足不温，大便多溏，舌淡，脉沉细。

二、护 理 措 施

1. 生活起居护理

（1）根据气候变化及时调整着装，如冬季户外活动时或是夏季空调房间内，都应该注意避免胃脘部受凉，既往有胃病患者应特别注意春秋季节天气变化时局部的保暖。

（2）保持心情舒畅、情绪稳定，避免过度焦虑等情绪状态，主动缓解各种压力。

（3）既往患有胃病者，生活要规律，特别是规律三餐进食时间和进食量，避免暴饮暴食和饥饱无常。

（4）虚证患者宜多休息以培养正气，避免劳累，以免过度劳动而耗伤人体正气。实证患者痛时注意休息，痛减后适宜适当活动。

2. 给药护理　寒邪犯胃或脾胃虚寒者，中药汤剂宜热服，以驱寒止痛。虚证患者汤药宜少量频服，并强调宜饭后服药。

3. 饮食护理

（1）各种原因引起的胃痛，可以给予清淡、易消化的饮食，忌食酒类、油脂类、辛辣食物。虚证特别强调以细、软、少量多餐为宜。

（2）寒邪犯胃患者，可多食生姜、红糖等。忌食用生冷的食物。

（3）食滞肠胃患者应限制进食，病情缓解后，再进食为宜。

（4）肝胃气滞患者宜多食理气和胃解郁之品，如萝卜、柑橘等。

（5）胃热炽盛患者多食蔬菜和水果，如西瓜、苹果等。

（6）胃阴不足饮食宜细软多汁，少食多餐。可多进滋养胃阴之品，如牛奶、豆浆、西瓜、藕等，可多饮水或果汁。

（7）脾胃虚寒饮食宜细软、温热，易消化、营养丰富的半流食或软饭，少量多餐，如各种营养粥、面条等。

4. 对症护理

（1）寒证胃痛发作时，局部适宜温热护理，如热水袋温熨、拔火罐、艾灸等。拔罐可选胃俞、脾俞；艾灸可选中脘、足三里。

（2）实证胃痛者按摩常取穴中脘、内关、足三里，用泻法；虚证胃痛者按摩常取穴中脘、脾俞、胃俞、足三里，用补法；肝胃气滞者可加用肝俞、期门、太冲等穴。

第四节　便　　秘

便秘是以大便秘结不通、排便间隔时间延长或排便艰涩不畅为主要临床表现的病证。外感寒热、饮食情志所伤、阴阳气血不足是引起便秘的常见病因，大肠传导失司是其基本病机。

一、基 本 证 型

1. 实秘

（1）肠道实热：大便干结，腹部胀满，按之作痛，口干口臭，舌苔黄燥，脉滑数。

（2）肠道气滞：大便不畅，欲解不得，甚则少腹作胀，嗳气频作，苔薄，脉弦。

2. 虚秘

（1）脾虚气弱：粪质并不干硬，虽有便意，但临厕无力努挣，挣则汗出气短，面色苍白，神疲，舌淡，苔薄白，脉弱。

（2）阴虚肠燥：大便干结，状如羊屎，神疲纳呆，腰膝酸软，口干少津，舌红少苔，苔少，脉细数。

（3）脾肾阳虚：大便秘结，甚则少腹冷痛，面色萎黄无华，时作眩晕，心悸，小便清长，畏寒肢冷，舌质淡，苔白润，脉沉迟。

二、护 理 措 施

1. 生活起居护理

（1）培养健康的生活方式，生活起居有规律，劳逸适度，每天坚持适量的运动。

（2）养成定时排便的习惯，保证定时如厕，时间充足，心情放松，环境私密，精神集中。

（3）年老体弱排便无力者平时加强腹肌的锻炼，提高排便时的辅助力量。

2. 给药护理

（1）实证患者遵医嘱服用中药或外用通便药物，便通即止。不宜长期使用，更不能滥用泻药，造成对泻药的依赖，导致便秘加重。

（2）脾虚气弱患者排便无力，平时可服用白术、山药，以增补气力；阴虚肠燥患者，适当增加服药次数，频频饮服持续缓慢给药，达到润肠通便的目的。

3. 饮食护理

（1）进食要规律，保证相应的进食量，不宜进食过少；平日宜多饮清水、蜂蜜水或果汁等。

（2）食物搭配要合理，多食富含纤维素食物如蔬菜、水果、全麦面包等。

4. 对症护理

（1）实证便秘者取穴天枢、曲池、太冲等，针刺疗法通便。

（2）虚证便秘者取穴天枢、上巨虚、大肠俞、足三里、八髎穴等，针刺疗法通便。并可按顺时针方向行腹部按摩以调畅气机，健脾助运。

第五节 积 滞

小儿积滞是指以不思饮食，食而不化，腹部胀满，大便不调为主要表现的一种疾病。多由内伤乳食，停聚不化，气滞不行所形成。

一、基 本 证 型

1. 乳食内积　食欲缺乏，或呕吐酸馊乳食，烦躁多啼，夜卧不安，小便短黄或如米泔，大便溏薄，舌红，苔腻，脉滑数，指纹紫红。

2. 脾虚夹积　面色萎黄，困倦无力，夜寐不安，不思饮食，腹满喜按，呕吐酸馊乳食，大便溏泄,舌淡,苔白,脉细。

二、护 理 措 施

1. 生活起居护理 居室宜卫生清洁、阳光充足、空气新鲜、温度适宜;按时作息,保证小儿充足的睡眠和适度户外活动;建立良好的进食环境,安静、快乐。

2. 饮食护理

(1)合理喂养,乳食宜定时定量,富含营养,易于消化,忌食肥甘炙煿、生冷瓜果等。

(2)根据小儿生长发育需求,调节饮食,逐渐添加辅食,避免小儿偏食、挑食,保证营养的均衡。

3. 对症护理 清胃经:揉板门,运内八卦,推四横纹,揉按中脘、足三里,推下七节骨,用于乳食内积证;补脾经:运内八卦,摩中脘,清补大肠,揉按足三里,用于脾虚夹积证。以上各证均可配合使用捏脊法。腹胀者,可按摩腹部。

第六节 痹 证

痹证是指以肌肉、筋骨、肢体关节疼痛、酸楚、麻木、重着、屈伸不利,甚或关节肿大灼热等为主要临床表现的病证。本病多因正气不足,卫外不固,感受风、寒、湿、热之邪,使气血运行不畅,经络痹阻所致。

一、基 本 证 型

1. 风寒湿痹

(1)行痹(风痹):肢体关节、肌肉酸痛,游走不定,多见于上肢、肩背。关节屈伸不利,或见恶风寒,苔薄白,脉浮。

(2)痛痹(寒痹):肢体关节疼痛较剧,痛有定处,得热痛减,遇寒痛增,关节不可屈伸,局部皮肤不红,触之不热,苔薄白,脉弦紧。

(3)着痹(湿痹):肢体关节重着、肿胀、酸痛或有肿胀,痛有定处,活动不便,苔白腻,脉濡缓。

2. 风湿热痹 关节红肿热痛,得冷则舒,得热则甚,痛不可近,关节活动不便,多兼有发热、恶风、汗出、口渴、烦闷,舌红苔黄燥,脉滑数。

3. 痰瘀痹阻 痹证日久,关节肿大,甚至强直畸形,屈伸不利,舌质紫暗,苔白腻,脉细涩。

4. 久痹正虚 骨节疼痛,时轻时重,腰膝软痛,形瘦无力,舌质淡,脉沉细无力。

二、护 理 措 施

1. 生活起居护理

(1)居室应避免潮湿,不要冒雨涉水,也不要汗出当风,应注意清洁卫生、居室通风、防潮防寒、燥湿调和、冷暖相济。

(2)增强体质,防止重感外邪,尤其要注意保温、防寒、避湿。

(3)对关节疼痛严重者建议其减少剧烈运动,适当休息以减轻不适。

2. 情志护理 此病证常反复发作且病程较长,患病初期由于关节疼痛和全身不适,易情绪低沉，这时要鼓励患者树立战胜病证的信心，积极配合各种治疗。病证后期常会出现关节变形、肌肉萎缩等后遗症，造成生活能力下降，患者容易产生悲观情绪，对生活失去信心，或是产生依赖他人照顾的思想，这时应鼓励患者尽量活动，消除由此而产生的不良情绪，增强生活自理能力。

3. 对症护理

（1）局部痛重者，可采用按摩、针灸或遵医嘱应用止痛药以缓解疼痛。针灸止痛：上肢取肩髃、曲池、尺泽、合谷、外关等穴，下肢取环跳、足三里、阳陵泉等穴。亦可局部按摩5～10分钟。

（2）痛痹可采用艾灸或隔姜灸；以温通经络，有较好的止痛效果。着痹配合按摩、梅花针等疗法，可以预防和治疗肌肉萎缩、关节畸形、缓解症状。

（3）痹证尤其是风寒湿痹，建议使用外用药物热敷、药熨、熏洗，或是药酒外涂，以温经通络，促进血液运行畅通，而达到消肿止痛的目的。在使用外用药熏洗时要注意药液的温度。

第七节 痛 经

妇女经期或经行前后，出现周期性小腹疼痛，或痛引腰骶，甚至剧痛难忍，影响生活和工作者，称为痛经，亦称经行腹痛。

一、基 本 证 型

1. 气滞血瘀 每于经前1～2天或月经期小腹胀痛或阵痛，拒按，可伴有胸胁乳房胀痛，经量少而经行不畅，经色紫黯有块，血块排出后痛减，经净疼痛消失，舌紫黯或有瘀点，脉弦或弦涩。

2. 寒湿凝滞 经前数日或经期小腹冷痛或绞痛，得热痛减，按之痛甚，经量少，经色黯黑有块，畏寒肢冷，面色青白，舌暗苔白腻，脉沉紧。

3. 气血虚弱 经后1～2天或经期小腹隐隐作痛，或小腹及阴部空坠，喜揉按，月经量少，色淡质薄，腰膝酸软，神疲乏力，面色不华，纳少便溏，头晕心悸，舌淡，边有齿痕，苔薄，脉细弱。

4. 湿热下注 经前或经期小腹疼痛拒按，有灼热感，或伴腰骶疼痛，平时小腹时痛，经来疼痛加剧。低热起伏，经色黯红，质稠有块，带下黄稠，小便短黄，舌红，苔黄腻，脉弦数或濡数。

5. 肝肾亏损 经期或经后，小腹隐痛喜按，月经量少，色淡质稀，头晕耳鸣，腰膝酸软，舌淡苔薄，脉沉细。

二、护 理 措 施

1. 生活起居护理

（1）保持环境整洁、舒适、安静，保持愉快心情，消除紧张、恐惧心理，避免不良情绪刺激；腹痛剧烈时应卧床休息，注意腹部保暖，可作腹部热敷。

（2）注意经期卫生，月经前后及经期不宜游泳、避免淋雨、涉水，禁止性交、盆浴。经期亦不宜参加剧烈运动或重体力劳动。

2. 饮食护理

（1）经前经期及经期饮食护理：经期或经前期应忌食生冷、酸醋等寒凉食物；寒湿凝滞患者，经期可适当服用红糖、大枣等。

（2）平时饮食护理：总体原则宜营养、清淡、均衡，避免饮食偏嗜，过寒过热。气血瘀滞患者，宜服红花每日口服少许。寒湿凝滞患者，平素应忌食生冷；湿热患者，平时不得过食辛辣或饮酒过度。气血亏虚患者多进食蛋、肉、乳制品和新鲜蔬菜；可常服生姜羊肉汤。肝肾亏损患者，注意多进黑芝麻、核桃等。

3. 对症护理

（1）针灸止痛：体针穴选中极、三阴交、气海、内关等，用泻法，宜针灸并用；寒湿凝滞患者：艾灸气海、关元等穴，以达到温阳祛寒、流通血脉，缓解疼痛的目的；耳针止痛取穴子宫、神门、内分泌、肝、肾，于经前3～5天作预防措施。

（2）贴敷或热熨止痛：用麝香痛经膏外帖上述穴位，痛经发作时帖敷，1～3天更换1次，痛经消失后除去；腹部热敷：食盐250～500g、葱白250g、生姜200g（切碎），烘热后入布袋中，热敷小腹，注意避免烫伤。

（3）按摩小腹缓解疼痛：具体方法是经前3天起，每晚用双手重叠，掌心向下压于小腹正中，做逆时针旋转按摩10分钟，同时从小腹至脐部推摩30～50次。

第八节 缺 乳

缺乳是指产后哺婴时乳汁甚少，甚至乳汁全无为主要临床表现的一类疾病，亦称"乳汁不行"，多发生在产后2～3个月至半年内。

一、基 本 证 型

1. 气血亏虚 产后乳少，甚或全无，乳汁清稀，乳房柔软，无胀满感，神疲食少，面色无华，舌淡苔少，脉细弱。

2. 肝郁气滞 产后情志不畅，乳汁涩少，浓稠，或乳汁不下，乳房胀硬疼痛，胸胁胀闷，食欲缺乏，或身有微热，舌正常，苔薄黄，脉弦细或弦数。

二、护 理 措 施

1. 生活起居护理

（1）创造温馨、舒适的环境。产后避免吹风受凉（如夏季空调）。产妇进行母乳哺喂时选择舒适体位，避免由于姿势不适产生疲劳。

（2）产妇注意休息，保证充足睡眠，每日不少于10小时，勿过度疲劳以免影响乳汁分泌。注意睡眠姿势，乳房胀痛时勿受压。

（3）适当活动，如做产后体操，有助气血通畅、调节情绪和机体复原。

2. 饮食护理 饮食富于营养，清淡，易消化，补充足量的水分，鼓励产妇服用富有营养的汤汁饮食以开乳源。忌酸涩、油腻、刺激性食物。

3. 情志护理 调畅情志，给予关怀、疏导，消除患者忧郁、恼怒等不良情绪。鼓励产妇不论乳汁多少都积极进行母乳喂养；进行母乳哺喂时保持良好的情绪状态，最好达到心情愉悦、放松、快乐的状态。

4. 对症护理

（1）嘱产妇及早哺乳，即使出现缺乳也应定时哺乳，若婴儿吸吮能力差，可用吸奶器或他人吸吮。

（2）哺乳前用温毛巾擦拭乳头、乳房。教会产妇自行按摩乳房的方法，如自乳房边缘向乳头方向按摩，也可用热毛巾热敷，以促进乳汁分泌。

（3）乳汁壅滞不出者，可采取局部按摩或挤压排乳的方法：推拿按摩取乳根、膻中、期门、肝俞、少泽等穴，患者多取仰卧位，单掌和多指摩擦胸腹数分钟；或用清洁的木梳顺乳腺管向乳头方向轻轻梳通，每天 2～3 次，每次 20 分钟，定时排空乳房，以免乳积化热，转变成乳痈；也可以用针刺通乳，取穴膻中、乳根，配少泽、天宗、合谷等，用补法，留针 20 分钟。

（王　琦）

1 Introduction of Traditional Chinese Medicine and Nursing Science of TCM

1.1 Traditional Chinese Medicine and Traditional Chinese Culture

Traditional Chinese Medicine (TCM) is such a broad and profound system that involves many disciplines. In *Lei Jing* (The Classified Classic) written by Zhang Jie-bin (1563-1640AD) in Ming Dynasty (1368-1644AD), it states that "Upward to the sky, astronomy has been discussed; downward to the earth, geography is involved; in the middle, personnel is being researched; in major aspects, changes of yin-yang are discussed, while in specific aspects, as small as insects, vegetation, music, rhythm, origins of *Xiang Shu* (image- numerology), as well as the ins and outs of the organs and channels are all in detailed statement." The all-encompassing TCM can be described as a microcosm of Traditional Chinese Culture (TCC). The unique TCM theory system was formed based on TCC. The elements of TCC contained in the theory of TCM also reflect the dominant thinking mode of TCM directly. TCM's contribution to the world is not only an original medical system but also an important part of TCC.

The contents of TCC are profound, including ancient Chinese philosophy, medicine theory, astronomy, geography, myths and legends, historical events, music, arts, customs, habits, etc. While the philosophy represented by Yin-Yang and the five phases, life cultivation that bases on Taoism and Taoist theory, *Yi* theory as the banner of astronomy and geography, the medical morals on the Confucianism and other theories that mix with all kinds of traditional theories, constitute the foundation of TCM theory and its cultural background. Only after getting familiar with TCC, you may comprehend TCM better, such as its historic process, philosophic system, thinking mode, value concept, etc. On the basis of well comprehension in the cultural connotation of TCM, you may use TCM techniques skillfully.

1.1.1 A Brief History of the Cultural Origin and Development of TCM

TCM plays an indelible historical role on healthcare, reproduction and prosperity in the five-thousand civilization of China. So far, there is no definitive conclusion about the origin of medicine. Generally, origin of medicine may involve instinctive medical behavior, theory, human labor, brain structure evolution, witchcraft, the sage, etc. Regarding to the basic view from current academia, "TCM originates from the sage", and "TCM originates from witchcraft" are two main viewpoints of the origin of TCM.

1.1.1.1   TCM Originates from the Sage

Our ancestors believed that medicine originates from the myth of the ancient times. According to the legend, Fu Xi, Shen Nong and Huang Di are considered as the pioneer of Chinese culture and medicine.

1.1.1.1.1   Fu Xi-Ancestor of the Chinese Humanities

It is recorded in *Di Wang Shi Ji* (*Age of Emperors*), Fu Xi created the ancient culture of the Chinese. In accordance with the changes of yin and yang in nature, he created the Eight Trigrams, that is, using eight symbols which are simple but having profound connotations to summarize and describe things in nature. It is said that Fu Xi also created Chinese medicine, made significant contribution in the prosperity and development of Chinese nation, thus Fu Xi is considered as the humanity ancestor of the Chinese.

----- Supplementary reading 1-1 --

Fu Xi's Eight Diagrams

In the legend, it is said that Fu Xi' appearance is human head with the snake body. By his sensitive sights, he observed the social facts and life acutely and held deep affections for the land. Owing to his super intelligence, Fu Xi recorded all his observations with mathematical symbols, which are the Eight Diagrams. In the ancient times, the diagram of dragon and horse originates from Tu-river, located in the east of Meng Jin meets the Yellow river. According to this diagram, Fu Xi draw out of the Eight Diagrams consisting of qián、duì、lí、zhèn、xùn、kǎn、gèn、kūn, known as "Fu Xi's Eight Diagrams". (Please see Figure 1-1)

Fu Xi observed things in the universe and applied yin-yang and the Eight Diagrams to explain the evolution of universe and humanity. By making fire, letting people get married, teaching people fishing and hunting, the history of primitive barbarism was ended.

1.1.1.1.2   Shen Nong-As a Founder of Agriculture, Courtesy and Music, Medicine

Shen Nong is the ancient emperor, whose tribe living in the south. Corresponding to the five-phase theory, south is fire, so Shen Nong is also called as Yan Emperor. Shen Nong represents the development of knowledge and the beginning of using nature source. Shen Nong is considered as the overlord of the world after Fu Xi and Nv Wa, who developed agriculture, courtesy and music, as well as medicine. As it is said in *Tong Wai Ji*, "people got sick and didn't know medicine. Yan Emperor tasted the vegetation and was poisoned 70 times a day. Then medical books were written to cure the patients, thus medicine started."

----- Supplementary reading 1-2 --

A Well Known Legend of Shen Nong

The most widely spread story about Shen Nong is "Shen Nong tasted hundreds of herbs". In the myths and legends, Shen Nong is described as head like the tau and human body, born with a transparent "crystal belly". Therefore, his organs were visible, and what he ate can be seen from the outside clearly. In ancient times, people didn't know farming, but feeding with wild fruits or raw animals, often got poisoned and cause death. In order to treat diseases and save lives, Yan Emperor, Shen Nong traveled all over the earth, tasted hundreds of plants to find the Medicinal properties. "Shen Nong was poisoned 70 times in a day while tasting various plants to find the edible herbs". In the process of tasting plants, Shen Nong found the herbs that can cure disease and have the function of health preservation. Thus, he is honored as "saint of herbs" by ancient people. (Please see Figure 1-2)

1.1.1.1.3 Huang Di (Yellow Emperor) -the Founder of Medicine

Huang Di is said as the overlord of the ancient China, in the first of the five emperors, whose last name is Gong Sun, born in the hill of Xuan Yuan. According to the historical records, Huang Di unified the tribes in China after Yan Emperor.

Huang Di is considered as the creator of Chinese culture, such as weapons, boats, arithmetic, rhythm, character, sericulture, bows and arrows, clothing, medicine, etc. It is said that the classics of TCM, such as *Huang Di Nei Jing* (*The Yellow Emperor's Inner Classic*) and *Huang Di Ba Shi Yi Nan Jing* (*The Yellow Emperor's Classic of Eighty-one Difficult Issues*), were written in Huang Di's name. In the legend, Huang Di and his minister Qi Bo, Bo Gao and Shao Yu talked about medical knowledge, thus, TCM is commonly known as "the art of Qi Huang" and Huang Di is respected as the founder of medicine as well. The saying "Shen Nong founds medical experience, while Huang Di creates medical theory" indicates that in Huang Di's age medicine began to transformed from empirical medicine to systemic rational medicine. (*Please see Figure 1-3*)

1.1.1.2 TCM Originates from Witchcraft

1.1.1.2.1 Witchcraft Culture

As one of the earliest forms of human culture, witchcraft culture has a long history and plays an important role in the history of human culture. Some scholars believed that witchcraft is the mother of institution, religion and science. It is considered as a versatile encyclopedia.

Early human beings knew little about the nature and regarded the nature with awe and wonder. Disease and death were completely beyond their understanding. At the same time, under great fears they imagined that the world was ruled by a supernatural force, hence, the concepts of "ghosts" and "god" came out. These concepts are the basis of the witchcraft.

Witchcraft reflects the desire of human to overcome the nature. The process of understanding the unknown things is from fear to worship and then trying to overcome the unknown. These phases may overlap and crisscross, but it is in line with the evolutionary process of human thinking and parallel to the progress of production, science and technology at that time.

1.1.1.2.2 *Zhu You* and TCM

In the thousands of years of TCM history, witchcraft has always existed. The most typical example is *Zhu You*. In medical literature from Han (206BC-220AD) to Ming (1368-1644AD) Dynasty, *Zhu You* is recorded as a medical practice together with other treatments.

Certain elements in *Zhu You* do have a scientific value if we analyze its content carefully. As a matter of fact, *Zhu You* is the forerunner of psychotherapy (suggestive therapy), *qigong* therapy and traditional Chinese sports therapy. Using today's theory to explain *Zhu You*, it is a technique that the practitioner achieves therapeutic results by using language or behavior to induce the patient into a certain psychological state. Because people believed that evil spirits were responsible for illness, *Zhu You* practitioners tried to induce their patients into believing they could overcome their fears with the guidance of *Zhu You* practitioners and drive the evil spirits out. Psychotherapy is dependent on the patients' subjective state of mind. Because the patient would show fear and awe towards those evil spirits, the practitioner would use that frame of mind and improve the patient's physiological status. *Qigong* therapy has the effects of regulating breathing, massaging internal organs and harmonizing qi and blood. The breathing mode in *qigong* therapy can also be traced back to *Zhu You*: one of the oldest breathing modes in *qigong* is expressed in six words (*chui*, *hu*, *he*, *xu*, *xi*, and *si*), which are originated from *Zhu You*. The unique traditional Chinese sports therapies such as *Dao Yin* and martial art are inherited by the movements of *Zhu You*. "Yu's Gait" is mentioned many times in documents on *Zhu You* unearthed from *Ma Wang Dui* (Han Tombs), which according to legend is how Da Yu (a legendary Chinese emperor who tamed the flood in ancient antiquity) would walk. It is a rhythmic way of walking and is similar to the steps in Waltz. This waking and dancing are in fact a form of physical exercise and have the effects of dredging channels and collaterals so as to relieve pain. Therefore, sports therapy is a component of *Zhu You*.

With the development of science medicine and witchcraft began to separate. Especially in the Spring and Autumn Period (770-476AD), under academic booming, the status of religious is no longer so sacred as pervious. People began to realize that medicine is more scientific, more practical, and more evidence-based comparing with witchcraft, so medicine finally replaced witchcraft and dominated in healthcare.

1.1.1.3   The Formation and Development of TCM Theoretical System

Although ancient people believed that medicine originates from ancient myth, which is actually comes from medical practice of our ancestors. The theoretical system of TCM originates from practice. TCM is a science based on long-term clinical practice.

1.1.1.3.1   A Brief History of the Development of TCM Theory

In ancient times, our ancestors had already found ways to relieve pain in tough environment. They found that certain food could relieve or cure certain illness, by hot sand and stone compressing the body or sharp stone puncturing the body can also relieve pain. With accumulation of these experiences, the earliest Chinese medicine appeared.

TCM is established on the basis of clinical experiences; meanwhile it was also influenced by the culture at that time and developed with the gradually gained experiences. After entering civilized society, especially in the spring autumn warring period, Chinese medicine began transformed into rational systemic medicine from empirical medicine.

In spring and autumn period (770-221BC), *Huang Di Nei Jing* (*The Yellow Emperor's Inner Classic*) represents the initial formation of TCM theoretical system. After four-hundred years practice, in Han Dynasty (201BC-220AD), *Shang Han Za Bing Lun* (*Treatise on Cold Damage and Miscellaneous Diseases*) written by Zhang Zhong-jing (150-219AD) refers as the saint of medicine established the basic principle of pattern differentiation. *Shen Nong Ben Cao Jing* (*Shen Nong's Classic of the Materia Medica*) lays the foundation of Pharmacy. During the seven hundred years from Jin Dynasty (265-420AD) to Five Dynasties and Ten Kingdoms, TCM theory system developed constantly. For example, the earliest extant acupuncture book, *Zhen Jiu Jia Yi Jing* (*The Systematic Classic of Acupuncture and Moxibustion*) was written by Huang Fu-mi (215-282AD) in West Jin Dynasty (265-316AD), while *Zhu Bing Yuan Hou Lun* (*Treatise on the Origins and Manifestations of Various Diseases*) is the earliest extant monograph on etiology and syndrome, written by Chao Yuan-fang (550-630AD). Sun Si-miao (581-682AD), the famous physician in Tang dynasty (618-907AD), devoted his lifetime to write the book *Bei Ji Qian Jin Yao Fang* (*Important Formulas Worth a Thousand Gold Pieces for Emergency*) and *Qian Jin Yi Fang* (*Supplement to Important Formulas Worth a Thousand Gold Pieces*), which give detailed accounts in clinical subjects, acupuncture, diet therapy, preventive medicine, and healthcare. In Song Dynasty (960-1279AD), the acupuncture bronze statue designed by Wang Wei-yi (987-1067AD) is one of the greatest innovations in the history of Chinese medicine education. During Jin (1115-1234AD) and Yuan era (1271-1368AD), the four famous physicians, Liu Wan-su (1110-1200AD), Zhang Cong-zheng (1156-1228AD), Li Dong-yuan (1180-1251AD) and Zhu Zhen-heng (1281-1358) leaded the academic contention. Through long time practices from Ming (1368-1644AD) to Qing (1616-1911AD) dynasty, Li Shi-zhen (1518-1593AD), a famous pharmacist in Ming dynasty, spent 27 years to write the book *Ben Cao Gang Mu* (*The Grand Compendium of Materia Medica*). In Qing Dynasty, the four famous books, *Wen Re Lun* (*Treatise on Warm-Heat Diseases*) dictated by Ye Gui (1667-1746AD), *Shi Re Tiao Bian* (*Systematic Differentiation of Damp-Heat Disorders*) by Xu Xue (1661-1750AD); *Wen Re Tiao Bian* (*Systematic Differentiation of Warm Diseases*) by Wu Tang (1758-1836AD), and *Wen Re Jing Wei* (*Warp and Woof of Warm-Heat Diseases*) by Wang Shi-xiong (1808-1868AD) signifies the rise of Febrile Disease theory. *Yi Lin Gai Cuo* (*Correction of Errors in Medical Works*) wrote by Wang Qing-ren (1768-1831AD), indicates the development of the blood stasis pathogenesis theory. The achievements in each clinical subject devotes to the development of Chinese medicine theory.

Among these monographs, *Huang Di Nei Jing* (*The Yellow Emperor's Inner Classic*) and *Shang Han Za Bing Lun* (*Treatise on Cold Damage and Miscellaneous Diseases*) have great impact on the formation and development of TCM systemic theory. *Huang Di Nei Jing* (*The Yellow Emperor's Inner Classic*) has provided guidance for TCM practice ever since its publication. It includes two parts, *Su Wen* (*Basic Questions*) and *Ling Shu* (*The Spiritual Pivot*). The essence of *Huang Di Nei Jing* (*The Yellow Emperor's Inner Classic*) lies in its theoretical framework including the holistic view of "heaven-man harmony", its logic tools of yin-yang and the five phases, and its core theories of *zang-fu* and channels. Thus a highly abstract, applicable and extremely powerful framework is established, which can be adapted to explain almost everything in the universe. The greatest achievement of *Huang Di Nei Jing* (*The Yellow Emperor's Inner Classic*) is its introduction of philosophy into empirical medicine. Without these philosophical concepts, the knowledge accumulated from experience would have been a pile of fragmented raw materials. It signifies that the ancient medical system in China had developed to the rational system medicine from empirical medicine.

Shang Han Za Bing Lun (*Treatise on Cold Damage and Miscellaneous Diseases*) was written by Zhang Zhong-jing in Eastern Han Dynasty (202 BC-9AD), an era of frequent wars and epidemics. There were over 10 widely spread epidemics in middle China and bodies were found everywhere on vast area of land. In less than 10 years, two thirds of Zhang Zhong-jing's family, with a total of 200 members, died of infectious diseases. Saddened and spurred by these events, Zhang Zhong-jing devoted himself to study medicine and published *Shang Han Za Bing Lun* (*Treatise on Cold Damage and Miscellaneous Diseases*), one of the greatest classics in the history of TCM. In this great book, vital link between TCM clinical practice and its theoretical framework in H*uang Di Nei Jing* (*The Yellow Emperor's Inner Classic*) are established. Under the umbrella of *Shang Han Za Bing Lun* (*Treatise on Cold Damage and Miscellaneous Diseases*), Zhang made different aspects of medicine into a coherent system of knowledge, from basic theories to treatment principles, and from prescriptions to material medics. In this book, the four diagnostic methods, the eight-principle pattern differentiation, causes of disease, treatments, prescribing medicines, acupuncture and external treatments all become one of branch under the TCM system of pattern differentiation and treatment. This great work signifies that a complete TCM theory system had been established, which has profound influence on future generations of practitioners and is the second landmark of TCM history since *Huang Di Nei Jing* (*The Yellow Emperor's Inner Classic*).

1.1.1.3.2 Achievements and Influence of TCM in History

There are many outstanding physicians and remarkable achievements in the history of TCM. For instance, Bian Que (407-310BC), a famous physician in the Spring-Autumn and Warring States era (770-221BC), used *Bian*-stone (a sharpened stone, the earliest form of needle), acupuncture, massage, herbs, hot compressing and other methods, achieved satisfactory effect in treating internal and external diseases, and diseases of women and children, as well as ear, nose and throat disorders.

During the Eastern Jin dynasty (316-420AD), Chinese physicians discussed several infectious diseases, such as smallpox, cholera, etc. For example, Ge Hong (284-364 or 343AD) describes the mites' lifestyle, transmission route, clinical characteristics, preventive measures and prognosis in great detail, which is 1600 years earlier than the similar studies abroad.

Variolation appeared in Ming dynasty (1368-1644AD) and effectively controlled the epidemic of smallpox, which is the pioneer of Modern Immunology.

----- Supplementary reading 1-3 ---

President Nixon's Visit to China Lead "Acupuncture Favor" in American

In some developed countries, it is popular to study, research and apply Chinese medicine, known as "Chinese medicine favor". In the 1970s, president Nixon visited China, Premier Zhou En-lai accompanied Nixon to observe thyroid ablation operation under acupuncture anesthesia. More than 30 members of Nixon's China-visiting group observed the whole process of the "right-superior pulmonary leucotomy" under acupuncture anesthesia. This operation was performed by Prof. Xin Yu-ling in the third affiliated hospital of Peking medical university. After returning home, American media publicized the mysterious acupuncture anesthesia, in succession arising American people's great interest in acupuncture again, the small needles of acupuncture shocked American and the world. Western scholars came to China to study and research TCM as finding a new continent to explore the treasure of TCM.

----- Supplementary reading 1-4 --

Cataract Extraction With a Metal Needle

In the treatment of cataract, metal needle is used rather early in the ophthalmological department of Chinese medicine. In the book Wai Tai Mi Yao (Arcane Essentials from the Imperial Library) written by Wang Tao (670-755AD) in Tang Dynasty (618-907AD), the treatment of cataract with "Jinbi" (made from metal, similar to surgical knife) is described in great details. Afterwards, this therapy gained great development under clinical practice and efforts of many ophthalmologists' in Chinese successive generations.

After 1950s, ophthalmologists of Chinese medicine conducted abundant clinical studies on cataract abaissement and successfully performed this operation for many cataract patients. Some domestic and important foreigners suffering from this disease accepted this therapy and recovered their sight. In 1972, premier Penm Nouth, the former Kampuchean prime minister accepted a successful abaissement performed by Tang You-zhi, a famous Chinese ophthalmologist, in Beijing 301 hospital and was cured. In August in 1975, a medical group with Prof. Tang being the lead adopted this therapy once again to treat chairman Mao Ze-dong's cataract and gained a great success.

1.1.2 TCM and the Ancient Chinese Philosophy

Philosophy plays an extremely important role in the ideology system of TCM culture. The relationship between TCM and the ancient philosophy is primarily manifested in original qi theory that explores the origin of the universe, yin-yang theory that observes the nature of life, and five-phase theory that explores the structure of life and the relationship.

In the process of formation and development of TCM, the philosophy thought had been melted into TCM, combined with the abundant medical knowledge and clinic experience, formed the unique TCM theory system and guided the clinical practice over a long period of time. Such as yin-yang, the five phases, qi, etc. gradually become a logic tool of TCM to explain medical problems. While on the other hand, philosophy is based on the specific subjects, and the TCM in turn enriches and develops the ancient philosophy in the process of setting questions with related philosophy of the human life activities, such as the action of qi, the relation between body and mind, the relations of man and the universe, and the theory of yin-yang and the five phases. For example, the interrelationships of the generation, restriction, subjugation and reverse restriction of five phases has been fully discussed in ancient literature of TCM.

1.1.2.1 Yuan Qi theory and the Holistic View of "Harmony Between Human and Nature"

1.1.2.1.1 The Origin of *Yuan* Qi (Original Qi)

Yuan qi (original qi) is an ancient Chinese philosophical concept, which refers to the generation and composition of the raw material universe. The explanation of *"yuan"* in *Shuo Wen Jie Zi* (*Elucidations of Script and Explications of Characters*) is the same as *"yuan"*, refers to the primitive elements of everything in the universe. The concept of qi is originated from "the theory of cloud qi" (cloud qi can be understood as "air"), as it is recorded in *Shuo Wen Jie Zi* (*Elucidations of Script and Explications of Characters*) "Qi refers to cloud qi". Cloud qi is the original meaning of qi. Our ancestor's understanding of qi had developed from the natural qi and breathing qi to the essential substance constituting everything in the universe. They believed that all formed substances are transformed from the non-substantial qi. The movement and changes of qi are the internal forces of the progressions and changes of all things in nature. This thought originates around the Prior Chin Dynasty (21st century BC-221BC), and has been developed during the War States Period (475-221 BC), Chin (221-207BC) and Han Dynasty (202BC-220AD). After being continuously supplemented by later ages from Jin Dynasty (265-420AD), this thought develops into a philosophical theory that has great influence on TCC and ancient technology.

1.1.2.1.2 The Connotations of Original Qi

(1) Qi is the Original Source of Everything in Nature

The basic views of original qi theory holds that qi is the original source constituting everything in the universe, as well as the source of spirit. *Su Wen* (*Basic Questions*) states that "when qi starts, things begin to transform and produce; when qi moves, things begin to grow; when qi spreads, things begin to reproduce; and when qi expires, things begin to die." Because of the existence of qi, its movement and changes, the heaven and earth could come forth, and everything in the world could be generated. So the heaven, earth, and everything in the world and together with human beings are all generated from qi. In ancient Chinese philosophy, the universe is known as *"tian di"*, *"tian xia"*, *"tai xu"*, *"huan yu"*, *"qian kun"*, *"yu kong"*, etc. The universe was called *"tai xu"* in *Huang Di Nei Jing* (*The Yellow Emperor's Inner Classic*) and holds the view that the vast universe was full of infinite original qi with capacity of generating and transforming.

(2) Qi is a Substance that is in Constant Movement and Changes

Qi is the essential substance with constant movement. The process of movement and change of qi is the course of development and transformation of things. qi can be divided into two categories: "Substantial" and "Non-Substantial". Substantial qi denotes the coagulative status of qi, which refers to the visible substance with all kinds of shapes and structures. Non-substantial qi refers to the essential substance with constant movement and changes distributed extensively in the nature. Although it is invisible, it could be recognized and mastered by observing the development and changes of substantial things. Substantial qi and non-substantial qi are in the process of inter-transforming all the time. Thus the constant movement and change of substantial qi and non-substantial qi result in the growing and transforming of everything in nature, as well as birth and perishing of life. Due to the movement of qi, there are various phenomena in nature.

Yuan qi (Original qi) theory views that the process of development and change of things as the course of "qi *hua*" (qi transformation). All kinds of changes in different aspects such as the shape, function and manifestation of everything in nature are resulted from qi *hua* (qi transformation). As the old saying "the activity of qi produces substance" and "substance could be transformed into qi" denote the inter-transforming process of substantial and non-substantial qi. The inter-transforming among substantial things, qi and the internal development and changes of the substantial things are all in the process and result of qi transformation. The inter-transformation of the healthy and morbid status of human beings is also the process and result of qi transformation. Therefore, qi transformation is considered as the internal mechanism of the development and changes of everything in nature.

(3) Qi is the Inter-media of the Heaven, Earth and Everything in Nature

Qi is not only the basic substance constituting everything in nature, but also the medium of the interaction and interrelationship of things in nature. Due to the existence and function of this medium, everything in nature could be integrated into a whole. It integrates the whole universe by the non-substantial qi (original qi) permeating in the space between the heaven and earth, including the relationship between human beings and nature. Meanwhile, the non-substantial qi disperses in the interior of thing, resulting in the universal inter-relationship and inter-sensitiveness among things. This function of qi forms the channel and medium for the universal relationship and mutual influence and transformation among things.

1.1.2.1.3   The Impact of Original Qi Theory on TCM

(1) The Impact of Original Qi on "Harmony Between Human and Nature" in TCM

The theory holds that qi is the original source of human life; qi is the essential substance constituting human body. As one of the organism in nature, human being is also created by the coagulation of qi from heaven and earth. Since human being is the superlative organism in nature, the qi constituting human body is called "essential qi" in nature.

Qi is the essential substance constituting human body and maintaining our activities. Concerning the structure of human body, qi not only constitutes the substantial organs of human body, but also permeates inside the whole body, circulates among all the organs, integrates each organic part of the body into a united whole. The smooth movement of qi inside the unity forms the close relativity between local and the whole body, internal structure and external functions. Hence, physicians can make a diagnosis of the nature and location of disorder by the method of "observe the external manifestation of the patient to know what is happening inside the body", and then decisions of the treatment and regulating methods come out.

As one of the organisms in nature, human beings also make the substance exchanges with everything in nature taking qi as the medium. The human being is the component of the substantial whole in nature, and the unity of human being and nature is therefore manifested this way. Based on it, the concept of holism "unity of human being and universe", "correspondence of human being and universe", and "unity of appearance and *shen* (spirit)" could be further illuminated, and play the guiding role and influence on the health care view in TCM "treatment corresponds to seasons", methods for differentiation of syndrome "observe the external manifestation of the patient in order to know what is happening inside the body", and treatment idea "treatment in accordance with individual physique".

1) The Connotation of the Holistic View of "Harmony Between Human and Nature"

"Harmony between human and nature" is one of the basic concepts of Chinese philosophy, the most significant feature of Chinese philosophy that different from the West. In the history of Chinese thought, "harmony between human and nature" is a fundamental belief. Ji Xian-lin (1911.8.2-2009.7.11), a renowned professor in Peking University, gave the following explanation: heaven refers to the nature; person means human beings; harmony, that is, mutual understanding and forming friendships. Oriental philosopher warned us that humanity is just a part of the universe, man and nature is closely related to each other. For instance, the laws of "generating in spring, developing in summer, harvesting in autumn and storage in winter" requires that influence of climates, seasons, and geography on human health should be taken into account in the treatment. Moreover, a variety of factors, such as, seasons, climates, time of conception, and parents' health, have impacts on the embryo and its development, leading to different individual constitution after birth. This is the constitution theory in *Huang Di Nei Jing* (*The Yellow Emperor's Inner Classic*) and the principle of "treatment according to each individual constitution" should be followed.

Moreover, human body is also considered as a small universe in TCM. Similarity of structure between human and nature is the most direct expression of the perspective in *Huang Di Nei Jing* (*The Yellow Emperor's Inner Classic*) that human and nature is a unit, and the structure of the human body corresponds to the structure of the heaven. The nature contains yin and yang while human have *zang* and *fu* organs; the nature contains four seasons while human has four limbs; the nature contains the five phases while human have five *zang* organs; the earth contains rivers while human have channels and collaterals. The category of the five phases in Chapter *Jin Gui Zhen Yan Lun* (*Sincere Remarks on the Synopsis of the Golden Chamber*) of *Su Wen* (*Basic Questions*) and *Yin Yang Yin Xiang Da Lun* (*Discussion on Correspondence of Yin and Yang*) of *Su Wen* (*Basic Questions*) exactly originates from the identity of the ways, status and the internal phenomenon of the things movements. Five-phase theory classify all kinds of things and phenomena into five categories, such as the directions, seasons, weather, and constellations in the heaven, the five creeds, five livestock, five sounds, five colors, five flavors, five smells in the earth, as well as five organs, five voices, five emotions, pathological changes, the locations of diseases of the human body. Therefore, the common features and similar interaction regularity of the same type of things and phenomena can be identified from their appearance.

----- Supplementary reading 1-5 --

"daily-rhythm", "monthly-rhythm" and "seasonal rhythm" in human body

Activities of human life cycle are influenced by the running period of the earth, the moon and stars. There are "daily-rhythm", "monthly-rhythm" and "seasonal rhythm" in human physiological and pathological cycle.

"Daily-rhythm" is the rhythm of human body with a cycle of 24 hours. "Daily-rhythm" in

TCM refers to the rhythm of the growth and decline of yin-yang in the body during the day and night, the running rhythm of wei qi (defensive qi) and ying qi (nutritive qi) of human body, the hour-rhythm of five zang organs, pulse rhythm, etc. Among these rhythms, the growth and decline rhythm of yin-yang in the body is the fundamental form of human activities, also known as generating, developing, harvesting and storage rhythm of the qi of the human body.

Monthly-rhythm, also named as month lunar rhythm, is the reaction of the body to the movement of the moon. It is closely related to the excess and deficiency of qi and blood in human body. Women's menstruation period is one month, just like the signs of sea tides, which has close relationship with the full and empty of the moon. Qi and blood in human body also have monthly-rhythm. In a word, the menstruation and the moon are synchronized with monthly rhythm cycle. It is believed that the rhythm of menstruation and moon are correlated with the tides in some way.

Seasonal rhythm reflects the seasonal changes of human body in different seasons. The pulses have different characteristics in the four seasons. The pulse are mainly wiry in spring, surging in summer, floating in autumn, deep pulse in winter, this is the so called seasonal pulse rhythm.

---

2) "Harmony Between Human and Nature" and Health Preservation

TCM believes that the most important principle of health preservation is conforming to nature and living in harmony with nature. The seasonal changes of yin-yang are the fundamental causes of the process of "generating, developing, changing, harvesting, storing" in nature. Everything in nature should follow the law of the nature, human daily life, emotional and mental health activities should also be compatible with natural law. Many chapters in *Huang Di Nei Jing* (*The Yellow Emperor's Inner Classic*) have discussed about health preservation conforming to the four seasons.

(2) Application of Original Qi Theory in Diagnosis and Treatment

Original qi theory influences the observation process of human activities. The foundation of the conception system of essence, qi and *shen* (spirit) is applied to explain the physiological and psychological phenomena of human beings and to illuminate human activity process. The substantial Qi including *yuan* qi (original qi), *zong* qi (pectoral qi), *ying* qi (nutritive qi), *wei* qi (defensive qi), qi of *zang-fu* organs and channels are produced by the interaction of congenital essence qi, acquired food essence, and clear qi from nature. Combined with blood, fluid, essence and other vital substance, the essential qi disperses and circulates throughout the whole body, promoting and inspiring the functional activity of all the organs of the body and maintaining a normal physical state.

TCM believes that all human activities are conducted by the essential qi. If the function of qi is normal, human would maintain a healthy condition, however, if qi is insufficient or excessive or abnormal, people will be in a pathological state. The conflict of *zheng* qi (anti-pathogenic qi) and *xie* qi (pathogenic qi) will result in the occurrence of illness. According to the classic statement in Chapter *Ju Tong Lun* (*Discussion on Pain Syndromes*) of *Su Wen* (*Basic Questions*), "All diseases are resulted from disorder of qi. Rage causes qi to rise up, joy causes it to move slowly, heat causes it to disperse, fright causes it to be deranged, overstrain and stress causes it to be exhausted, and worry causes it to be stagnated." Therefore, in clinical diagnosis of TCM, much attention is paid on the dysfunction of qi and location of disorder. As well as in the treatment, the methods of promoting qi, nourishing qi, descending qi and regulating qi are greatly stressed, until the relative balance state of qi is achieved.

1.1.2.2 Yin-Yang Theory

1.1.2.2.1   The Concept of Yi-Dao and Yin-Yang

The initial concept of yin-yang is very primitive, which is originated from pictographic characters, corresponding to the two sides of sunshine. The side facing sunshine refers to yang, while the other side back to sunshine refers to yin. Later by extension, it indicates the two inter-opposing aspects within every object or phenomenon.

Yin-yang theory originates from ancient astrology and astronomy. In Han Dynasty (202BC-220AD), the concept of yin and yang has permeated into philosophy, natural sciences, and social and political theory, etc. almost all fields. It has profound impact on the formation and development of ancient Chinese astronomy, meteorology, mathematics, chemistry, medicine and other natural disciplines.

The book "Zhou Yi" (*I Ching*) summarizes yin-yang theory from the view of philosophy, pointing out "Alternating between yin and yang is called Tao", and viewing yin-yang as the source and general law of the movement and development of everything in nature. The relationship between yin and yang are considered as the following: opposition and restraint, mutual permeation, inter-consuming-supporting and inter-transforming. Thus, yin and yang become a pair of independent philosophic concept and is widely applied in the process of observing and reforming the nature. A man named as "Bo Yang-fu" in the eight centuries B.C. used to explain the earthquake by yin and yang, and he attributed the cause of earthquake to the uncoordinated movements of the yin and yang inter-opposing substance inside the earth.

1.1.2.2.2   The Application of Yin-Yang Theory in TCM

Yin-yang theory is applied to describe the organic structure of the body, TCM holds that the inter-opposing-dependent relationship of yin-yang manifests among all the organic systems inside the human body. All its organs and tissues can be divided into some parts, which are not only mutual independent but also mutual dependent, so all its organs and tissues including *zang-fu*, meridians and organic structure possess their own qualities, namely yin and yang respectively, thus according to the relationship within all the upper and lower, internal and external, exterior and interior, anterior and posterior organic structures, it could be further observed and analyzed by the opposing-uniting view of yin and yang.

The physiological activities and physiologic functions of each organ of human body possess its special quality of yin and yang respectively, and they are mutual related and dependent, to maintain and coordinate the human activity together. The functional activity of the human being is the process of regulating yin and yang to the dynamic balanced state, and once this kind of balance were being disturbed, then it must result in the abnormal condition of the human body. So dysfunction of yin and yang is one of the basic pathogenesis for disease. Yin-yang theory is applied to analyze the yin and yang property of pathogenic factors, as well as in clinical diagnosis, treatment and the medication.

----- Supplementary reading 1-6 ---

Ba Gua (the Eight Diagrams)

The Eight Diagrams is one of the most significant inventions in the history of ancient China civilizations. It is applied to clarify the multilevel and the universal significance of yin and yang, as the old saying "Yi-Tao to the yin and yang". The explanation of yin and in yang in Shuo Wen Jie Zi (Elucidations of Script and Explications of Characters) states that yin and yang were initially refers to "dark" and "light". The alternation of light and dark formed time sequence, which is associated with the orientation, thus the origin of the Eight Diagrams has close relationship with time sequence and orientation.

The Eight Diagrams represents the systemic changes of yin and yang in nature. "—" represents yang, while "- -" represents yin. Three of these symbols compose eight forms, which is called the Eight Diagrams. Each Diagram represents a certain thing. Qián represents heaven, kūn) represents earth, kǎn represents water, lí-represents fire, zhèn represents thunder, gèn represents mountain, xùn represents wind, duì-represents marsh. The corresponding the five phases of the eight diagrams are stated as the following: metal to qián and duì, wood to zhèn and xùn, earth to kūn and gèn, water to kǎn. (Please see Figure 1-4)

Coordinating with each other, the eight diagrams generate into sixty-four hexagrams, which are applied to symbolize a variety of nature and personnel phenomena (Table 1-1).

Table 1-1　The symbolized things of the eight diagrams

name of hexagrams	nature	body	animal	direction	seasons	yin-yang	the five-phases	five organs
qián	heaven	head	horse	northwest	Among autumn and winter	yang	metal	Large intestine
duì	marsh	mouth	sheep	west	Autumn	yin	metal	Lung
lí	fire	eye	pheasant	south	Summer	yin	fire	Heart/small intestine
zhèn	thunder	foot	dragon	east	Spring	yang	wood	Liver
xùn	wind	thigh	rooster	southeast	Among spring and summer	yin	Wood	Gall bladder
kǎn	water	ear	pig	north	winter	yang	Water	Kidney/bladder
gèn	mountain	hand	dog	northeast	Among winter and spring	yang	Earth	Stomach
kūn	earth	abdomen	Cattle	Southwest	Among summer and autumn	yin	Earth	Spleen

1.1.2.2.3　Five-phase Theory

The concept of "the five phases" originates from the idea of "the five directions" of Yin and Shang Dynasties (17th century BC-11th century). According to the recordation in "*jia gu wen*" (inscriptions on bones or tortoise shells of the Shang dynasty), the people of the Yin Dynasty named the realm of the Shang Dynasty as "Middle Shang", and paralleled by the five directions. After the five directions theory, "the five materials theory" turned up, which classified all the substantial substance into the five categories, named as wood, fire, earth, metal and water. After that, people abstracted their characteristics from the five kinds of concrete materials, wood, fire, earth, metal, water and they classified all these, according to their natures, by using analogy. Thus five-phase theory ascends to the philosophic conception, and it classifies all kinds of things and phenomena in nature into five categories by using analogy and deducing, and explains the law for the occurrence, development, changes of all kinds of things and phenomena by applying the relationship among the five phases.

Five-phase theory is applied in explaining the physiological function and characteristics of internal organs. The interaction among the five phases: inter-generation and inter-restriction, inhibition and generation, predominance and retaliation, over-restriction and reverse, and the abnormal change of promotion, mother to child and opposite are used to explain mutual influence of the five *zang*-organs, the transmission and changes of diseases, and the relationship among the diseases and the nature, which is applied as the guidance in diagnosis and treatment.

----- Supplementary reading 1-7 --

The Four Liquid Equilibrium Theory in the Western Medicine

Around 460-371 BC, Hippocrates, a great physician in the ancient Greek, created the four liquid equilibrium theory of human body, known as the "father of medicine." in the west. "Four liquid" equilibrium theory is developed on the basis of the four elements theory of Empedocles. Empedocles believed that the four basic elements composed the world are air, water, fire and earth. These four elements are corresponded to blood, mucus, yellow bile and black bile. The balance and movements of these four fluids in the body are applied to illustrate the physiological and pathological phenomena of human body. If the four fluids sustain in an equilibrium condition, the body will be in a healthy state. If the imbalance of four fluids is temporary, it tends to restore balance.

1.1.3 TCM and the Ancient Chinese Science, Religions, Military and Geography

Huang Di Nei Jing (*The Yellow Emperor's Inner Classic*) commands the future generations who study medicine should "not only understand astronomy and geography, but also well known of sociology." It indicates that there is a closely linked relationship among TCM and natural science, the humanities social sciences. Multi-disciplinary knowledge is involved in the famous book, *Huang Di Nei Jing* (*The Yellow Emperor's Inner Classic*), such as astronomy, geography, mathematics, religion and military, etc.

1.1.3.1 TCM and the Ancient Astronomy in China

Medicine is closely linked with astronomy. The astronomy has a long history same as mankind. "When Fu Xi, an archaic emperor in Chinese history, governed his country, and he always faced upward to learn from the sky, faced downward to learn from the earth, researched the accord of the pattern of animals with different areas, and learned from things nearby and in distant, and finally invented the theory of Eight Diagrams to explain everything on earth."

1.1.3.1.1　Achievements of Chinese Ancient Astronomy

China is one of the countries of the earliest and fastest development of astronomy in the world, and Chinese ancient astronomy plays an important role in the history of astronomy development. Chinese ancient astronomy originates in primitive society. There were astronomical officers who engaged in observing astronomical phenomenon and editing the calendar that were specialized during the age of *Yao* emperor (24th century B.C). The historical records show that the history of astronomical observation lasted for a long time.

(1) Chinese Ancient Astronomical Apparatus

Scientists in China also gave great contributions to inventing the astronomical apparatus. The apparatus, named "*hun yi*", is invented for measuring the location of celestial bodies 2000 years ago. Afterwards more than 10 astronomical apparatus are invented or modified, such as "*jian yi*", "*gao biao*", "*yang yi*" and so on.

(2) Chinese Ancient Calendar

Ancient people observed location and changes of the sun, the moon, stars and planets with the main purpose to master the regularity of the movement of celestial bodies to identify four seasons and draw up calendar for the work and living.

The calculation of "*jie qi*" (solar term) is the main content of ancient calendar. *jie qi* is the calendar that shows relation between weather changes and agriculture, which is a precious heritage of science. It is formally confirmed calendar with 24 *jie qi*, which are fixed clearly of their astronomical position in calendar, in 104 B.C. Apart from *jie qi*, ancient calendar also includes distribution of days in each month, arrangement of month and embolism of month, the time of eclipses, prediction and calculation of the astronomical events, calculation and prediction of the five major planets, etc.

The 24 Solar Terms are Spring begins, The rains, Insects awaken, Vernal Equinox, Clear and bright, Grain rain, Summer begins, Grain buds, Grain in ear, Summer solstice, Slight heat, Great heat, Autumn begins, Stopping the heat, White dews, Autumn Equinox, Cold dews, Hoar-frost falls, Winter begins, Light snow, Heavy snow, Winter Solstice, Slight cold, Great cold. (*Please see Figure 1-5*)

(3) Stem and Branch (*Gan Zhi*) Theory

Heavenly stems (*tian gan*) and earthly branches (*di zhi*) is a symbol for sequential system. Heavenly stems are used to describe gravitational influence of the Sun on the Earth's cycle, and the five phases, wood, fire, earth, metal and water are used to represent their phase characteristics. The twelve earthly branches are used to describe the impact of moon on the cycle of the earth receiving the sun's radiation, with three-yang and three-yin and six natural factors to indicate their phase characteristics.

"Heavenly Stems" and "Earthly Branches" are like a tree through the ages, supporting our understanding of the changes of everything in nature, while the understanding of the rules is simple and definite: the six heavenly stems and five earthly branches constitute a cycle of sixty. Yang heavenly stems and yang earthly branches combine together, while yin heavenly stems and yin earthly branches combine together, and then the combination of yin and yang, thus the sixty calendar are formed in an alternating turns, which consists the Image-Number expression of time and space. Then the sexagenary sequence of the heavenly stems and earthly branches is formed, starting with "*jia zi*" to the sixtieth "*gui hai*".

"Ten Heavenly Stems": (yang) *jia*、(yin) *yi*、(yang) *bing*、(yin) *ding*、(yang) *wu*、(yin) *ji*、(yang) *geng*、(yin) *xin*、(yang) *ren*、(yin) *gui*.

"Twelve Earthly Branches": (yang) *zi*、(yin) *chou*、(yang) *yin*、(yin) *mao*、(yang) *cheng*、(yin) *si*、(yang) *wu*、(yin) *wei*、(yang) *shen*、(yin) *you*、(yang) *xu*、(yin) *hai*.

A recurring sixty-year can be calculated by grouping 10 stems and 12 branches into the same polarity (yin or yang). For example, 5 yang heavenly stems combine with 6 yang earthly branches (5×6) + 5 yin heavenly stems combine with 6 yin earthly branches (5×6) = A Cycle of Sixty Years calendar (sixty Chinese Zodiac Years).

The interrelationship among the heavenly stems and earthly branches for counting the years, months, days and hours become the strong basis of the theory of traditional Chinese time-biomedicine, such as "doctrine of circuit and qi", "*Zi Wu Liu Zhu* (the ebb and flow of midnight and midday)" and "correspondence between heaven and humankind".

"*Jia zi*" means the beginning of the universe, with ascending strength and function, while "*gui hai*" represents an end, expressed by cold water's freezing, which is the most scientific exploration of the rules of things movement in nature by ancient people, as well as a specific product of the concept of "unity of human and nature".

There is similar concept of twelve earthly branches in India's ancient astronomy, but they use twelve animals for representation. With the integration of Buddhism, Chinese Zodiac is used to represent the twelve earthly branches.

----- Supplementary reading 1-8 --

The Origin of Chinese Zodiac

In order to let people including the people who were lack of money to study and illiterate people to remember the reign of his birth, the ancient literati use the most simple chronology by animals to help them to remember, later named as "Lunar Year". The cycle of Zodiac is 12 years. Each person has an animal zodiac at his birth. The twelve Zodiacs are rat, ox, tiger, rabbit, dragon, snake, horse, sheep, monkey, rooster, dog, pig, which is not only a Chinese folk method of calculating age, but also an ancient chronology. (Please see Figure 1-6)

1.1.3.1.2 Seasonal Health Preservation and the Ancient Astronomy

In remote antiquity, people worked and rested following natural principles, as the old saying "go to work when sun is rising up while have rest when sun is setting down". Then it leads to the formation of holistic concept, which includes "regarding human body as a whole and interacting with the surroundings", the physiological rhythm, circulation of qi and blood are consistent with natural changes. In order to keep healthy, people have to follow the astronomical principles. Human survives depending on the material supported by the qi of heaven and earth and have to comply with the seasonal changes of yin and yang. Health preservation in four seasons means living according to the biological rules such as generating in spring, developing in summer, harvesting in autumn and storage in winter. The changes of four seasons have great influence on human body in many aspects, such as spirit, qi and blood, five *zang*-organs, metabolism of body fluid, diseases, etc. The physiological activities of five *zang*-organs have to follow the seasonal change of yin and yang to keep balance and harmony with external surrounding. For example, during spring and summer, qi and blood move to the superficial part of the body, with the manifestation of loose skin, profuse sweating, etc. While in autumn and winter, qi and blood tends to go to *zang-fu* organs, with the manifestation of dense skin, less sweat and polyuria. Therefore in the health preservation, people have to follow this change and don't go against it, as the old saying "strengthen yang in spring and summer while nourish yin in autumn and winter".

1.1.3.2 TCM and the Ancient *Shu Shu* (skill number)

The method of *shu shu* (skill number) is a method of mathematics, which is considered as the minimum requirement of scientific knowledge that possesses exactness. Since there are essential difference of the application between the ancient Chinese technical territory and modern science, the application of the technique is called *shu shu* (skill number) instead of *shu xue* (mathematics). The ancient Chinese *shu shu* (skill number) was once at the advanced level all over the world.

There are many descriptions of numbers and quantity in TCM. *Yi Jing* (*The Book of Changes*), one of the sources of Chinese culture, is a book that is full of mathematics symbols, which is considered as an academic system of "generate from numbers, succeed in figures, and is flexible to the numbers". The combinations and changes of *yang yao* (—) and *yin yao* (— —), are the linguistic stating of mathematics in fact. Thus, the ancient Chinese mathematics is called "study of *shu shu*".

The applications of "study of *xiang shu*" in TCM also have the same features mentioned above. For instance, it is stated in Chapter *San Bu Jiu Hou Lun* (*Discussion on the three parts and nine sub-parts of pulse*) of *Su Wen* (*Basic Questions*), "the numbers of heaven and earth begin from one and end in nine". Number 1 and 9 are taken as the name of measurement to classify and mark the phenomena of life, similar to the labels. In details, "one indicates sky, two indicates earth, three indicates human, and three times three is nine that is corresponding with the number of the nine prefectures. Hence, there are three parts in the pulse, and each of them has three sub-parts that are the foundations to distinguish the death and survival of the patient, diagnose the diseases, adjusting deficiency and excess to cure disease."

Chapter *Wu Chang Zheng Da Lun* (*Discussion on the energies of the five phases' motion*) of *Su Wen* (*Basic Questions*) discusses the five phases with numbers, "the number of wood is eight, fire is seven, earth is five, metal is nine and water is six". While in Chapter *Xuan Shu* of *Tai Xuan*, numbers are used to discuss the five element, direction and four seasons, "number one and six belong to water, two and seven belong to fire, three and eight belong to wood, four and nine belong to metal, and five belongs to earth". In addition, those also include the information such as yin-yang, directions, climate and terrain, etc. Thus, the numbers become the symbols of these elements.

1.1.3.3   The Influence of Confucianism on TCM

Confucianism refers to the thoughts of Confucius (551-479BC), Meng Ke (372-289BC), Xun Kuang (313-238BC) as the representatives, advocating "courtesy and music", "benevolence", "royalty and forgiveness", "doctrine of mean thought", asserting "rule of virtue" and "policy of benevolence" in politics and stressing on ethics and moral in education. Confucianism is an important part of TCC and has great influence on TCM, stated as the following aspects:

1.1.3.3.1   Confucianism Promoted the Formation of the Core Values of TCM

Firstly, the mean thought of Confucian is an important part of TCM theoretical system. The framework of TCM theory consists of Confucianism, Taoism, Yin-Yang theory, etc. while the mean thought of Confucian have great impact on the formation of the values and thinking mode of TCM. Secondly, "benevolence" and "filial piety" advocates respect for others and self cultivation, which have a positive impact on the ethics, medical sociology and medical behavior of TCM. Thirdly, Confucian advocated systematic study and extensive reading. Having insatiable desire to learn and tireless in teaching others are the fine tradition of Confucianism, which impels TCM doctors to learn widely from others and strive for perfection, such as Zhang Zhong-jing, Sun Si-miao, Li Shi-zhen, etc. devoted their lifetime to pursuit the profound medical knowledge and techniques.

1.1.3.3.2   Confucianism Promotes the Development of TCM in the Following Aspects

Confucianism promotes the development of TCM education. The medical education system in the ancient times has a close relationship with the educational system of Confucianism.

Confucianism enriches TCM theoretical system. Yin-yang, the mean thought of Confucian and the holistic view mentioned in *Zhou Yi* (*I Ching*), *Lun Yu* (*the Analects of Confucian*), *Li Ji* (*The Book of Rites*) are important parts of TCM.

Confucianism promotes the formation of the unique research methods and thinking modes of TCM. Confucianism stresses on thinking in images other than abstract thinking, understanding human being from the macro function. The theoretical system of humanistic philosophy has been formed gradually on the basis of human and nature harmony and analogy of similar things by *xiang* (image), with the characteristic of holism and pattern differentiation.

1.1.3.4   The Influence of Religions on TCM

There are various religions that are popular in Chinese history. As the main traditional religions, Taoism and Buddhism, both have greatly influence on the development of Chinese history, TCC and TCM.

1.1.3.4.1   The Influence of Taoism on TCM

Formed in East Han Dynasty, 1800 years ago, Taoism is the only religion that originated in China, based on showing respect to ghosts and spirits, believing the folk legend of various mysteries, aiming at achieving longevity and keeping young, pursuing happiness at present life that come from Lao Zi (About 571 BC-471 BC) and Zhuang Zi (369 BC-286 BC). Mixed with the procedures of Buddhism and Confucius, absorbing part of the thought of Buddhism and

Confucius, Taoism put philosophy, legends and witchcraft together to form a complicated system.

Tao is the core of Taoism. Tao scholars believe that there is a rule that the diversity of things in nature have to follow, which is named as "*tao*". Everything in nature originates from *tao*. "One generates two, two to three, three to hundreds of thousands of things." "*De* (moral)" embodies the humanities, human relations and feelings of *tao* while *De* (moral) has to tally with the rules of *tao*. Human should follow the rules of *tao*. Taoism believes that life is the most important thing in nature, moral is the most important thing to the individual. Thus we should emphasize on external form and internal spirits, humanity and health. Good health and moral cultivation are important to human life. Taoism holds that the longevity comes from mutual actions of health and spirits.

As the old saying "medicine and Taoism are of the same origin", the Taoist ritual, practice, alchemy, medicine and food, etc. have a close relationship with TCM. The health preservation methods of Taoism have contributed greatly to the development of TCM, such as *qigong*, diet therapy, sexual health keeping, drugs and other healthcare techniques.

1.1.3.4.2 The Influence of Buddhism on TCM

The influences of Buddhism on TCM are mainly in medical morals and health preservation. The tenets of Buddhism are to persuade people to be good at keeping healthy spirit and mind. Many monks, nuns and believers tend to have a longevity life. Meditation in Buddhism is similar to *qigong*, so the books of Buddhism, which refers to the relationship between ways of static sitting (meditation) and health preservation, which is not only a way of Buddhist practice, but also a way of *qigong* training. *Chan* with static sitting plays a certain role in the history of Chinese *qigong*. The majority of Buddhism requires Buddhist to follow vegetarianism and is encouraged to practice hard, since vegetarian is good for both the body and the mind, which objectively have dietary therapeutic effect. There are very strict arrangements for rest and work in temples, such as reading the classics, working, doing exercises, etc. Many temples have the traditions of martial arts practice to protect the temple, which are good for health. In addition, the environment of the temple is beautiful, most of the buildings in the temples are high, wide, surrounding by green trees, and air is fresh, which is good for health. Above all, Buddhism have optimistic influences on the development of TCM healthy preservation in many aspects, such as medical moral, spirit, psychology, *qigong*, food nourishment, exercise, environment and personal hygiene, etc.

1.1.3.5 The Influence of Chinese Ancient Military Thoughts on TCM

Military and TCM have the common principles, as the old saying "The prescription of herbs was similar to resorting to arms." So doctors in past dynasties often used the military theories to draw the inspiration of clinical thinking, which have great contributions in development of TCM.

The explanation of how to choose the time of acupuncture in *Huang Di Nei Jing* (*The Yellow Emperor's Inner Classic*) is cited from "the art of war", that is avoid the excess and face the deficiency. As it is stated in Chapter *Ni Shun* (*Treatise on the agreeableness and adverseness*) of *Ling Shu* (*The Spiritual Pivot*), "according to 'the art of war', one must not make a head-on attack to the approaching army which is irresistible, and one must not launch an attack to a strong and grand battle array of the enemy". In Chapter *Ci Fa* (*Treatise on the techniques of acupuncture*) of *Ling Shu* (*The Spiritual Pivot*), it is recorded that "don't prick when the patient is suffering from excessive heat, don't prick when the patient has profuse sweating, don't prick when the pulse of the patient is confusing and when the disease is contrary to the pulse". The similar writing can be found in the military conflicts chapter of "the art of war". *Huang Di Nei Jing* (*The Yellow Emperor's Inner Classic*) cites the rules of wars to explain the conflicts between anti-pathogenic qi and pathogenic factors to guide the acupuncture treatments. Ancient doctors hold that the conflict between anti-pathogenic qi and pathogenic factors is the same as battle of the war. When one bout finished, another bout would continue.

"Using herbs in a prescription is similar to using soldiers", that is the enemy of war refers to the opposite side, while during the treatment it refers to the pathogenic factors. Strategist mention tactics and emphasize on the strategy while doctors stress on medical techniques and therapeutic methods. The ancient military theory shows the instinct thinking of the traditional Chinese thinking modes, such as "improving the occasion", "looking one way and rowing another", "avoiding the mightiness and attacking the weakness", "distributing the soldiers to surround", etc. There are great similarities between the clinical thinking of TCM and the military theory, so it is not difficult to understand why strategists and doctors shared the same opinions and application. Many clinical miracles have been created by doctors in the past dynasties under the strategists' theory.

----- Supplementary reading 1-9 --

There was a patient who suffered from constipation in Song Dynasty (960-1279AD). He was treated by many famous doctors but had no effect. One doctor named Shi only prescribed an herb, Zi Yuan (Radix Asteris), which is commonly used for cough. The miracle came after a while. The reason is that the lung and the large intestine are exteriorly-interiorly related, the constipation in that patient was caused by failure of lung qi to descent. Zi Yuan (Radix Asteris) was used for regulating lung qi to promote the bowel movement, so the constipation was eliminated. There is a method named as "opening-teapot" in the treating principles of TCM, which is applied to treat edema and retention of urine through regulating lung's function.

There was a case recorded in the book TCM aesthetics: the patient found his right hip point limited in flexing position when he got up in the morning, he couldn't move it even with strong external force. So he was sent to doctor with stretcher and treated with medicine, massage and Tuina and physiotherapy, but no effect. The author of the book TCM aesthetics inserted the needle in the patient's shoulder, when the needle was penetrated into the body about 2cm depth, the patient extended his right leg suddenly and jumped on the ground, recovered immediately after withdrawing of the needle.

Clinical thinking of TCM are very similar to the war, just do unconsciously. Everyone knows it but often inhibited by some common theory. Applying military theory frequently may inspire your stiff thought, thus you may use the TCM theory freely, which you recite very well.

1.1.3.6   The Influence of Chinese Ancient Geography on TCM

The relationship of geography and medicine is very close, since different terrain leads to different geographic surrounding and different life customs, and there are many obvious differences in time, temperature, quantity of raining, landscape, etc. Terrain is the earth for the birth of culture and the cradle of civilization. Natural conditions are formed by geographic surrounding, which will directly influence human in physiology, psychology, world view, methodology, etc.

China is a big country with lots of different landscapes such as plain, mountainous region, hill, desert, altiplano, island, etc. So the onset of diseases and treatments for disorders are different because of different natural conditions in different areas. It is requested that health preservation, prevention of disease, treatment and rehabilitation in TCM should in accordance with the local conditions. The Chapter *Yi Fa Fang Yi Lun* (*Discussion on discriminative treating for patients of different regions*) of *Su Wen* (*Basic Questions*) records different geographic landscapes, products and situations of people in east, west, south, north and center of China, shows us the influence to the physiology, personality and diseases and give the different medical therapies. For example, the people who live in the east of China are easy to suffer from carbuncles and ulcers, so the operation with *bian shi* (stone knife) should be given; in the west, the most common disease happen to the internal organs, stronger herbs should be given; in the north, *zang-fu* organs are easy to be attacked by cold and lead to abdominal distention, so moxibustion should be given; in south, more arthritis due to wind and dampness, so *tui na* (Chinese medical massage) and massage are often applied.

In addition, the dosage and property of the herbs should be selected in accordance with different regions. Large dosage should be given in north because of severe cold while lighter in south because of the extreme heat. *Fu zi* (Radix Aconiti Lateralis Preparata) and *xi xin* (Herba Asari) are commonly used in southwest because of dampness but should gave great cares for application in the areas in the below the south bank of Yangtze River because of damp-heat. In TCM, the genuine medicinal materials are very important. In addition, there are different therapies to treat diseases in different areas such as folk therapy, local medicine etc.

----- Supplementary reading 1-10 ---

Achievements of Ancient Chinese Geographical

Chinese made great achievements in the research of geography in ancient time. Maps and the theory of mapping appeared quite early with quite a lot geographical documents. Chinese had developed geographical concepts from 11th to 8th century B.C. with the map to indicate the distribution of areas and to national management of administration. Shan Hai Jing (the classics of mountains and seas), published 2500 years ago, contributes to ancient geography, history, mythology, nationality, zoology, botany, mineral resources, medicine, religions and so on. This book describes the national geography systematically with the marks of mountains. There are 460 mountains and 260 rivers listed in this book with the records of more than 140 plants, 112 animals and many of minerals, which is the earliest mineral literature in the world.

At the beginning of 6th century, Shui Jing Zhu (Notes for classic of rivers), a national geographic work with completely and colligated description of the outline of rivers and landmarks, which covers 1252 rivers in the whole country. The records of this book include drainage areas of rivers, geographic situations of rivers and historic stories of rivers with the choosing of typical affairs.

At the beginning of 17ᵗʰ century, Ming Dynasty, Xu Xia-ke (1587-1641), a geographer, had spent 30 years traveling the half of China, who was engaged in scientific observation of geography and exploration since he was 22 and wrote the famous book Xu Xia Ke You Ji (Xu Xia-ke's travel notes). Xu Xia-ke (1587-1641) was the first scientist who proposed the conception of watershed and drainage areas in the world and the first person who pointed out that the drainage areas of Yangtze River as twice as that of Yellow River. He was also the first scientist who made systemic observation of rocky physiognomy with more than 300 caves personnel exploration and description. All of those made Xu Xia-ke (1587-1641) famous in the history of science and culture as one of the creators of modern geography.

1.1.4 Differences and Integration of TCM and Western Medicine

1.1.4.1 The Similarities and Differences of TCM and Western Medicine in Understanding Disease

The fundamental difference between TCM and Western medicine is the understanding methodological differences. The method used in TCM is observing the natural and personnel phenomena by sensory organs directly, from the concrete to the abstract image, then from abstract thinking to the philosophical understanding of specific unknown phenomenon. Western medicine is experimental science established on analytical methods. The methods of experimental analysis in western medicine and systematic thinking methods of TCM are different medical theory to illustrate the same body, which reveal the many aspects of the body, allowing people to have a comprehensive understanding of the physiology of the body.

1.1.4.1.1 TCM Focus on Functional Relationship

Starting with observing the life phenomena, TCM pay less attention to the internal structure, but tends to understand the law of functional changes in terms of natural integrity instead. The Chapter *Wu Chang Zheng Da Lun* (*Discussion on the energies of the five elements' motion*) of *Su Wen* (*Basic Questions*), states that "when qi starts, things begin to transform and produce; when qi moves, things begin to grow; when qi spreads, things begin to reproduce; and when qi expires, things begin to die." TCM holds that the physical body is formed during qi transportation and transformation, which is the basic life function of human. Life is a type of vital functional state of man in the nature, mixing with other varieties of factors. The manifestations shown in the changes of qi of human body can reflect the functional state of the whole body, that is "the disorders of internal organs will definitely manifest in externally".

The *zang-xiang* (visceral manifestation) theory of TCM establishes a unique body system on the basis of functional relation according to the changes of *xiang* (manifestations). *Xiang* means manifestation, *zang* (internal organs) is located interior but manifests exterior. The *zang-xiang* (visceral manifestation) theory describes the inter-promoting and interacting relationship among *fu*-organs, the interior-exterior relationship among *zang-fu* organs, orifice-opening relationships between internal organs and five sensory organs and the subordinate relationship between *zang-fu* organs and channels. It doesn't refer to the movement and function of one specific organ, but to deduce the interrelationship among the functional system through the external *xiang*. Frijof Capra from the United States points out that "Chinese concepts on the body are always about the function and the relationship among different parts, but not much about its accurate structure." Functional changes are also observed and researched in TCM.

The understanding and treatment of TCM are based on the functional system. The morbid state in TCM refers to functional disorder of *zang-fu* organs and qi, blood resulting from yin-yang imbalance and disorder of qi activity, not of the organic pathological changes. The treatment of TCM also targets on regulating function and promote the inherent production and transformation. Medications or other therapies may not directly act on the target point of the disease, but to maintain yin-yang balance by regulating its functional state to keep healthy. However, TCM realizes that functional abnormalities are frequently the prelude of organic disease, as it is said "discomforts of the body are all caused by the disorder of qi activity." Therefore, functional regulation can be regarded as a preventive measure for organic disease.

1.1.4.1.2   Western Medicine Focus on Substantial Structure

The publication of "the structure of human body" by Andreas Vesalius from Belgium in 1543 indicates that the modern development of western medicine has started. Western medical system is established on the basis of structural study. With further knowledge from human body to tissues, cells, and molecules or even gene, the focus on life understanding of western medicine has been guided by the reductionism all the time, aiming to explain the nature of life from gene or even more microcosmic level.

Western medicine classifies the organs and tissues into several major systems based on the structure of human body according to their structural liaison and similarity. Based on the structure of human body, the study on human physiology and pathology is carried out, focused on the organic changes of anatomical structure, localization and pathological anatomy of the affected areas within the framework system. Therefore organic pathological changes are the major concern of western medicine, while functional changes are considered as subordination. Western medicine maintains that organic pathological changes are the general and basic structures of disease, some scholars even believe that any functional changes can be proved with organic changes of the body.

1.1.4.2   The Unique Thinking Mode of TCM

Due to the difference ways of thinking, many people feel particularly difficult at the early stage of learning TCM. After achieving a conversion or communication of the two ways of thinking, learning TCM will be very interesting. There are many factors that may affect on the way of TCM thinking, however, to analyze ultimately, the basic category is attributed to *xiang* (phenomenon) and *yi* (idea). The thinking mode guiding TCM scholars is instinct thinking. This mode uses analogue, determination of etiologic factors and deduction based on differentiation. It emphasizes on affiliation of surface and essence. TCM focuses on the thinking way of "comparing phenomenon to get similarities", the thinking way mainly manifests as dialectic logic. Among TCM learning methods, observation and thinking, the perceptual and the rational can't be separated. The combination of the perceptual and the rational is called savvy or instinct. Therefore, the results of TCM thinking are material and nonobjective, natural and vivid.

1.1.4.2.1 Analogy of Similar Things by *Xiang* (Phenomena)

The concept of *xiang* (phenomenon) originates from *Yi Jing* (*The Book of Changes*), which states that "saint used to assimilate the profound truth in universe to some very concrete images, because all profound truths must have external appearance, we term this kind of condition as '*xiang*'". "*Xiang* in *Yi Jing* are all expressed as phenomenon, what is *xiang* (phenomenon), it is just the image (*Xi Ci Xia* <part II of notes for *Yi Jing* >). TCM gives a definition to *xiang* (phenomenon) from the aspect of medicine, that is "since there are some invisible *zang-fu* organs inside human body, there must be some visible conditions manifested in the external appearance". "The appearance manifests outside is just the *xiang*", which can manifest the condition of "internal *zang-fu*". Although five *zang*-organs and six *fu*-organs dwell inside human body, we could still observe their functions and characters, and people could speculate the nature of *zang-fu* organs by the observed functional characters. Therefore, *zang-fu* theory of TCM is also termed as "*zang-xiang* theory". The method of TCM "*wei xiang*" is established on the basis of the disciplinary relationship between the internal part with external part of human body depending on the observation, comparison, analysis on intact human being to study the laws of its physiology, pathology and treatment, and it is a kind of an indirect method of understanding the object by the principle of internal-external relationship, so it pertains to holistic system method. The concept of "Method of *wei xiang*" is close to that of "method of black box" in cybernetics.

The four diagnostic methods of TCM is the clinical application local "*xiang*" manifested the holistic changes, which rely on sensory organs' observation of the vital information of the patients by the physicians. The commonly used local diagnostic methods are pulse diagnosis, inspection on face, auricle, nose, tongue diagnosis, and inspection on infantile superficial venule of index fingers, etc. The principle of these diagnostic methods is mainly from the statement "*zang-fu* organs inside the body, the manifestations are in the exterior", the local exterior changes can manifest the function of the whole. Thus, the local parts for diagnosis or treatment are termed as "*xiang*" of the whole.

The theories of "regarding human body as a whole and interacting with the surroundings" in TCM compare human with many natural phenomena, such as comparing qi and blood circulation with the tide, which will be subjected by sun and moon, coldness and warmth, day and night, etc. This kind of analogy emphasizes the uniting between the body and nature of moving laws. The ancient people analogized the human body as "the microcosm", the nature as "the macrocosm", and searched for the methods of recognition for the scientific knowledge of human body from the nature in appreciation and understanding.

(1) Comparing the Similarities Between the Function of Human Body and the Social Phenomenon.

In Chapter *Ling Lan Mi Dian Lun* (*Discussion of secret classics*) of *Su Wen* (*Basic Questions*), it analogizes the internal organ's function with the official ranks in similarity, such as heart is crowned king; lung is premier; liver is general; spleen and stomach are officials of the granary. This is because the characteristics of the function of internal organs are similar to the features of the function of official ranks. This kind of similar relation also displays in the composition of formulas, the herbs aimed at the cause of disease or the main disease symptom are called the principal herbs, the herbs that are assisting and cooperating with the principal herbs act as the ministerial herbs, the herbs that are treating the secondary symptoms or giving dual attention to accompanied diseases are called the adjuvant while agitating herbs and guiding herbs are messenger herbs.

(2) Comparing the Natural Objects with the Anatomy and Physiology of Human Beings

The Chapter *Wu Zang Sheng Cheng Pian* (*Generation of five zang organs*) of *Su Wen* (*Basic Questions*) compares qi and blood circulation in the human body with the waxing and waning of tides. In *Mai Jing* (*The Classics of Pulses*), according to the similarity between the lack cycle of moon and the menses periods of women, the phenomenon of the menses periods of women is named as menstruation. In *Zhong Zang Jing* (*The Classic of Internal Zang Organs*), Hua Tuo (145-208AD) links lung shape to the canopy of internal organs that covers all internal organs. Interior of lung is empty like honeycomb without the lower aperture that is full after inspiring and empty after expiring. Moreover, many names of the acupoints of the human body are named according to the characteristics of locations and the similarity of natural objects. For instance, location of *da ling* (PC 7) is like mountains. Location of *tai yuan* (LU 9) is like a valley.

(3) Comparing the Similarities of the Pathogenic Factors with That of the Pathological Results

TCM holds that natural factors are necessaries for human's surviving, but which become the pathogenic factors when they surpass the normal degree. The pathogenic factors affect the human body usually resulted in similar characteristics of pathogenic factors. For instance, the characteristics of the pathogenic dampness are flowing downward, heaviness and turbid. When dampness invades human body, similar characteristics are also displayed, such as edema, heaviness in the limbs, asthenia, and head heaviness as being wrapped, etc. Likewise, the characteristics of the fire is tending to flame and consume body fluid, and invades by summer heat, the body displays fever, blush, dry mouth and less urine.

1.1.4.2.2 Surmising the Interior From Observing the Exterior

"Surmising the interior from observing the exterior" is a method of extrapolating the interior change through the observation of external representation. It is the foundation of TCM understanding method, practicing method, philosophical method, etc.

The ancient people discovered that there were corresponding relations between the exterior representation and internal organs during the long time practice, as well as the changes of internal organs of the body, as the old saying "inner place possesses variously, certainly it forms various external manifestations". In Chapter *Wai Chuai* (*Determination from outside*) of *Ling Shu* (*The Spiritual Pivot*), it states that the sunlight emerges the shadow, rapping gong and drum sends out sound, which is applied to explain that there is a causal association between the phenomenon and the essence of things. Reasons can be extrapolate from the results and results can be found from reasons.

The method of "surmising the interior from observing the exterior" is similar to the theory of "Black Box" in modern cybernetics. Without opening the black box, merely by means of importing message to "Black Box" and read the feedback messages that come out, then comparatively study the similarities and differences of the importing and outputting information. The situation inside the black box could be obtained, as well as the movements and changes. Since this method doesn't disturb or destroy the inherent relation of the objects itself, so the inherent characteristics and the changes of the objects can be observed. Therefore, this method has advantage in researching the complex phenomenon, especially in the process of life compared to other methods.

1.1.4.3 The Basic Characteristics of TCM

1.1.4.3.1 The Basic Thoughts of Pattern Differentiation

Pattern differentiation is the process of thinking to differentiate the causes of different syndromes and taken out appropriate treatment, based on the theory of TCM, applying the diagnostic methods such as inspection, auscultation-olfaction, interrogation and palpation, combined with comprehensive analysis of the physiological characteristics of the patient as well as climate, geography, lifestyle factors, etc.

----- Supplementary reading 1-11 ---

In the Three-State Period (220-280AD), administer Ni Xun and Li Yan went to see doctor Hua Tuo (145-208AD), both suffering from headache and fever. After diagnosis, Hua Tuo (145-208AD) said: "dispersing method should be used for Ni Xun, while sweating method should be used for Li Yan." Some people didn't understand. Hua Tuo (145-208AD) explained that "Ni Xun suffered from exterior entity, the evil qi accumulated in the body, like the accumulated water in the mountain, reducing method should be used to disperse the evil pathogen. While Li Yan suffered from inner entity, easily to get excessive fire flowing up, just like the earth qi stagnation, sweating method should be used to disperse the evil pathogen." Different prescriptions were given to them and both were recovered the next day.

1.1.4.3.2 The Basic Principle of Causative Treatment of TCM

The principle of seeking the initial cause (the root) in treating disease is the most distinctive feature of TCM. As it is stated in Chapter *Ci Fa Lun* (*Discussion on Needling Techniques*) of *Su Wen* (*Basic Questions*), "pathogenic factors can hardly attack the body if the anti-pathogenic qi is strong". The anti-pathogenic qi refers to the self-defending ability of the body, including the tissue structure, substance and functional activity, while pathogenic qi refers to various pathogenic factors. The occurring and developing of the disease is depended on the final result of the struggle between pathogenic qi and anti-pathogenic qi. Sufficient anti-pathogenic qi is the inherent foundation to defend against disease. To seek the initial cause in treating disease means to understand the key factors in the struggle between pathogenic qi and anti-pathogenic qi, with the purpose of invigorating anti-pathogenic qi and improvement of the self-defending and restoration ability of the body. The principle should be applied in all aspects of TCM health prevention, health preservation and treatment.

1.1.4.3.3   The Principle of Regulating Yin and Yang

TCM believes that illness is the dynamic imbalance of yin and yang, manifesting as maladaptive of the changes in external environment, disorder of the spirits and dysfunction of the *zang-fu* organs. As it is stated in *Sheng Qi Tong Tian Lun* (*Discussion on the Human Vital Energy Connecting with Nature*) of *Su Wen* (*Basic Questions*), "If yin and yang keep balance mutually, the spirit will present, if yin and yang were separated, the primordial qi will disappear." "Adjusting the yin and yang can make the spirit present" is stated in Chapter *Gen Jie* (*Root and Knot*) of *Ling Shu* (*The Spiritual Pivot*). The Chapter *Zhi Zhen Yao Da Lun* (*Discussion on Essentials*) of *Su Wen* (*Basic Questions*) points out that to cure is to "observe the place of yin and yang carefully, then adjust it, take peace as the purpose.", and also give definitely explanation on the treatment "make the cold heat up, make the hot cold, make the warm cool, make the cool warm, make the dispersion come together, make the suppressant spread, make the dry moist, make the fast slow down, make the strong and tough soft, make the fragile hard, make the lack excessive, make the excessive decrease, each part keeps its level of qi, and must keep peace, then the disease goes away, all in all, this is the main principle of treatment." The treatment of TCM mainly includes "regulation and recuperation". Regulation means harmonizing and adjusting, recuperation means supplementing, reducing, and removing the obstruction. By using Chinese herbs and acupuncture, TCM aims to harmonize qi, blood and yin-yang, regulating the physiological function of *zang-fu*, with the purpose of increasing self-defending ability and remove the soil on which disease depended. Above all, it is clear that resuming the balance of yin and yang in the body is the basic principle of TCM treatment.

1.1.4.4   Integration and Development of TCM and Western Medicine

TCM is being integrated into the current culture, science and technology development, its practical value, advantages and potential development is more prominent, as the statement in "Science and Technology Development Strategy Study of TCM Modernization" by the Ministry of Science and Technology and State Administration of TCM of China, "to develop TCM according to its own development law, meet the development requirement of the times, make full use of modern scientific technology, inherit and carry forward its advantage and characteristics and eventually to make novel innovations and upgrading in both theory and practice and turn it into medical theoretical system with modern science and technology level."

Ilya Prigogine (1917-2003), the inventor of western dissipative structure theory pointed out that the academic thinking of ancient china focused more on integrity and naturalness, or on coordination and harmony. The development of modern science and the research on physics and mathematics in the last decade such as the Rene Thom's catastrophe theory, renormalization group, and bifurcations all conform to ancient Chinese philosophy. German sinologist Manfred Porkert believed that "TCM is an induction-comprehensive science and western medicine is a causal analysis science. TCM and western medicine can provide reliable and significant information from totally different aspects, just as two mountaineering teams may climb to the mountain peak from either the southern aspect of from the northern aspect. However, considering their own limitations, the two systems are supposed to complement each other.".

In the long period ahead, TCM and western medicine will develop following their own respective tracks in the course of mutual exchange, infiltration, supplement and integration. Dr. Joseph Needham (1900-1995), a historian on world science and technology thought that "the more biological features a science has, the longer time it takes to form worldwide natural science unity". We believe that TCM and western medicine, sharing the same research object, will reach the dialectal unity of reductionism and holism through the mutual merging and development by unremitting efforts of different generations, which will in turn make a new medical system on human health and disease with unity of function, structure and metabolism.

(Ma Xueling)

1.2　Brief History of TCM Nursing

The formation and development of TCM Nursing has a long history. Since the ancient times, treating diseases with TCM has incorporated medicine, Chinese materia medica and nursing together. Though the nursing science of TCM hasn't developed into an independent subject in the past, there is abundant knowledge of the theories and techniques of TCM nursing displayed in different categories of medical literatures in past dynasties.

1.2.1　Ancient TCM Nursing

1.2.1.1　From Warring States Period to East Han (475 BC-220AD)

Huang Di Nei Jing (*The Yellow Emperor's Inner Classic*) is the earliest extant medical classic in China that comparatively expounds the system of TCM. It consists of two books, *Su Wen* (*Basic Questions*) and *Ling Shu* (*The Spiritual Pivot*). It systematically expatiates on the theories of human physiology and pathology, as well as diagnosis, prevention and treatment of diseases. It is a stable foundation for the establishment and development of theoretical and clinical system of TCM. In the aspects of TCM nursing, it expounds syndrome nursing, dietary nursing, daily life nursing, emotion nursing, life cultivation and rehabilitation nursing, medication nursing and nursing techniques such as acupuncture and moxibustion, *tui na*, *dǎo yǐn* (도引), hot compressing and fumigating and steaming therapy, etc. Therefore *Huang Di Nei Jing* (*The Yellow Emperor's Inner Classic*) also establishes the foundation of TCM nursing. For example, *Su Wen* (*Basic Questions*) points out that for daily life nursing one should "abide by the rule of yin and yang and the principle of nature, regulate the diet and the living habit and avoid overstrain", which is not only the principle of health cultivation and disease prevention, but also the method of self-nursing. *Huang Di Nei Jing* (*The Yellow Emperor's Inner Classic*) also indicates the concept of "adapting to the variation of the season and following the rules of nature." It points out the law of life cultivation according to seasonal variation that also embodies the concept of holism that human beings are integrated into the nature. In terms of nursing of visceral diseases, *Huang Di Nei Jing* (*The Yellow Emperor's Inner Classic*) states that "when the spleen is sick, one should neither eat warm or hot food or overeat, nor stay in damp place or wear wet clothes"; "when the lung is ill, one should neither eat cold food nor wear less clothes". In the aspect of dietary nursing, it points out the diet taboos of visceral diseases that "liver disease patients should avoid pungent food, heart disease patients should avoid salty food, spleen disease patients should avoid acid food and kidney disease patients should avoid bitter food." *Huang Di Nei Jing* (*The Yellow Emperor's Inner Classic*) also gives high light on mental and psychological nursing which is regarded as an important factor attached to the progress and prognosis of diseases. It emphasizes that bad mental stimulation will cause qi and blood disorder in the body, visceral dysfunction, and induce or exacerbate diseases. For example, "rage causes qi to rise up", "over joy causes qi to move slowly", "grief causes qi to be consumed", "great fear causes qi to sink", "great fright causes qi to disarranged", "over-thinking causes qi stagnation". In addition, many special nursing methods noted in *Huang Di Nei Jing* (*The Yellow Emperor's Inner Classic*) such as acupuncture and moxibustion, *dǎo yǐn* (导引), *tui na* (Chinese medical massage) and hot compressing are still applied in the clinical nursing up to the present.

Shang Han Za Bing Lun (*Treatise on Cold Damage and Miscellaneous Diseases*) is the most influential masterwork of clinical medicine in China written by a famous physician Zhang Zhong-jing (150-219AD) of the late East Han dynasty (25-220AD). This work sums up clinical experience of many doctors before the East Han dynasty (25-220AD). It not only establishes the foundation of the system of treatment based on syndrome differentiation of TCM, but also expounds the theory and methods of nursing based on syndrome differentiation of disease and starts the clinical nursing based on syndrome differentiation. In the aspect of nursing techniques and manipulations, it expounds in detail the fumigating and steaming therapy, smoke fumigating therapy, medicated hip bath therapy, needle-cauterizing therapy, spot ironing therapy and feet-soaking therapy. Especially the medicated clyster therapy initiated by Zhang Zhong-jing (150-219AD), such as the honey suppository and pig's bile enema, fully reflects the advanced level of nursing of the East Han dynasty. In the aspect of emergency nursing, the way to treat the self-hanging person recorded in the book is similar to the modern pneumatogenie. In terms of medication nursing, *Shang Han Za Bing Lun* (*Treatise on Cold Damage and Miscellaneous Diseases*) also expatiates herbal decocting methods, precautions for decoction, effect watching after decoction taking and diet taboos. One can find these nursing requests in the annotations of many prescriptions of this book, such as *Da Qing Long Tang* (大青龙汤, Major Green Dragon Decoction), *Wu Ling San* (五苓散, Five Substances Powder with Poria), *Shi Zao Tang* (十枣汤, Ten Jujubes Decoction), *Da Cheng Qi Tang* (大承气汤, Major Purgative Decoction), *Gan Cao Fu Zi Tang* (甘草附子汤, Licorice and Aconite Decoction), *Fang Ji Huang Qi Tang* (防己黄芪汤, Stephania Root and Astragalus Decoction). For example, in the annotation of *Gui Zhi Tang* (桂枝汤, Cinnamon Twig Decoction), it notes that "one may use seven litres (1 ancient litre is equal to 1.5 kg) of water to decoct the herbs with slight fire and stop decocting when the decoction becomes three litres, then get rid of the dreg and drink one litre." It requires that after taking the decoction one may "eat one litre hot gruel to help exert the power of the decoction" and "keep warm with quilt for about two hours and mildly sweat all over to get better effect," but the diaphoresis "should not be too heavy, or the illness wouldn't be cured." In the aspect of diet taboos after dosing it advises that after taking *Gui Zhi Tang* (桂枝汤, Cinnamon Twig Decoction) one should "keep away from the food that is raw and cold, sticky and slippery, meaty and starchy, pungent and spicy, alcoholic and milky or effluvial". *Shang Han Za Bing Lun* also has a special chapter dealing with diet nursing. For example, the taboos of eating bird, beast, fish, worm and for eating fruit, vegetable, paddy, the taboos of visceral illness, seasonal food taboos, cold and hot food taboos and food taboos of pregnant women. It clearly points out that diet should be decided by syndrome differentiation. It indicates that "some food you eat is good for your body, while some is harmful. Fit food benefits the body, while harmful food leads to illness." In food sanitation, it warns that "stale meal, rotten meat and olid fish is harm for the body", "eating too many plums will injure the teeth", "the meat must be rotten and inedible if it floats on water", "the meat with white dots on it is inedible". In the aspects of treatment and nursing, *Shang Han Za Bing Lun* (*Treatise on Cold Damage and Miscellaneous Diseases*) emphasizes the viewpoints of prevention in advance when illness doesn't occur, treatment at early stage when illness occurs and prevention from further progressing and advancing of illness. It says that "it is better to reinforce the spleen for treatment of a liver disease since the liver disease often affects the spleen."

Hua Tuo (145-208AD), a noted physician of the late Han and Three Kingdoms period, is the founder of surgery and medicinal physical training. He adopts the essence of the "*dǎo yǐn* (导引)" of forerunners and invents the *Wu Qin Xi* (five mimic-animal games) which imitates the motions of the five animals of tiger, dear, bear, monkey and bird. He holds that for keeping fit one "should have moderate labor but should not overstrain, because movement promotes easy digestion and smooth blood circulation. And people can avoid diseases just as the door hinge never gets worm-eaten." *Wu Qin Xi* (five mimic-animal games) exercises are helpful for digestion, promoting qi and blood circulation, reinforcing constitution and decreasing morbid rate. *Wu Qin Xi* (five mimic-animal games) is the earliest health-care and surgical nursing method in the world that integrates medicine, nursing and physical training together. The other great contribution of Hua Tuo (145-208AD) is the invention of the *Ma Fei San* which is used as the general anesthetic in surgery. During the operation, the students of Hua Tuo (145-208AD) and the relatives of the patients were guided to do much nursing work. So Hua Tuo (145-208AD) can be regarded as the earliest expert of surgical nursing in China.

1.2.1.2　Wei, Jin, Northern and Southern Dynasties (220-581 A.D.)

In *Mai Jing* (*The Pulse Classic*) written by Wang Shu-he (201-280AD) of the Jin dynasty (265-420AD), the names of the pulses are ruled and summed up to 24 pulses. It deeply expounds the theory of pulses, compares the biological and pathological pulse conditions of different visceral organs and analyses the syndromes indicated by the pulses of all kinds of miscellaneous diseases, and diseases of pediatrics and gynecology. It clearly brings forward the theories that examine the pulse only at *cùn kǒu* (wrist pulse) and each of the six regional pulses corresponds to one of the *zang-fu* organs and reveals the pathological changes of the corresponding organs. It makes the pulse examination become important means of observing state of illness in clinical nursing.

Zhou Hou Bei Ji Fang (*Emergency Formulas to Keep Up One's Sleeve*) written by Ge Hong (284-364AD) of the East Jin dynasty (316-420AD) is the integration of emergency, contagion, internal medicine, surgery, gynecology, ophthalmology, otorhinolaryngology, psychoneurosis and traumatology and orthopedics. Many emergency treatments of all these branches noted in this book involve nursing requests. For example, it points out that heavy bleeding patients caused by the trauma were inhibited from drinking water or taking spicy food and should stay in a quite surrounding, avoiding too much physical movement and emotional wave. In the prescription for ascites, it notes that "it is good for the patients with ascites to abstain from the salt and they should often eat bean meal, drink soybean milk and eat carp." The book also has the earliest record about smallpox in the world.

The extant earliest monograph of surgery in China is *Liu Juan Zi Gui Yi Fang* (*Liu Juan-zi's Ghost-Bequeathed Formulas*) of the Northern and Southern dynasties (420-589AD). It records that one should keep the surroundings sanitary and quiet while pushing back the prolapsed intestines of the patients of abdominal traumatism. Besides, one should also pay attention to keeping the herbal paste wet in using external plastering therapy and change the herbal paste when it turns dry. All of these are noticeable issues in nursing.

1.2.1.3 Sui, Tang Dynasties and the Five Dynasties Period (581-960AD)

Zhu Bing Yuan Hou Lun (*Treatise on the Origins and Manifestations of Various Diseases*) compiled by Chao Yuan-fang (550-630AD), a renowned doctor of the Sui dynasty (581-681AD) describes causes, pathogens, manifestations, diagnoses, prevention and nursing of many kinds of diseases and also records many methods of life cultivation and *dǎo yǐn* (导引) exercises. For example, in the part of diabetes mellitus, it notes that "this disease is caused by eating too much greasy and tasty food, the patients must be always indulging in fatty and delicious food." In surgery, this book introduces diet nursing after the operation of intestinal anastomosis. In gynecology nursing, Xu Zhi-cai (492-572AD) of the North Qi dynasty (550-577AD) summarizes the "Cultivating Methods for Ten pregnant Months" which emphasizes dietary nursing, daily life style and emotion regulation during gestation period. They play positive roles in safeguarding the body and mind of pregnant women and protecting the fetus and preventing miscarriage. He also introduces nursing methods for the breast carbuncle during the lactation. It suggests that one may "use hands to twiddle and squeeze the milk out of the breast and ask other people to help suckle the breast," in order to discharge the stagnated milk and disperse the breast carbuncle. This kind of nursing method is in use up to the present. In pediatrics, he advocates that on mild and windless days one may make the infant gambol in the sunlight so as to keep him healthy and endurable to the wind and cold and avoid illnesses.

The masterpiece of *Qian Jin Yao Fang* (*Important Formulas Worth a Thousand Gold Pieces*) compiled by Sun Si-miao (541-682AD) of the Tang dynasty (618-907AD) expatiates on the content of nursing, dietotherapy and health cultivation, and attaches importance to health care and treatment of women and children. The book insists that dietotherapy has precedence over medicine therapy. In this book there is dietotherapy as well as medicine therapy for treatment of all kinds of diseases. For example, let the patients eat animal's liver to treat blurred vision, eat grain husk porridge to prevent and treat beriberi, and take *Gua Lou* (Trichosanthes Ririlowii Maxim) to treat diabetes. For the nursing of diabetes mellitus, Sun Si-miao (541-682AD) advocates the importance of diet. He pointed out that "the three noticeable things are alcohol, sexual intercourse and salty or starchy food." For the nursing manipulation technique, he initiates using thin shallot tube as the catheter. It is more than 1,200 years earlier than the urethral catheterization using rubber tube invented by Frenchmen. His proposition of prevention first is quite clear. He protests that "the lofty doctors treat the patients when his disease is still in latent period". He enlightens people that one should "remember not to spit at random" and "should not share clothes, towel, comb, pillow and mirror with others" so as to prevent contagion.

In this book, Sun Si-miao (541-682AD) writes two pieces respectively named "how does the divine doctor study the medicine" and "the divine doctor should be accomplished and honest" specially focusing on the virtue of the doctor. He emphasizes the importance of the virtue of the doctor, which suggests that the doctor should treat the patients equally without discrimination whether they are poor or wealthy. The doctor should be serious, religious and wholehearted while treating patients. He admonishes that the doctor should never regard the medical practice as the means of capturing lucre. The doctor should also have an elegant appearance and a sense of social responsibility.

Wang Tao (670-755AD), another famous doctor in Tang dynasty, compiles an integrative magnum opus named *Wai Tai Mi Yao* (*Arcane Essentials from the Imperial Library*), which dissertates nursing measures such as observation of the state of illness, diet nursing, and daily life regulation of many diseases, including exogenous febrile disease, tuberculosis, malaria, smallpox, cholera. For example, about the observation of the state of patients with phthisis, he pointed out that in the afternoon the symptoms of tidal fever, night sweat and flushed face may appear, which are signals of aggravation of illness when accompanied by increasing thinness, red-black excrement or ascites. The book also has the particular description of observation of jaundice. It writes that one may "immerse a piece of silk in the urine everyday and mark the date on the silk and the gradual fading of the urine-immersed silk means recovering." In addition, the book notices that the urine of the patients with diabetes mellitus is sugary, and diabetes mellitus can be treated by dietotherapy and daily life regulation.

1.2.1.4   Song, Jin, Yuan Dynasties (960-1368AD)

After the Song dynasty (960-1279AD), the development of paper making industry and typography gives advantage to the compilation and generalization of medical masterpieces. Different medical schools create an active atmosphere and contend for their own unique academic views.

Among the famous "four physicians in the Jin and Yuan dynasties", Li Dong-yuan (1180-1251AD) creates the theory of the spleen and stomach. He attaches importance to regulating and nursing the spleen and stomach. He puts forward a series of propositions about nursing of the spleen and stomach. For example, one should "never eat after rage," "never eat when feeling sleepy," and one should "have a little movement after meal." He thinks much of the regulation and nursing of the diet, overstrain and emotion. In his monograph of *Pi Wei Lun* (*Treatise on the*

Spleen and Stomach), there are many chapters about nursing of the spleen and stomach, such as "The Theory of Indications and Contraindications of Dosing", "The Theory of Cultivating Mind to Modulate and Nurse the Spleen and Stomach". He emphasizes regulating the diet and life style and brings forward many dietary suggestions such as eating warm food, eating less, eating nourishment. Liu He-jian (1120-1200AD) advocates the theory of pathogenic fire and claims that "all the six climatic factors can be transformed into fire." Therefore he prefers to use cold cool medicine and prescriptions for treatment of the disease, and this is later known as "the School of Cold Medicine." Zhang Zi-he (1156-1228AD) holds that "illness is mainly caused by invasion of pathogenic qi, once the pathogenic qi is dispelled, the illness disappears." He raises the three therapies of "diaphoresis, emesis and purgation" and is regarded as the spokesman of "the School of Eliminating Pathogen." Zhu Dan-xi (1281-1358AD) founds the theory of nourishing yin. He believes that "yang is ever excessive while yin is ever deficient", and fathers the rule of nourishing yin and reducing fire. He puts forward many valuable suggestions of nursing and health care. For example, one is inadvisable to be excessively fed and warmed in childhood; and one should get married at a mature age in order that yin can be fully grown. Zhu Dan-xi (1281-1358AD) also thinks much of nursing and health care of the elderly and the infantile.

The book of *Ben Cao Yan Yi* (*Extension of the Materia Medica*) records the relationship of the salt and the illness that "the patients with edema ought to abstain from salt", which is consistent with the modern nursing theory of diet that the patients with edema should eat meal free of salt or with a bit salt.

Fu Ren Da Quan Liang Fang (*The Complete Compendium of Fine Formulas for Women*) compiled by Chen Zi-ming (1190-1270AD) dissertates the dose plan of the pregnant women of their different pregnant months, the nursing methods of parturition and post partum, and taboos of food and medicine.

Wai Ke Jing Yi (*Quintessence of External Medicine*) written by Qi De-zhi has the special chapter discussing nursing. It firstly brings forward the notions that the surroundings of the sickroom should be peaceful, and that one should "just visit and greet the patient briefly and not stay long and talk much to tire the patient."

The physicians in the Jin and Yuan Dynasties attach great importance to health cultivation, health care and diet regulation. One representative bookmaking of nutriology of TCM is *Yin Shan Zheng Yao* (*Principles of Correct Diet*). It puts forward taboos of life cultivation, gestation and lactation, as well as many kinds of edible recipes of rare food. It records a lot of medicinal and healthy diet, including soup decoction, dietotherapy, and vegetable food. It summarizes and advances the valuable experience of diet nursing by inheriting the ancient tradition of combination of diet, invigorant and medicine. When it records each food, the book emphasizes its edible and tonic values related to the medicinal effect. For example, *Ku Dou Tang* (苦豆汤, Sophora Alopecuroides Decoction) can be used to "invigorate the kidney, strengthen the waist and knees, warm and coordinate the center qi." The chicken cooked with *Sheng Di Huang* (Rehmannia Glutinosa Libosch) can be used to "cure pain of the waist and back, heal deficiency of the marrow and remedy fatigue and lassitude." The Crucian carp soup can be used to "treat weakness of the spleen and stomach and heal the patients long affected with diarrhea." These foods can be used to strengthen the body and prolong life, which are delicious foods as well as fine medicine for preventing and treating illnesses. The book advances the nursing demand about the sanitation of diet. It advocates that one "shouldn't eat until feeling hungry and should never overeat", "shouldn't sleep when fully satiated and should never eat too much especially in the nighttime", "shouldn't eat insanitary or rotten food", should drink moderately "shouldn't get heavily drunken", and should pay attention to sanitation of the mouth, "should gargle with warm water after meals and should brush the teeth before sleep".

1.2.1.5 Ming and Qing Dynasties (1368-1840AD)

The Ming Dynasty (1368-1644AD) makes great progress in technology and culture and acquires prominent achievements in many other aspects. There appear many medical inventions and creations of great significance. The nursing science of TCM therefore gets further development and obtains outstanding accomplishments.

Wu You-ke (1582-1652AD) puts forward the preeminent original idea about the etiology of contagion in his work *Wen Yi Lun* (*Treatise on Pestilence*). He believes that the special pathogens of pestilence are "pestilential qi". The infection is spread through the mouth and nose. Anybody, whether old or young, weak or strong, may contract pestilence once contacting the pestilential qi. It records the characteristics of many contagions such as black plague, smallpox, diphtheria. It writes about the principles and methods of treatment and nursing for pestilence. Besides the basic principles of treatment and nursing, it holds that "it is important to dispel the exogenous evil as early as possible" and use the method of purgation to eliminate the pathogens for the proposition of "dispelling as early as possible." When eliminating the pathogens, one should "differentiate the deficiency or excess of the body, assess the degree of the pathogen, and observe the emergency of the illness." In aspect of nursing, it particularly describes the nursing demand for the pestilence. In terms of the diet nursing of pestilence, it holds that the pestilential pathogen is yang evil which is prone to consume body fluid. About how to complement liquid in time, it brings forward the advice that "when the patients are seriously thirsty and desiring for ice drink, one may supply them with rations no matter what season it is", "one may give the patients half of the capacity that they ask for, and give them the rest later on." For the patients with polydipsia caused by inner heat, one may give them "the juice of pear, lotus root, sugar cane and watermelon to meet their needs at intervals". The purpose is to clear heat, relieve thirst and generate liquid.

Ben Cao Gang Mu (*The Grand Compendium of Materia Medica*) compiled by Li Shi-zhen (1518-1593AD), a famous physician and pharmacist of the Ming Dynasty, is a significant magnum opus of Chinese pharmacy. Li Shi-zhen (1518-1593AD) picks and processes herbal medicines in person. He not only visits and treats the patients but also decocts the herbs and feeds the decoction to the patients, and guides his disciples or the kinfolks of the patients to do the nursing job.

Zhang Jing-yue (1563-1640), another famous doctor, writes in his work *Jing Yue Quan Shu* (*The Complete Works of [Zhang] Jing-yue*) that "the patient with exogenous febrile disease has the tabus of diet......One shouldn't force the patient to eat if he has no appetite, and constrained diet may aid the evil." This illuminates the importance of diet nursing. At that time there is already the specific cognition that pestilence is a contagious illness. For example, Hu Zhengxin, a famous physician, says that "the family whose member has contracted plague should braise the clothes of the patient in the container, and then the other members of the family can be free of the plague." This explicitly points out that the clothes of the contagious patients should be disposed with the method of steam sterilizing.

Leng Qian of the Ming Dynasty (1368-1644AD) puts forward "sixteen appropriate points for life cultivation" in his book *Xiu Ling Yao Zhi* (*The Keystone to Prolong and Cultivate Life*), which says that the hair ought to be combed more; the face ought to be washed more; the eyeballs ought to be moved more; the ears ought to be flipped more; the tongue ought to support the maxilla frequently; the teeth ought to knock frequently; the saliva ought to be swallowed frequently; the turbid qi ought to be breathed out frequently; the back ought to be warmed always; the chest ought to be protected always; the abdomen ought to be massaged frequently; the anus ought to be pinched frequently; the extremities ought to sway frequently; the skin ought to be bathed with hands or dry towels frequently; and one should shut the mouth when relieving the bowels. All the above sixteen points are experiential principles for health cultivation. They are still of significant and instructive values for nursing and life cultivation to this day.

In the Qing Dynasty (1616-1912AD), after the Opium War, much western modern medicine come in China and give impact to the development of TCM. The theory of *Wen Bing* (seasonal febrile disease or warm diseases) gradually grows up. For example, the famous physician of warm diseases, Ye Tian-shi (1666-1745AD) illuminates the rules of appearing and advancing of the warm diseases in his masterwork *Wen Re Lun* (*Treatise on Warm-Heat Diseases*). He puts forward the principle that treatment and nursing should be decided by syndrome differentiation of the four stages of the warm diseases which are named respectively defensive level, qi level, nutrient level and blood level. He says that in terms of the pregnant woman with warm disease, one should "lay the mud from the bottom of a well or the blue cloth wet by cold water over the abdomen" to protect the fetus. In terms of the senile illness, he suggests that the diet should be of "plain taste," "alcohol, meat and food with excessively rich taste" should be strictly avoided. In the aspect of emotion he protests that "one should be sure to be pleased" and "abstain from getting angry." In the aspect of observation of state of illness, he emphasizes observation of the tongue and teeth and the differentiation of macula and anthema. Besides, he insists on carrying out mouth nursing while estimating the degree of the illness and speculating the prognosis of the illness by observing the tongue appearance. He also puts forward the view that "the invigorator or tonic is what the patient wants to eat" and advises to use the weighty and strong-flavored food which is thought to contain blood and meat.

There are frequent epidemic diseases in the Qing Dynasty (1616-1912AD). Therefore, in terms of the prevention of plagues, besides dosing the healthy people in advance, much more importance is attached to carrying out the measures of seclusion and disinfection. For example, *Zhi Yi Quan Shu* (*Cyclopedia of Treatment of the Plagues*) mentions that "one should not get near to the bed of the contagious patients in case of contracting the dirty evil, should not mourn the dead near his coffin in case of contacting the fetor, should not eat the meals of the family whose member falls into the plague and should not collect the clothes of the contagious dead."

The monograph of nursing *Shi Ji Yao Yu* (*Essential Content about the Nursing of Illness*) written by Qian Xiang, a famous physician of the Qing Dynasty (1616-1912AD), records dietary nursing, daily life nursing and nursing of the old patients. It records the "*Shi Sou Chang Shou Ge* (The Ballad of Longevity of Ten Old Men)" that introduces the experiences of ten centurial old men about prolonging life, preventing illness and postponing consenescence. It holds that to acquire longevity one needs to regulate daily life and diet, cultivate temperament, and pay attention to physical exercises.

1.2.2 Modern TCM Nursing Science

With the development of science and technology, TCM have made great progress in scientization and modernization in recent decades. The TCM and pharmacology have not only inherited the traditional method of TCM but also combined the modern diagnostic means and advanced medical equipment. This largely improves curative effect of TCM. The modern hospitals of TCM are set up one after another. There appears strict division of the work between the doctor and the nurse. In all hospitals of TCM and wards of TCM in general hospitals, there appears a professional branch engaging in TCM nursing.

TCM nursing becomes more and more mature and perfect under this situation. In the early 1960's, the training class of TCM nursing was held in Nanjing for the first time. The first systematic monograph of TCM nursing, *the Illness TCM nursing*, published in Nanjing in 1959 symbolizes the science of TCM nursing coming into new times. In June 1984, the Chinese Nursing Academy convened a forum on nursing science of TCM and combination of TCM and modern medicine. At this meeting, the Nursing Learning Committee of TCM and Combination of TCM and Modern Medicine of the Chinese Nursing Academy came into existence. Since then, TCM nursing science developed gradually and become mature. Many kinds of monographs of TCM nursing were published one after another. From 1996 to 2001, the Xueyuan Publishing Company formally published a series of five teaching materials of TCM nursing for the institutions of higher learning of TCM. They are Basic Nursing of Traditional Chinese Medicine, Medical Nursing of Traditional Chinese Medicine, Surgical Nursing of Traditional Chinese Medicine, Gynecological Nursing of Traditional Chinese Medicine, and Pediatric Nursing of Traditional Chinese Medicine. This set of learning materials is the only one published formally for higher education of TCM. In 2005, the Institute of National Higher Education of TCM was entrusted by the State Administration of Chinese Medicine to compile 21 books of the New Century Nursing Learning Materials for Nursing Majored Students of National Universities of TCM published by China Press of TCM.

Presently, the procession pursuing TCM nursing is ever expanding. There emerge large numbers of experts with senior professional titles. The scientific research of TCM nursing has gained new development while its academic and researching atmosphere is more and more active and its academic level is higher and higher. Academic activists of TCM nursing preside over all kinds of scientific research projects, holding in-depth discussion about development of TCM nursing. These all help improve the theories of TCM nursing to be more systematic, perfect and abundant. TCM nursing is gradually growing up into an independent and complete scientific system.

The education of TCM nursing is also progressing rapidly. The multi-level, multi-route and multi-mode educational system of TCM nursing is developing national wide. All kinds of education of TCM nursing at master, bachelor, higher vocational, technical secondary, amateur training, correspondence teaching and short-term training levels, are bringing up all types of nursing personnel that are fit for the clinical nursing needs.

Since 1977, the Chinese Nursing Academy and the branch academies of different areas have resumed academic activities successively. They conduct many nursing exchanges and hold all types of special training classes and seminars. Since 1980, the international nursing communication activities have been more and more frequent. In 2002, National Higher Institute of Nursing Education of Chinese Medicine Research Association was established and many TCM nursing education academic activities have been carried out since then. Therefore the advancement of TCM nursing also receives the attentions from the international nursing circles. Many nursing delegations from different countries come to visit or investigate the nursing work in China. This not only improves the international communication, widens the vision and activates the learning atmosphere, but also spreads the influence of TCM nursing all over the world.

(Ma Xueling)

2 Fundamentals of TCM Nursing

2.1 Basic Theories of Chinese Medicine

Theoretical framework of TCM Nursing originates from TCM basic theories. This chapter introduces theories of yin-yang, five-phase, and visceral manifestation and their significance and application in nursing. Theories of yin-yang and five-phase are also ancient philosophical basis of TCM while theory of visceral manifestation is how TCM understand human physiology.

Basic theories of TCM also include etiology, disease mechanism, therapeutical principles and methods. These are how TCM interprets pathology and will be explained in following chapters on nursing of specific diseases. For complete introduction of TCM basic theories, please refer to matching textbook.

2.2.1 Yin–Yang Theory

2.2.1.1 Basic Meanings of Yin and Yang

Originally, the words yin and yang were used to describe the sides of a mountain that predominately faced away or towards the sun respectively. In other words, the side facing the sun pertains to yang while the side facing away from the sun is yin. Yang is associated with such qualities such as brightness and warmth while yin is associated with the opposing characteristics of darkness and cold. Further expansion of this logic leads to the division of everything in the universe into yin or yang. The concept of yin-yang is then abstracted into a general division of any given thing (including living things, inanimate objects, feelings, actions, etc.) into two polar attributes which are related to each other.

Generally speaking, things that bear the properties of being warm, bright, active, external, rising, strong, invisible and functional pertain to yang; while those that bear properties of being cold, dim, static, internal, descending, weak, visible and organic pertain to yin. Qi, the fundamental unit of the universe, is also categorized into yin (heavy and turbid aspect) and yang (light and clear aspect). The concept of yin and yang is thus deemed to be associated with all natural phenomena (Please see Table 2-1 for examples of yin-yang categorization).

In yin-yang theory, everything has an intrinsic yin aspect and yang aspect which are opposite to each other. The opposition is manifested in its mutual restraining and opposing actions. For example, warmth and heat can dissipate cold while cold can bring down high temperature. Changes and development of natural phenomena are also the results of such mutual restraining and opposing relations. For example, yang qi is exuberant in summer yet yin qi starts to grow gradually after summer solstice to restrain excessive yang qi; yin qi is prevailing in winter yet yang qi begins to recover after winter solstice to inhibit cold yin qi. Dynamic changes of yang and yin qi lead to the changes of four seasons with cold, heat, warmth and cool properties.

Meanwhile, yin and yang are also interdependent. Either party's existence is prerequisite to the other party. Properties yin and yang represent, such as heaven and earth, superior and inferior, mobile and static states, cold and heat, deficiency and excess, are not only opposing each other but also mutually dependent. Yang is rooted in yin while yin is also rooted in yang. Yin cannot generate without yang while yang cannot generate without yin. Yang is within yin while yin is within yang. Yin and yang are two divided from one and integrated as one as well. Deficiency of either one will eventually leads to the deficiency of the other. It is called "solitary yang cannot grow and lone yin cannot increase".

Table 2-1　Examples of Yin-yang Categorization

Category	Yang	Yin
Time	Day	Night
Space	Heaven	Earth
Season	Spring, Summer	Autumn, Winter
Temperature	Hot	Cold
Weight	Light	Heavy
Speed	Fast	Slow
Motion	Up and out, vigorous	Down and in, subtle
Brightness	Light	Dark
Sex	Male	Female
Tissue and organs	Skin, hair	Bone, tendon
Disease	Acute	Chronic

2.2.1.2　Interaction and Relation of Yin-yang

Yin and yang are interdependent. This means that the condition of one will affect the other. They are interdependent and mutual opposing at the same time. None of them could exist without the presence of the other as they are both the premises for each other. For example, the upper pertains to yang while the lower pertains to yin. There would be no upper part if there were no lower part and vice versa. Heat is yang while cold is yin. There would be no heat if there were no cold. Furthermore, yin and yang could convert into each other under certain extreme circumstances, which are often interpreted as "things will develop in the opposite direction when they become extreme". The waning and waxing of yin and yang is the pre-phase of conversion between yin and yang as it is changes of quantity to prep for changes of quality (See Figure 2-1).

The mutual opposing, interdependent and converting relations between yin and yang provides approaches to interpretation of anatomy, physiology, pathology and clinical practice of diagnosis and treatment.

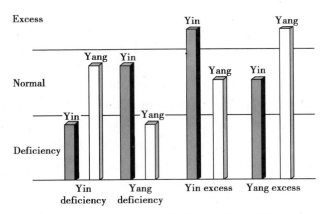

Figure 2-1   Waning & Waxing of Yin and Yang

A patient diagnosed with an excess of yang will have yang-type symptoms such as high fever, restlessness, red complexion, rapid pulse, or yellowish tongue coating since an excess of yang leads to heat. The heat of excess yang can damage the cool water of yin and can be seen when the patient has symptoms like dry mouth and throat, thirst, dry tongue. Other typical manifestations of yin-yang excess and deficiency (See Table 2-2).

In clinic every patient may present with a different syndrome, or usually a combination of syndromes, because every patient is different. Even for one patient, depending on the development of the disease, life style modifications adopted, or environmental changes, the diagnosis will also have to be modified and refined at each specific stage. The diagnosis of yin or yang is based on an integrative and insightful analysis of all the symptoms and signs of each individual patient.

Table 2-2   Typical Manifestations of Yin-yang Excess and Deficiency

	Typical Manifestations
Yang excess	Fever, aversion to heat, thirst, desire for cold drinks, reddish complexion, restlessness, yellowish-colored sputum, dark-colored urination, constipation, red tongue, yellowish tongue coating, rapid pulse
Yin excess	Aversion to cold, no thirst, desire for warm drinks, thin and watery sputum, loose stool, pale complexion, light-colored tongue, whitish tongue coating, slow or tense pulse
Yang deficiency	Preference for warmth, cold limbs, pale complexion, spontaneous sweating, fatigue, shortness of breath, loose stool, enlarged and light-colored tongue, whitish tongue coating, deep, slow and weak pulse
Yin deficiency	Thirst, dry mouth and throat, hot feeling in the soles and palms, afternoon tidal fever, night sweating, red tongue with little coating, rapid and thready pulse

2.2.1.3 Application of the Yin-yang Theory in TCM Nursing

The imbalance between yin and yang is considered as the root cause of the occurrence, development and change of diseases, therefore the basic principle of clinical treatment and nursing should be regulating yin and yang by reinforcing the deficient and reducing the excess so as to restore the relative balance between yin and yang.

2.2.1.3.1   Therapeutic Principle for Relative Excessiveness of Yin or Yang

Excessiveness of yin or yang is a condition of predominant pathogenic qi. Yang predominance leads to yin disease.

Exuberance of yang heat may easily consume yin fluid. Therefore excess-heat pattern should be treated by restricting yang with cold or cool medications, by treating the hot with coldness or "treat heat with cold".

Predominance of yin results in cold and makes yang suffer. Exuberance of yin cold may easily damage yang qi. Therefore excess-cold pattern should be treated by restricting yin with warm hot medications, by treating cold with hot or "treat cold with heat".

2.2.1.3.2   Therapeutic principle for relative deficiency of yin or yang

Deficiency of yin or yang presents with either yin deficiency or yang deficiency. It may be directly treated by the method of nourishing yin or warming yang.

In case of deficiency-heat pattern caused by yang hyperactivity due to deficient yin failing to restrict yang, the methods of nourishing yin and strengthening water instead of heat-clearing ones should be used to restrict up-flaring fire caused by hyperactive yang.

In case of deficiency-cold pattern caused by excess of yin due to deficient yang failing to check yin, the methods of strengthening yang and supplementing fire instead of acrid dispersing ones should be applied to dispel pathogenic yin cold.

According to the theory of interdependence of yin and yang, the methods of "seeking yin from yang and seeking yang from yin" may also be considered for treatment of deficiency of yin or yang. When yang-warming medications are used, yin-nourishing medications may be prescribed as a subsidiary method. When yin-nourishing medications are adopted, yang-supplementing medications may be prescribed meanwhile as a subsidiary method. The purpose is to bring into full play the generating action of mutual generation of yin and yang.

2.2.2   Five–Phase Theory

Five-phase theory postulates that everything in creation can be categorized with these basic parameters: Wood, Fire, Earth, Metal and Water. Five-phase thinking provides the basis for describing the development of forms, systems, and events. All phenomena in the universe are the products of the movement and mutation of five qualities: wood, fire, earth, metal and water.

Five phases are not just the materials that the names refer to, but rather metaphors and symbols for describing how things interact and relate to each other. Five phases actually refer to the movement and transformation of these five phases as well as their relationships. In TCM, five-phase theory has had considerable influence in physiology, pathology, diagnosis, treatment and nursing.

2.2.2.1   Basic Meanings of Five Phases

In Chinese language "*wu*" refers to five categories of things in the natural world, namely wood, fire, earth, metal and water; "*xing*" refers to the movement and change. So "*wu xing*" actually refers to the movement and change of the five elements.

Ancient Chinese people recognized in their long period of life practice that wood, fire, earth, metal and water are essential materials in human life, so they are called the "five materials". By taking the knowledge of the five materials as the basis, five-phase theory extracts and deduces the attributes of the five elements so as to explain the movement and change of inter-promotion and inter-restriction among all things and phenomena in nature.

TCM applies the laws of the five phases in characteristics, categorization and promotion-restriction relation to summarize functional attributes of the *zang-fu* organs, explain the inner relations among the five *zang* system, expound human physiology, pathology as well as mutual relation between the human body and the outer environment, and guide treatment based on pattern differentiation for the purpose of disease prevention and treatment.

2.2.2.2   Characteristics and Categorization of the Five Phases

2.2.2.2.1   Characteristics of the Five Phases

The characteristics of the five phases were developed by ancient people through extraction and sublimation based on the simple recognition of the five materials of wood, fire, earth, metal and water. They are generally used to analyze the attributes of various things in the five materials, and study the interrelations of the five materials themselves. The understanding of the characteristics of the five phases is of more abstract and extensive significance compared with the understanding of the five phases.

Wood: Ancient people stated that "wood is characterized by bending and straightening". This means that the stem and branches of the trees can bend and strengthen, and can grow upward and outward. Therefore, it is extended that anything that has the function or property of growing, developing and flourishing can be attributed to wood.

Fire: Ancient people stated that "fire is the flaming upward". This means that the fire has the characteristics of warmth, heat and ascending. Therefore, it is extended that anything that has the function or property of warmth, heat and ascending can be attributed to fire.

Earth: Ancient people stated that "earth is the sowing and reaping". This means that people can grow seed and gain crops on the earth. Therefore, it is extended that anything that has the function or property of generating, holding and receiving can be attributed to earth.

Metal: Ancient people stated that "metal is the working of change". This means that the metal can follow the man to change its shape. Therefore, it is extended that anything that has the function or property of clearing, descending and astringing can be attributed to metal.

Water: Ancient people stated that "water is the moistening and descending". This means that the water has the property of moistening and downward going. Therefore, it is extended that anything that has the function or property of cold and coolness, moistening and downward going can be attributed to water.

2.2.2.2.2   The Structural System of the Five Phases

The characteristics of the five elements are the basis for categorization of the five elements. The property and function of a thing is compared with the characteristics of the five elements to decide the property of the thing in the five elements. However, things similar to the five elements in property and function are not the five elements themselves. For example, a thing similar to the wood in property pertains to the wood and a thing similar to the fire in property pertains to the fire. For another example, the east, where the sun rises, is full of vital energy and similar to growing, developing and flourishing of wood in property, so the east pertains to the wood. The south, where it is hot and plants are flourishing, is similar to burning and up-flaring of fire in property, so the south pertains to the fire.

Taking the correspondence between man and the universe as the guidance principle, the five elements as the center, the space structure as the five directions, time structure as the five seasons, and human body structure as the basic framework, the theory of the five elements can serve to categorize all things and phenomena in nature as well as human physiology and pathology by comparing their properties and functions with the characteristics of the five elements (Table 2-3).

Table 2-3   The Structural System of the Five Phases

Nature						
Five Notes	Five Flavors	Five Colors	Five Transformations	Five climates	Five Directions	Five seasons
Jue (*mi*)	Sour	Blue-green	Germinate	Wind	East	Spring
Zhi (*sol*)	Bitter	Red	Grow	Summer-Heat	South	Summer
Gong(*do*)	Sweet	Yellow	Transform	Dampness	Center	Late summer
Shang (*re*)	Acrid	White	Reap	Dryness	West	Autumn
Yu(*la*)	Salty	Black	Store	Coldness	North	Winter

Human body						
Five phases	Five *zang*	Five *fu*	Five sensory organs	Five constituents	Five emotions	Five humors	Five states of pulses
Wood	Liver	Gallbladder	Eye	Tendon	Anger	Tear	Wiry
Fire	Heart	Small intestine	Tongue	Vessel	Joy	Perspiration	Surging
Earth	Spleen	Stomach	Mouth	Muscle	Excessive thinking	Saliva	Moderate
Metal	Lung	Large intestine	Nose	Skin & hair	Grief	Snivel	Floating
Water	Kidney	Urinary bladder	Ear	Bone	Fear	Spittle	Deep

It can be seen from the above table that all changing things and phenomena in nature can be categorized into the system of the five elements of wood, fire, earth, metal and water while various tissues and functions of the human body can be summarized into the five physiological systems centered round the five *zang* organs.

2.2.2.3   Application of the Five-Phase Theory in TCM Nursing

2.2.2.3.1   Deciding Therapeutic Principles and Methods

According to the promotion relationship among the five elements, the therapeutic principles can be tonifying the mother and reducing the child; and the therapeutic methods can be replenishing water to nourish wood, mutual promotion of metal and water, reinforcing earth to strengthen metal, and assisting fire and strengthening earth.

According to the restriction relationship among the five elements, the therapeutic principles can be checking the strong and strengthening the weak; and the therapeutic methods can be inhibiting wood to assist earth, banking up earth to treat water, assisting metal to subdue wood, and reducing the south and tonifying the north.

2.2.2.3.2　Checking Disease Transmission

By the promotion, restriction, subjugation and violation relationships among the five elements, TCM can not only deduce and summarize the law of disease transmission, but also decide measures for disease treatment of prevention. For example, a liver disease may easily affect the spleen, so strengthening the spleen should be suggested for treatment in order to prevent transmission of the liver disease to the spleen.

2.2.2.3.3　Guiding Psychotherapy

Psychotherapy is mainly indicated for emotional disorders. TCM holds that the five emotions of sorrow, fear, anger, joy and thinking originate from the five *zang* organs and among the latter there are relations of promotion, restriction, subjugation and violation, so there are also these relations among the five emotions. By application of the promotion, restriction, subjugation and violation relationships among the five elements, the emotional disorders can be regulated and cured. For example, sorrow is the emotion of the lung, and the lung pertains to metal while anger is the emotion of the liver, and the liver pertains to wood; since metal restricts wood, sorrow can serve to check anger.

The laws of promotion and restriction among the five elements are of some significance to guide clinical treatment and nursing. But they are not suitable for all diseases. Flexible application is recommended for concrete conditions in clinical practice.

2.2.3　The Theory of Viscera and Their Manifestations

Zang refers to internal organs inside the body. *Xiang* means image or phenomenon. When used together, *zang xiang* refers to internal organs and the external manifestations of their physiological and pathological states. Therefore, *zang* is the intrinsic base of *xiang* and *xiang* is the external manifestations of *zang*.

According to their characteristics, the internal organs can be divided into *zang* organs, *fu* organs and extraordinary *fu* organs.

Zang organs include the heart, lung, spleen, liver and kidney, collectively called the five *zang* organs; their common functions are to produce and store essence-qi, meanwhile store spirit, and their characteristics are that "they can be full of essence-qi instead of containing food".

Fu organs include the gallbladder, stomach, small intestine, large intestine, *sanjiao* and the urinary bladder, collectively called the six *fu* organs; their common functions are to receive, digest and transmit the food, and their characteristics are that "they can be full of food instead of storing essence-qi".

The extraordinary *fu* organs are the brain, marrow, bone, vessel, gallbladder and uterus. Their physiological characteristics are to store the essence-qi like the five *zang* organs, but their shapes are mostly hollow like the six *fu* organs, thus being called "extraordinary *fu*-organ".

Only the five *zang* organs and six *fu* organs are discussed in this section.

The organs of the organ manifestations doctrine are not exactly the same as those of modern anatomy, they are not simply organs in anatomy, but they also refer to physiological functions.

2.2.3.1   Heart and Small Intestine

2.2.3.1.1   Heart

The major functions of the heart are to govern blood vessels and house spirit. The heart and small intestine form interior-exterior relationship through the mutual connection and affiliation of their meridians. The heart plays a dominant role in the vital activity of the whole body, so it is called the "monarch" and "dominator of *zang* and *fu* organs".

(1) Major Functions

1) Governing blood vessels

This includes two aspects of producing blood and circulating blood in the vessels.

a. The heart produces blood

Blood is mainly generated from nutritive qi and body fluid, and the action of heart yang is necessary for nutritive qi and body fluid to generate blood or change them into blood.

b. The heart circulates blood

Heart qi can drive and regulate circulation of blood within the vessels. The heart and blood vessels form a continuous circulatory system in which continuous flow of blood in the vessels depends upon the action of heart qi.

Therefore, if heart qi is sufficient and the function of the heart in governing blood vessels is normal, then the complexion will be rosy and lustrous, and the pulse will be even, moderate and forceful.

On the contrary, insufficiency of heart qi will be manifested as palpitation, pale complexion and weak pulse; or in severe cases there will appear stagnation of qi and blood, obstruction of the vessels, chest oppression, stuffiness and stabbing pain, dark and gray complexion, cyanosis of the lips and tongue, and irregular pulse as well.

2) Housing spirit

This means the heart has the function of dominating mental activities such as psychology and emotion, and life activities of the whole body.

When the function of the heart in housing spirit is normal, there will be high spirit, clear consciousness, sharp thinking and acute response. On the contrary, if the function is insufficient, there will appear clinical manifestations of palpitation, amnesia, insomnia, and dreamful sleep.

If the heart is attacked by phlegm, there will appear coma, dementia, improper action; when phlegm-fire disturbs the heart, restlessness, delirium and madness will appear, and even endanger the life in severe cases.

The functions of housing spirit and governing blood vessels of the heart are closely related. Blood is the major material basis for mental activities, and mental activities can regulate and influence blood circulation. If the heart fails to govern blood vessels, such symptoms as insufficiency of heart blood or heat in blood will inevitably lead to disorder of heart spirit; contrarily, dysfunction of the heart in housing spirit may also result in anomaly of blood flow.

(2) Relations of the Heart with Emotion, Fluids, Constituent and Orifice

1) The heart is associated with joy in emotion

Generally speaking, appropriate joy is a reaction of the body to an optimal stimulation, and it is good for the heart in governing blood. However, over-joy may make the heart spirit injured and lax, leading to clinical manifestations such as poor concentration, even endless joy and mental disorder.

2) The heart is associated with sweat in fluids

Sweat is transformed from body fluid, and body fluid shares the same source of food-essence with blood, and the two can transform themselves into each other. The body fluid, as it permeates into the vessels, will become blood; while blood, as it permeates out of the vessels, will become body fluid. So there is a saying that blood and sweat share the same source. Furthermore blood is governed by the heart, so when the heart blood is abundant, body fluid will be ample, and sweat will have its source for production. In addition, the heart houses spirit, and the production and secretion of sweat are regulated by the heart spirit.

3) The heart is associated with vessels in constituent and manifests on the face

The heart is associated with vessels in constituent as the blood vessels of the whole body are dominated by the heart. When the heart qi is sufficient, the pulse will be moderate and forceful with an even rhythm. If the heart qi is insufficient, the pulse will be fine and forceless.

"It manifests on the face" means the state of the physiological function of the heart may be reflected as the changes of color and luster in the face. When the heart qi is sufficient and blood vessels are full of blood, the face will be rosy and lustrous; if the heart qi is insufficient, the face will get pale or dark and gloomy; if the heart blood is deficient, the face will become lusterless with less brilliant; and if the heart blood gets stagnated, the face will get cyanotic.

4) The heart is associated with the tongue in orifice

This means the tongue is the outer reflection of the heart. When the functions of the heart in governing blood and housing spirit are normal, the tongue will be light red and moist, soft and flexible, with acute sense of taste and fluent speech. If the heart gets disordered in governing blood, the heart yang gets short, the tongue will be pale and enlarged and tender. If the heart blood is deficient, the tongue will become deep red, thin and shrunken. If the heart fire is flaming up, there will be red tongue, even with prickles. If the heart blood gets stagnated, the tongue will become dark and purplish or with bruises. If the heart fails to house the mind, there may be symptoms of curled tongue, stiff tongue with dysphasia or aphasia.

2.2.3.1.2 Small Intestine

The small intestine is located in the abdomen. Its upper end connects with the stomach, and its lower end connects with the large intestine. The major physiological functions of the small intestine are to dominate reception and digest the chyme, and separate the clear from the turbid.

(1) The small intestine governs reception and digestion of the chyme

The small intestine accepts the chyme sent down by the stomach and holds it for a longer time so as to facilitate further to digest it into the essence. If the small intestine functions abnormally in reception of the chyme, it will result in abdominal distention and ache. If it functions abnormally in digestion of the chyme, it will lead to indigestion, diarrhea or extremely with indigested food.

(2) The small intestine governs separation of the clear from the turbid

The small intestine separates its digested food into two parts of essence and waste, and absorbs the essence and sends the waste down into the large intestine. At the same time of absorbing food, the small intestine also absorbs a great amount of water and sends the waste down into the urinary bladder.

If the small intestine functions normally in separation of the clear from the turbid, metabolism of food and water would be in order. If the small intestine functions abnormally in separation of the clear from the turbid, it may lead to mix-up of the clear and the turbid manifesting as sloppy stool and scanty urination.

2.2.3.2 Lung and Large Intestine
2.2.3.2.1 Lung

Lung is located at the highest position among internal organs and covers the others; it is thus called the "canopy". Because its lobes are delicate and communicate with the outside environment, it is subject to invasion of external pathogens, hence there is the name of "delicate viscus".

The major functions of the lung are governing respiratory qi and qi of the whole body, governing diffusion, purification and down-sending, regulating waterways and connecting with vessels. The lung and large intestine form exterior-interior relationship through connection and affiliation of their meridians.

(1) Main Functions

1) Governing qi

Qi of the whole body is governed and managed by the lung, including two aspects of governing respiratory qi and whole body qi.

a. The lung governs respiratory qi

The lung possesses the actions to exhale the turbid qi in the body and inhale the clear air of nature so as to achieve qi exchange between the interior and exterior of the body and maintain the normal metabolisms of the body.

b. The lung governs qi of the whole body

The lung has the actions to govern the production and circulation of qi of the whole body. It includes two aspects as follows:

Lung embodies the production of qi of the whole body, especially the ancestral qi (*zong qi*). The ancestral qi, which forms and accumulates mostly in the chest, is mainly produced by combination of the clear air inhaled by the lung and with the food qi transformed and transported by the spleen and stomach. The main functions of the ancestral qi are going up through the throat and helping the lung to respire, and going into the heart channel and assisting the heart to circulate blood. The lung governs the qi of the whole body through promoting the production of ancestral qi.

Lung regulates the movement of qi of the whole body. The process of the lung's respiratory movement is the upward, downward, inward and outward movement of qi. Thus inhalation and exhalation of the lung in rhythm plays an important role in the movement of qi of the whole body in all directions.

Generally speaking, the abnormality of the lung in governing qi may manifest as two aspects: one is the disorder of respiratory function, such as difficulty in breathing, shortness of breath, cough with chest oppression; the other is the disorder of the lung in governing qi of the whole body, manifesting as lassitude, faint low voice, slack circulation of blood, and disturbance of body fluid metabolism as well.

2) Governing dispersing, depurative and descending function

The lung dominating dispersing implies that lung-qi can disperse upwards and outwards, whereas the lung governing depurative and descending function signifies that lung-qi can go downward and keep the respiratory tract pure and clear.

The physiological function of lung-qi in dispersion mainly embodies three aspects: exhaling turbid qi in the body, dispersing defensive qi to the body surface (to warm the muscle and skin, guard against exogenous pathogens, regulate opening-closing of the striae to control the excretion of sweat) and transporting food essence and fluid generated by the spleen outward to the surface of the body.

Therefore, if lung-qi fails in dispersion, there will appear cough, asthma, intolerance of cold, spontaneous sweating, susceptibility to colds, retention of phlegm, edema, etc.

The physiological function of lung-qi in depurative and descending function also embodies three aspects: inhaling the clear air from nature; next, distributing food essence and fluid generated by the spleen downward and inward to other organs and tissues; and eliminating the foreign body in the lung and respiratory tract so as to keep the respiratory tract intact and smooth. Therefore, if lung-qi fails in this function, there will be shallow breathing, chest oppression, cough with wheezing and panting, or difficulty in urination, retention of phlegm and edema, or constipation.

Under the normal physiological conditions, dispersing and depurative descending function of the lung-qi depend upon each other and restrict each other. When the lung-qi disperses and descends normally, the respiration will be even and free; under the pathological conditions, the coordination of the two aspects gets disturbed, there will appear disorders of "failure of lung-qi in dispersion" and "failure of lung-qi in depuration and descent", manifesting as chest distress, cough, panting, retention of phlegm and other morbid fluids.

3) Regulating waterways

This means the lung possesses the actions to dredge and regulate distribution, circulation and excretion of water in the body.

Lung-qi not only diffuses the fluid upward and outward to the skin and body hair and disperses to the body surface, but also diffuses the defensive qi to control the opening and closing of the interstices, regulating excretion of sweat, at the same time, part of the water can be excreted through respiration; purification and descent of the lung-qi not only transmits (transports) the water downward to the lower and the internal, but also can transmit the turbid liquid produced by metabolism of the organ into the kidney as the source of urine formation, meanwhile, it can help push the large intestine to pass stool out with water.

Only when the lung functions properly in regulating waterways can the water metabolism be kept normal. Contrarily if the lung's function of regulating waterways is disordered, it will lead to accumulation of water manifesting as disorders of water metabolism, dampness, phlegm retention and fluid stagnancy.

4) Connecting and regulating all meridian vessels

Qi and blood of the whole body converge in the lung through the meridian vessels. Qi exchange is carried out through the lung's function of inhaling the clear and exhaling the turbid. By the diffusing and descending motion of lung-qi, the lung assists the heart in promoting blood circulation, the blood richly containing clear qi goes through the vessels again to the whole body. Meanwhile, lung governs regulating means that lung can aid the heart in regulating qi, blood, fluids and functions of internal organs.

Therefore when the lung-qi is sufficient, the production and flow of qi will be normal, ensuring smooth blood circulation. On the contrary, if the lung qi gets declined and fails to assist the heart in promoting blood circulation, the blood will not flow smoothly, thus there will appear the signs of qi deficiency and blood stasis marked by chest oppression, palpitation, cyanotic lips and purplish tongue.

(2) Relations of the Lung with Emotion, Fluids, Constituent and Orifice

1) The lung is associated with anxiety in emotion

The major influence of sorrow and anxiety is continuous consumption of qi, so called "grief consumes qi".

The lung governs qi, so over sorrow and anxiety may cause deficiency of lung qi manifesting as shortage of breathing. Meanwhile, if the lung qi gets deficient, human tolerance to negative stimulation will decrease, and thus it is more likely to lead to emotions of sorrow and anxiety.

2) The lung is associated with snivel in fluids

Snivel is the nasal discharge, and lung opens at the nose. When the essential qi in the lung is sufficient, the snivel moistens the nasal cavity and does not flow outward, meanwhile can protect against external pathogens so as to help the lung to breathe. If the lung is invaded by cold pathogen, it will cause thin nasal discharge; if the lung is invaded by heat pathogen, it will cause yellow and stick nasal discharge; if the lung is invaded by dryness pathogen, it will cause dry nose.

3) The lung is associated with the skin in constituent, manifesting on the hair

The skin and hair are on the surface (exterior) of the body. The lung possesses the physiological function of diffusing the defensive qi and transporting the essence of food and water as well as body fluid onto the skin and hair, warming, nourishing and moistening the skin and hair, meanwhile regulating body temperature through sweat excreting and resists external pathogens.

Therefore the lung is closely related with skin and hair. When the lung-qi is sufficient, the function of the lung in diffusing defensive qi and transporting essence onto the skin and hair will be normal, then the skin will be compact and the fine hair be lustrous, body's protection against external pathogens will also be strong; on the contrary, if the lung-qi gets declined and fails to diffuse the defensive qi and essence onto the skin and hair, there will occur profuse sweating, being rather easily subject to catching cold, or haggard skin and hair.

4) The lung opens at the nose

When lung qi diffuses smoothly, the nose will be normal in ventilation and smelling, free from nasal congestion with keen smelling. On the contrary, if lung qi fails in diffusion, it will manifest as nasal obstruction, running nose, sneezing, itching and sore throat, hoarseness, or loss of voice. Since the lung opens at the nose, external pathogens often invade the lung through the nose and mouth.

2.2.3.2.2　Large Intestine

The major function of the large intestine is to transform and transport the waste. The large intestine receives the food residue from the small intestine by its separation, and reabsorbs the extra water in the waste so as to make the waste become solid stool; then conveys the stool down and discharges it out of the body via the anus.

If the large intestine functions abnormally in conveyance and transformation of waste, there will be abnormality in quality and quantity of stool and frequency of defecation. If the large intestine reabsorbs too much water in the food residue, there will be symptoms such as constipation. If water is not properly absorbed, there will occur diarrhea, or thinness of stool.

2.2.3.3　Spleen and Stomach

2.2.3.3.1　Spleen

The main physiological functions of the spleen are to govern transporting and transforming, send up the useful essence and control blood. The spleen and stomach form the exterior-interior relationship through the mutual affiliation and connection of their meridians.

The spleen transforms food into essence, thus provides substantial basis for postnatal life activity and production of qi and blood, it is thus called "acquired constituent" and "the source of qi and blood formation".

(1) Major functions

1) Governing transformation and transportation

The spleen can digest food, absorb essence (nutrients) of food and water, and then transport them to the whole body. Spleen has two functions: transforming and transporting food and water, and transforming and transporting body fluids.

a. Transforming and transporting food

The spleen can promote food digestion and essence absorption and further distribute the essence. Digestion takes place in the gastrointestinal tract, but it must depend on the transformation of the spleen to make the food transform into essence; and the essence again must depend on the transportation of the spleen to be absorbed and transported to the whole body, all of which is based on spleen qi.

When spleen qi is strong, sufficient transforming from food and water to essence through digestion and absorption could be achieved, and enough nourishment such as essence, qi, blood and fluid could be produced, so that the organs, meridians and collaterals, four limbs and skeleton, as well as sinews, muscles, skin and body hair could be fully nourished.

Contrarily, if the spleen's function in transforming and transporting food and water decreases, there may appear such qi and blood deficient symptoms as abdominal flatulence, sloppy stool, poor appetite, lassitude and emaciation with yellowish complexion.

b. Transporting and transforming body fluid

The spleen has the functions of absorbing and transporting body fluid, which include two aspects.

On one hand, the spleen qi can transform water into body fluid through its absorption, transforming and transporting functions; meanwhile, it is distributed to all parts of the body to moisten and nourish the body.

On the other hand, it can also timely transport the surplus water in the body into the lung and kidney where the surplus water, through the qi transformation of the lung and kidney, is transformed into sweat and urine to be discharged out of the body to keep the balance of body fluid metabolism.

Therefore, if the spleen qi is sufficient, it can not only guarantee the function of transforming and transporting body fluid to be normal, but also prevent pathological products such as excessive water, dampness, phlegm and retained fluid from appearing.

If spleen qi is deficient, the function of the spleen in transporting and transforming body fluid declines, body fluid stagnates in the certain parts of body, and thus the pathological changes such as retained phlegm, edema, and dampness-turbidity appear.

2) Governing ascent of the clear

The spleen qi goes upward and thus transports essence of water and food up to the heart, lung, head and eyes; and maintains the positions of the internal organs relatively fixed.

This function can be divided into two aspects as follows:

a. The spleen sends up the clear up to the heart, lung, head and eyes

The spleen can send up essence of water and food up to the heart, lung, head and eyes so as to moisten and nourish the clear orifices, meanwhile, nourish the whole body through the heart and the lung producing qi and blood.

If the spleen qi fails to raise the clear, then there can appear symptoms of dim complexion, dizziness and vertigo; if the spleen loses its power to lift yang qi, there can appear symptoms of abdominal distention with chronic diarrhea.

b. The spleen can also maintain the position of the internal organs

Owing to the ascent of the spleen qi, the positions of the organs are kept relatively fixed which rely on the essence of water and food coming from transformation and transportation of the spleen.

If spleen qi is insufficient, it not only cannot send up the clear, but also sink down, resulting in such symptoms of prolapse of internal organs as gastroptosis, hysteroptosis and chronic diarrhea with prolapse of the rectum.

3) Governing control of the blood

The spleen governs the action of keeping blood circulating within the meridian vessels and preventing it from leaking.

When the spleen qi is strong and healthy, it can control blood circulating within the meridian vessels without escaping and bleeding, contrarily, if the spleen is too insufficient to transform and transport, securing and governing function of qi and blood will be deficient, then it will cause bleeding.

(2) Relations of the Spleen with Emotion, Fluids, Constituent and Orifice

1) The spleen is associated with thinking in emotion

Over thinking may lead to qi stagnation and melancholy, thus it will influence the functions of the spleen in transformation and transportation, and sending up the clear, then there may appear symptoms of poor appetite, distension and stuffiness of the epigastrium, dizziness and vertigo. Therefore there is the saying that "over thinking leads to qi stagnation and melancholy".

2) The spleen is associated with saliva in fluids

Saliva is the secretion in the mouth. When the spleen functions normally in transformation, transportation and raising of the clear, the body fluid will go up to the mouth, forming sufficient saliva to help swallow and digest food.

If there is disorder of the spleen and stomach, it will lead to acute increase of excretion of saliva drooling out of the mouth.

3) The spleen is associated with the muscles in constituent, governing the four limbs

When the spleen functions normally in transformation and transportation, the muscles and four limbs can get enough nourishment of the food essence, which is the source of qi and blood, then the muscles are well developed, thick and strong, the four limbs are nimble and forceful.

If the spleen's function in transformation and transportation gets disordered, it will lead to the inadequate intake of the transformation into qi and the blood, and the muscles and four limbs will lose their nourishment, causing extenuation of the muscles and flaccidity and weakness of the limbs, even atrophy.

4) The spleen is associated with the mouth in the orifice, manifesting on the lips

When the spleen qi is sufficient in transformation and transportation, appetite, taste and color of lips will be normal.

If the spleen fails in normal transformation and transportation, there will appear poor appetite, or some abnormal sensations of tastelessness, or greasy, sweet tastes of the mouth and abnormal color of lips such as purple and pale with no luster.

2.2.3.3.2　Stomach

Stomach is responsible for receiving, digesting and transforming water and food. The stomach is concerned with descending and the stomach qi is normal when there is harmonious down-bearing.

(1) The stomach governs intake and decomposition (of food)

Stomach would receive the food first and then preliminarily transform them into chyme for further digestion and absorption. The dysfunction of the stomach in receiving and transforming food and water will be characterized by loss of appetite, abdominal distention and pain, food stagnation or acid regurgitation and polyorexia, while its normal function will bring about a good appetite.

(2) The stomach governs descending and dredging of stomach qi

This means the stomach is characterized by descending stomach qi. It's normal for the stomach qi to descend. Food enters the stomach, after being received, transformed and preserved for a while, it would be reduced to chyme. Then the chyme is forced downward into the intestine by the stomach qi to be further digested and absorbed. The small intestine would separate the refined matter from the feces. The refined matter would be distributed to the whole body by the transformation and transport of spleen, while the feces would descend to large intestine and finally be transported out in wastes. If the stomach (qi) fails in dredging and descending, the stomach qi gets stagnated, it will lead to epigastric distention, or pain, gingivitis and foul breath, constipation. If the descending function is abnormal, there may be such symptoms of adverse rising of the stomach qi as nausea, vomiting, acid regurgitation and hiccup.

2.2.3.4 Liver and Gallbladder

The major functions of liver are governing the free flow of qi, and storing the blood. The liver and gallbladder form the exterior-interior relationship through the affiliation and connection of their meridians. The liver is characterized by ascent and movement of qi, and liver qi tends to be flourishing and free from obstruction, therefore the liver has the name of "resolute organ".

2.2.3.4.1 Liver

(1) Major Functions

1) Governing the free flow of qi

Liver dredges the routes and regulates the movement of qi so as to ensure smooth flow of qi, blood, body fluid, and to regulate functions of the spleen and stomach in transformation and transportation, secretion and excretion of bile, emotional activities, as well as ejaculation of men and menstruation of women. The major effects of dredging and regulating are as follows:

a. Regulating and smoothing qi movement

If the liver functions normally in regulating qi movement, the qi flow will be smooth, with harmony of qi and blood, smoothness of meridians and collaterals and normal activities of the organs. Hypofunction of liver in regulating and smoothing qi movement will lead to obstructed qi movement, manifesting as distending pain and discomfort of the chest, two breasts or lateral parts of the lower abdomen, hypochondria, as well as pathological symptoms of blood circulation and body fluid metabolism. On the other hand, hyperactivity of liver in regulating and smoothing qi movement will result in ascent of qi, with pathological changes of adverse rise of liver qi manifesting as distending pain of the head and eyes, red face and eyes, irritability, or even adverse rising of blood following qi with hematemesis and hemoptysis.

b. Promoting circulation of blood and body fluid

If qi flows normally, blood will circulate soundly. On the contrary, if qi gets stagnated, blood and body fluid will get stagnated. The liver can regulate and dredge the activity of ascending, descending, inward and outward movement of qi. If the liver functions normally in governing the free flow of qi, circulation of blood and distribution of body fluid will be smooth. On the contrary, if liver qi gets stagnated, it will lead to disturbance of blood and body fluid circulation. For example, longtime stagnation of qi will lead to blood stagnation or tumor. If liver qi rises adversely, it will force blood to go upward and lead to bleeding like hematemesis and hemoptysis, even faint and unconsciousness. Besides, the abnormality of the liver in governing the free flow of qi may also lead to disturbance of body fluid metabolism causing pathological changes of water dampness and retention of phlegm and fluid.

c. Promoting transformation and transportation of the spleen and stomach

On the one hand, when the liver functions normally, qi flows freely and smoothly, spleen qi which can raise the clear, and stomach qi can direct the turbid downward, then the foodstuff can be properly digested, absorbed and excreted. As the liver functions abnormally, it will not only affect the spleen in sending up the clear manifesting as dizziness and vertigo in the upper part and diarrhea in the lower part of the body, but also affect the stomach in sending down the turbid manifesting as hiccup and eructation in the upper, epigastric distention and fullness in the middle, and constipation in the lower.

On the other hand, when the liver functions normally in governing the free flow of qi, the bile will be normally secreted and excreted, thus it is conducive to the spleen's transformation and transportation and the stomach's decomposition. If the liver qi gets depressed, it will affect the secretion and excretion of the bile, resulting in pathological changes of distension, fullness and pain in the hypochondrium, bitter taste in the mouth, indigestion, even jaundice when bile overflows to the skin.

d. Regulating mental activity

If the liver functions excessively in transformation and transportation with hyperactivity of qi, it will lead to irritability and headache. If the liver functions insufficiently in governing the free flow of qi, the liver qi will be stagnated, giving rise to depression, melancholy and sentimentality.

e. Regulating ejaculation of men and menstruation of women

When the liver functions normally, the qi movement will be free and smooth, the ejaculation in men will be smooth and proper, and the menstrual cycle in women will be regular as well. Contrarily, if the liver's function gets abnormal, the qi movement will get disordered, then the ejaculation will become unsmooth and improper, and the menstrual cycle will become disturbed and obstructed.

2) Storing the blood

Liver can store the blood, regulate blood volume and prevent bleeding. It can be expressed in three aspects.

Firstly, the liver can store certain amount of blood to check yang qi of the liver to prevent its over-rise, and thus to maintain the normal process of flow of the liver qi. Next, the liver can regulate the amount of blood demanded by every tissue according to the physiological conditions of the body. As a person is in movement, his blood will circulate through the meridians and collaterals, and as he is at rest, his blood will return to the liver. Thirdly, the function of the liver storing a certain amount of blood helps to hold blood within the vessels to prevent it from losing unduly.

Therefore if the liver fails to store blood, it will not only lead to shortage of liver blood and over rise of yang qi manifesting as dizziness, numb limbs and tense tendon, scanty and light-colored menses, amenorrhea, irascibility, susceptibility to rage; but also may result in various kinds of bleeding.

(2) Relations of the Liver with Emotion, Fluids, Constituent and Orifice

1) The liver is associated with anger in emotion

On one hand, over anger easily injures the liver, leading to abnormal dredging and regulating function of the liver with liver qi hyperactivity and blood ascending adversely along with rising of qi, red face and eyes, vexation and irritability, even haematemesis, nose bleeding, sudden coma, and unconsciousness. On the other hand, if the liver fails to dredge and regulate qi and blood flow, it will also lead to improper emotions, manifesting as depression or impetuousness and irritability.

2) The liver is associated with tear in fluids

When the qi and blood of the liver is harmonious, the tear can moisten the eyes and does not flow out. On the contrary, if the liver blood gets deficient, dry and uncomfortable feelings in the eye will appear; in case of invasion of wind and fire in the liver meridian, red eyes and aversion to light and epiphora will appear, and in case of dampness-heat in the liver meridian, too much secretion in the eye will occur.

3) The liver is associated with tendons in constituent, manifesting on the nails

Jin in TCM is often translated as tendon yet it refers to both ligament and sinew. If the liver blood gets deficient, the tendons will lose their nourishment, the numbness of the limbs will be unable to flex, even tremors of the hand and foot will appear. If heat damages the liver meridian, impairment of liver-yin, loss of nourishment in tendons, and such wind-like shaking symptoms as convulsion of four limbs, stiff and hard neck, and opisthotonus will appear.

4) The liver is associated with eyes in orifice

If the liver blood is insufficient, the eyes will be dry and uncomfortable with blurred vision or night blindness; flaming of liver fire will cause redness, swelling, hotness, and pain of the eye; and excessive liver yang due to liver yin deficiency may cause dizziness and vertigo.

2.2.3.4.2 Gallbladder

The major function of the gallbladder is to store and excrete bile. When the liver functions normally in governing the free flow of qi, the secretion and excretion of bile is proper, the digestion and absorption of the food will be normal. On the contrary, if the liver functions abnormally, the secretion and excretion of bile is obstructed, it will affect the digestion and absorption of the foodstuff, there may appear distending pain in the hypochondrium, abdominal distention, and poor appetite, nausea, vomit. If the bile goes adversely upward, there may occur bitter taste in the mouth, or vomiting with bitter liquid yellowish and green in color; if the bile spreads out from the bile tract, there may appear jaundice all over the body such as skin, face, and eyes.

2.2.3.5 Kidney and Urinary Bladder

2.2.3.5.1 Kidney

The major functions of the kidney are storing essence, governing water and governing qi reception. The kidney and urinary bladder form the exterior-interior relationship through mutual connection and affiliation of their meridians. The kidney stores the innate essence, which is the origin of life, so it is called "the foundation of congenital (prenatal) constitution".

(1) Major Functions

1) Storing essence

Kidney stores essential qi. It prevents qi from escaping, and promotes individual growth, development and reproduction and modulates visceral activities of the whole body. The kidney is the root for storage, being in charge of storing essence. The essence stored in the kidney includes "congenital essence" and "acquired essence". The congenital essence comes from the reproductive essence of one's parents and provides the original substance to compose embryo, also called "reproductive essence". The acquired essence comes from the water and food essence transformed and transported by the spleen and stomach. After birth, the water and food essence is stored in every *zang-fu* organs, so is called "visceral essence". After supporting the functions of every *zang-fu* organs, the residual part of the visceral essence is transported into the kidney to supplement and nourish the congenital essence. The congenital essence and the acquired essence combine with each other to form the kidney essence. The kidney essence is the material basis for generation of kidney qi.

The physiological effects of the essential qi in the kidney are mainly to promote the growth, development, reproduction and modulate activities of the whole body. There is a life law of birth, growth, prime, aging and death in human body, and the whole process of life is influenced by qi of the kidney-essence.

When the essential qi is sufficient, the growth, development and reproduction will be normal and sound. Contrarily, if the essential qi gets deficient, there could be poor development in children, early senility, hyposexuality, amenorrhea and sterility in adult. So taking good care of essential qi is of great importance to maintaining health, preventing premature senility, and prolonging life.

The kidney essence can transform into kidney qi, and the kidney qi can present with physiological effects of two respects of kidney yin and kidney yang. The kidney yin has the effect of moistening, calming and inhibiting; while the kidney yang warming, propelling and exciting. The kidney yin and kidney yang restrict each other and depend on each other to maintain the balance of yin and yang of every *zang-fu* organs. In case of kidney yin deficiency, there may appear internal heat with restlessness in palms, soles and the chest, sore and weak feeling of the waist and knees, tinnitus, dizziness, nocturnal seminal emission, red tongue with lack of moisture; and if kidney yang is deficient, there may occur cold body and limbs, cold pain and weakness of the waist and knees, clear urine with increased volume, or inhibited urination, enuresis, sexual hypofunction and edema as well as pale tongue.

2) Governing water

Kidney controls and regulates the distribution and excretion of water in the body so as to balance water metabolism. The whole process of water metabolism is concerned with a series of physiological activities of several organs, however the essential qi in the kidney plays a controlling and regulating role. If the steaming and transformation of essential qi in the kidney get disordered, it will lead to disorders of production and discharge of urine, resulting in pathological phenomena of inhibited urination, edema, enuresis and urinary incontinence.

3) Governing qi reception

Kidney receives the fresh air inhaled by the lung so as to keep the depth of respiration. The respiratory function of the body is governed by the lung, but it must be achieved through the absorption and storage of the kidney qi to keep a certain depth. There is the saying "The lung is the ruler of qi and the kidney is the root of qi". The lung governs exhalation of qi and the kidney governs absorption of qi. When the essential qi in the kidney is sufficient and with ability to receive qi, the respiration will be even and harmonious. On the contrary, if the essential qi in the kidney gets deficient and with no power to receive qi, then lung qi cannot go down, but float upward, manifesting as pathological phenomena of tachypnea, dyspnea on exercise, or dyspnea with prolonged expiration, and decompensation.

(2) Relations of the Kidney with Emotion, Fluids, Constituent and Orifice

1) The kidney is associated with fear in emotion

Great fear makes qi sink. If a person is in a state of great fear, the kidney qi will fail to go up and conversely go downward, thus the kidney qi cannot normally spread, the symptoms of incontinence of urination and stool will occur.

2) The kidney is associated with spittle in fluids

Too much or prolonged excretion of the spittle will be apt to consume the kidney essence. So health preservation specialists suggest that one should touch the palate with the tongue for a while until spittle is full of the mouth, then swallow it down to nurture the essential qi in the kidney, this is so called "drinking nourishing nectar".

3) The kidney is associated with the bone in constituent, generating marrow, and manifesting on the hair

When the kidney essence is sufficient, the bone will be strong and firm with teeth solidity, so tooth is called the surplus of the bone. If the kidney essence gets deficient, the bone marrow will be short, and the bone has less nourishment, then there may appear stunt, weak bone with no strength, delayed closure of the fontanel in children; weak waist and knees, inability to walk in adults; and fragile and weak bone subject to fracture, flexible teeth in the elderly people.

When kidney qi is abundant, the hair will be dense and jet black with luster; contrarily, as the kidney qi gets deficient, the hair will lose its nourishment, leading to grey with falling off, dry with no luster.

4) The kidney is associated with the ear and two yin organs (genital and anus) in orifice

When the essential qi in the kidney is sufficient, the sea of marrow will get nourished and the hearing will be sharp. On the contrary, if the essential qi in the kidney gets deficient, the sea of marrow will lose its nourishment, leading to blunt hearing, tinnitus, or even deafness. Two yin organs are genital and anus. The genital has the function of urination and reproduction, and the anus is the passage to discharge feces.

The reproduction function of human beings depends upon the abundance of the essential qi. The discharge of urine and feces is closely related to qi transformation of the kidney. Therefore there is the saying "the kidney is in charge of urine and feces" and "the kidney opens at the two yin organs".

2.2.3.5.2 Urinary Bladder

The major function of the urinary bladder is to store and discharge urine. The urine is produced from the water under qi transformation of the kidney, and then poured into the bladder for storage.

If kidney qi is sufficient, the bladder closes and opens orderly, then the function of storing and discharging urine will be normal. If the essential qi fails in transformation due to deficiency, the urinary bladder will also have difficulty in qi transformation, leading to obstruction of urination, even the retention of urine. If the kidney qi fails in fixation due to deficiency, the urinary bladder will be unable to control, and symptoms such as frequent urination, enuresis, and urinary incontinence will appear.

2.2.3.6 Pericardium and *Sanjiao*

2.2.3.6.1 Pericardium

Pericardium in TCM is referring to the outer membrane that encloses the heart, whose function is to protect the heart by undertaking pathogens invading the heart.

In the theory of visceral manifestation, the heart, the monarch organ, is so important that it can never be invaded by any pathogens. Therefore, the pericardium serve as the frontier protection for the heart, which often manifests as disorders of consciousness, as the heart fails to store the spirit. In warm diseases by external pathogens, warm pathogen invades inward, leading to coma, high fever, delirium and other symptoms of disturbed heart spirit. These manifestations are often summarized as heat entering the pericardium.

Actually, if the pericardium is affected, its clinical manifestation will be identical to those of heart disorders. Therefore, similar treatment methods based on similar pattern differentiation is often applied in the management of pericardium and heart diseases.

2.2.3.6.2 *Sanjiao*

Sanjiao, or three *jiao*, refers to upper, middle and lower *jiao*. As for the Chinese character *jiao*, there are still controversies about its explanation. Some experts think that *jiao* means an organ, some say it is about the food-ripening function, while others argue it means segments, referring to the three sections that the human body can be divided into: upper, middle and lower *jiao*.

Huang Di Nei Jing (*The Yellow Emperor's Inner Classic*) was the first book using the term *sanjiao* and explaining its function. *Sanjiao* was also categorized in this classic as one of six *fu* organs and considered sharing an interior-exterior relation with the pericardium. However, the definition of *sanjiao* was not definite in the Inner Classic and *Nan Jing* (*The Classic of Difficult Issues*) stated that *sanjiao* 'has a name without a form'. The focus of controversy in the following centuries has been the nature of *sanjiao*. However, there has been a consensus on the function of this organ. The major functions of *sanjiao* are governing qi movement and water passages.

1) *Sanjiao* governs qi movement and transformation

Sanjiao is the passage for ascending, descending, exiting and entering of qi movement and also the venue of qi transformation. In other words, the qi movement throughout the body in the organs is through the passages of *sanjiao*. *Sanjiao* governs qi movement and transformation of the whole body.

2) *Sanjiao* serves as the passage of water metabolism

Sanjiao is the passage for water movement and metabolism. It is where water ascends, descends, exits and enters the body.

2.2.3.7 *Zang-fu* Pattern Differentiation and TCM Nursing

Zang-fu organs are an organic whole as constituents of the human body. The inter-promoting, inter-acting, over-acting and counter-acting relationships exist among the five-*zang* organs. Meanwhile, the *zang*-organs are internally-externally connected with the *fu*-organs. The meridians connect all the five-*zang* and six-*fu* organs, four limbs, bones and joints, five sensory organs, nine orifices and the body surface.

Clinical manifestations resulting from the functional disorders of the *zang-fu* organs can be identified in the *zang-fu* pattern differentiation. The *zang-fu* pattern differentiation is an approach to specify the disease location and nature according to the physiological functions and possible pathological changes of the *zang-fu* organs. It is the core of pattern differentiation and treatment for traditional Chinese internal disease and essential elements of pattern differentiation for TCM nursing.

Basic theories of TCM are theoretical foundation for TCM nursing. Under the guidance of TCM basic theories, TCM nursing is characterized by holistic nursing and nursing based on pattern differentiation. It includes knowledge and techniques involved in various nursing practices including disease prevention, health preservation, nursing care and rehabilitation. TCM nursing has its unique clinical feature and adjuvant effects.

(Li Xiaoli)

2.2 Channels, Collaterals and Acupuncture Points

2.2.1 Channels and Collaterals

2.2.1.1 Concept of Channels and Collaterals

Channels and collaterals, or "*Jing Luo*" in Chinese, are the pathways run through the body that transport qi and blood, and link the internal *zang-fu* organs with the surface and other parts of the body. "*Jing*", the Chinese name for "channels" means "path", "route", or "longitudinal main line". The term "*Jing*" refers to the channels in general and comprises the main part of the channel system. The channels travel at deeper level of the body and perform an extremely important role of linking and integrating the interior with the exterior and the upper with the lower. "*Luo*", the Chinese name for "collaterals" means "network", refers to the smaller branches of the channels. The collaterals run superficially and enmesh the body horizontally like a network.

2.2.1.2 Composition of the Channel System

The channel system is composed of the channels, collaterals and affiliated channel sinews and cutaneous regions which link the main channels with the surface of the body. The channels mainly include twelve regular channels, eight extraordinary vessels and twelve divergent channels. The collaterals mainly include fifteen collaterals, superficial collaterals and minute collaterals. (Please see Figure 2-2)

2.2.1.2.1　Twelve Regular Channels

The twelve regular channels are the dominant part in the channel system, which pertain to the *zang-fu* organs internally and connect to the extremities and joints externally. The twelve regular channels include three yin channels of hand, three yang channels of hand, three yin channels of foot and three yang channels of foot. They are the major pathways for qi and blood circulation.

The twelve channels have their own starting and terminating points, running regions; connecting orders; certain regularities in distribution and course in the limbs and trunk. They have direct connection and affiliation relationships with *zang* and *fu* organs within the body, and have external-internal relationships among themselves. The twelve channels are the necessary passages for qi and blood circulation.

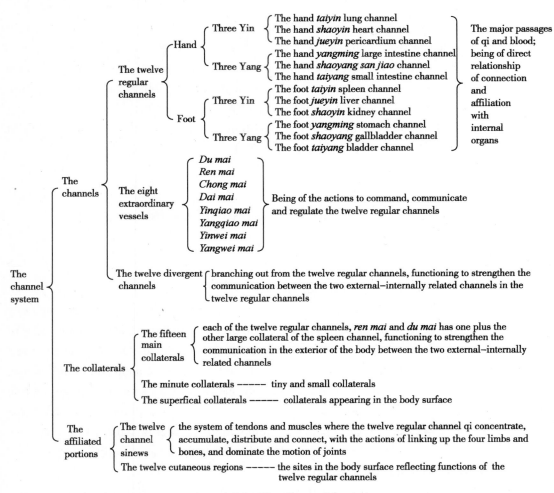

Figure 2-2　The Channel System

(1) The Nomenclature of the Twelve Regular Channels

The nomenclature of the twelve regular channels is based on three factors, which are hand or foot, yin or yang, and *zang* or *fu* organs. Hand or foot refers to the channel running on the upper or lower limbs respectively along their external pathways. The channels run on the upper limbs are named Hand channels, while those run on the lower limbs are named Foot channels. The second factor, Yin or yang indicates the channel's yin or yang property and the amount of yin qi or yang qi it carries. Yin channels travel on the medial side of the body, while yang channels on the lateral side. The yin and yang are then further divided into three yin and three yang categories in order to differentiate the amount of yin qi or yang qi of the channels. The channels that carry the most abundant yin qi are called *taiyin*, or Greater Yin. The channels that carry the lesser amount of yin qi are called *shaoyin*, or Lesser Yin. The ones that carry the least yin qi are called *jueyin*, or Terminal Yin. Similarly, the channels that carry the most abundant yang qi are called *yangming*, or Bright Yang. The channels that carry a lesser amount of yang qi are called *taiyang*, or Greater Yang. The ones that carry the least amount of yang qi are called *shaoyang*, or Lesser Yang. The third factor, *zang* or *fu* organs indicates the *zang* or *fu* organ to which the channel pertains to (see Table 2-4).

Table 2-4　Nomenclature and Classification of the Twelve Channels

	Yin channel (pertains to *zang* organ)	Yang channel (pertains to *fu* organ)	Running route (Yin channel on the medial side, Yang channel on the lateral side)	
Hand	*Taiyin* lung channel	*Yangming* large intestine channel	Upper limb	Anterior line
	Jueyin pericardium channel	*Shaoyang* sanjiao channel		Middle line
	Shaoyin heart channel	*Taiyang* small intestine channel		Posterior line
Foot	*Taiyin* spleen channel	*Yangming* stomach channel	Lower limb	Anterior line
	Jueyin liver channel	*Shaoyang* gallbladder channel		Middle line
	Shaoyin kidney channel	*Taiyang* bladder channel		Posterior line

(2) Distribution of the Twelve Regular Channels on the Surface of the Body

The superficial pathways of twelve regular channels are distributed symmetrically on the head, the trunk and the four limbs.

The terms for the orientation of the human body used in locating the distribution of channels and acupuncture points are not the same as those used in modern anatomy. For example, the palmar side of the upper limb, or the flexional side, is called the medial side. The dorsal side or the extensional side of the upper limb is called the lateral side. The side of the lower limb closer to the midline is called the medial side, while the side of the lower limb away from the midline is called the lateral side.

The twelve channels in the body basically run vertically. With an exception of the foot *yangming* stomach channel, all yin channels run on the medial side of the limbs and chest-abdominal parts of the trunk, and all yang channels run on the lateral side of the limbs and back parts of the trunk. The hand channels run in the upper limbs, and foot channels run in the lower limbs.

In the four limbs, yin channels run on the medial side and yang channels on the lateral side. There are three yin channels on the medial side, so are there three yang channels on the lateral side. On the medial side of upper limb, *taiyin* channel runs in the anterior, *jueyin* channel in the middle, and *shaoyin* in the posterior. On the lateral side of upper limb, *yangming* runs in the anterior, *shaoyang* channel in the middle, and *taiyang* channel in the posterior. On the medial side of lower limb, in the region 8 *cun* below the medial malleolus, *jueyin* channel runs in the anterior, *taiyin* channel in the middle, and *shaoyin* channel in the posterior; in the region 8 *cun* above the medial malleolus, *taiyin* channel runs in the anterior, *jueyin* channel in the middle and *shaoyin* channel in the posterior. On the lateral side of lower limb, *yangming* channel runs in the anterior, *shaoyang* channel in the middle and *taiyang* channel in the posterior.

In the head and face, *yangming* channels run in the face; *Taiyang* channels run in the zygomatic regions, vertex and posterior side of the head; *Shaoyang* channels run on both lateral sides of the head. But not all yin channels arrive at the neck and chest. Some of them run in the deeper parts of the head and face or even to the vertex. Among them, the hand *shaoyin* heart channel and the foot *jueyin* liver channel run up to the eye connector; the foot *jueyin* liver channel meets the *du mai* at the vertex; the foot *shaoyin* kidney channel runs up to the root of the tongue, and the foot *taiyin* spleen channel connects with the root of the tongue and scatters its collaterals over the lower surface of the tongue.

In the trunk, the three yang channels of hand run in the scapular regions. Among the three yang channels of foot, *yangming* channel runs in the ventral part (chest and abdomen), *taiyang* channel runs in the dorsal part (back side), and s*haoyang* channel runs on the lateral sides. The three yin channels of hand all run out from the axilla. All of the three yin channels of foot run in the ventral part.

(3) The Exterior-interior Relationship of the Twelve Regular Channels

The twelve regular channels connect to *zang-fu* organs. Among them, yin channels pertain to *zang*-organs and connect to *fu*-organs. The yang channels pertain to *fu*-organs and connect to *zang*-organs. The twelve regular channels form six pairs of exterior-interior relationship, namely: the hand *taiyang* small intestine channel and the hand *shaoyin* heart channel exterior-interiorly relate with each other, so do the hand *shaoyang saojiao* Channel and the hand *jueyin* pericardium channel, the hang *yangming* large intestine channel and the hand *taiyin* lung channel, the foot *taiyang* bladder channel and the foot *shaoyin* kidney channel, the foot *shaoyang* gallbladder channel and the foot *jueyin* liver channel, the foot *yangming* stomach channel and the foot *taiyin* spleen channel. The exterior-interior relationship of the twelve regular channels can be strengthened by the divergent channels and collaterals which facilitate the communication between the inner and the outer parts of the body.

(4) Running Direction and Connection of the Twelve Regular Channels

The three yin channels of hand in the twelve channels run from the internal viscera of the thoracic cavity to the ends of fingers, and connect with the three yang channels of hand there. The three yang channels of hand run from the ends of fingers to the head and face, and connect with the three yang channels of foot there. The three yang channels of foot run from the head and face to the ends of toes, and connect with the three yin channels of foot there. The three yin channels of foot run from the ends of toes to the abdomen and thorax, and connect with the three yin channels of hand in the viscera of the thoracic cavity. In this way, the hand channels connect at the hand and the foot channels connect at the foot, yang channels connect at the head, and yin channels connect at the viscera in the thoracic cavity. Thus the twelve channels form a circulatory cycle in which "yin and yang channels communicate with each other". (Please see Figure 2-3)

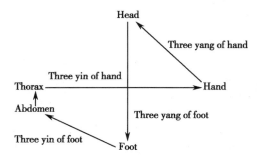

Figure 2-3　Regularity in Course and Connection of the Twelve Regular Channels

There are three models of connection in the twelve channels.

1) The exterior-interiorly related yin and yang channels connect with each other at the ends of limbs. There are altogether six pairs of exterior-interiorly related yin and yang channels. Among them, the exterior-interiorly related three yin channels of hand and three yang channels of hand connect at the ends of upper limbs, and the exterior-interiorly related three yin channels of foot and three yang channels of foot connect at the ends of lower limbs.

2) The yang channels of hand and foot with the same name connect in the head and face. There are three pairs of yang channels of hand and foot with the same name. For example, the hand *yangming* large intestine channel and the foot *yangming* stomach channel connect at the side of nose wing; the hand *taiyin* small intestine channel and the foot *taiyang* bladder channel connect at the inner canthus; and the hand *shaoyang sanjiao* channel and the foot *shaoyang* gallbladder channel connect at the outer canthus.

3) Yin channels of foot and hand connect in the thorax. The yin channels of foot and hand are also called "channels with different name". There are three pairs of them. They connect in the viscera of the thoracic cavity. For example, the foot *taiyin* spleen channel and the hand *shaoyin* heart channel connect in the heart; the foot *shaoyin* kidney channel and the hand *jueyin* pericardium channel connect in the chest; and the foot *jueyin* liver channel and the hand *taiyin* lung channel connect in the lung.

(5) Flow of Qi in the Twelve Regular Channels

The twelve channels are the main pathways for circulation of qi and blood. They communicate with each other from the head to the foot, connecting in a fixed order. The flow of qi and blood within them also follows a definite order.

Since qi and blood of the whole body are produced by foodstuff essence through transformation and transportation of the spleen and stomach, the flow of qi and blood within the twelve channels starts from the hand *taiyin* lung channel that originates from the middle energizer, in turn it flows to the foot *jueyin* liver channel, then it runs back to and starts again from the hand *taiyin* lung channel. It is thus communicated from the head to the foot, and there is no end. The following figure shows its flow order (Please see Figure 2-4)

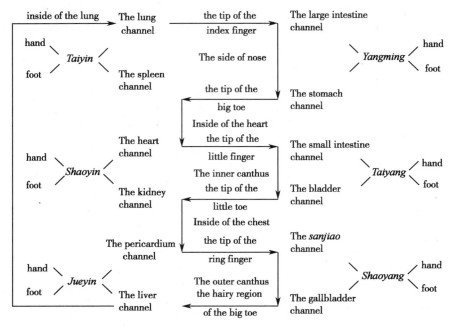

Figure 2-4   Flow of Qi in the Twelve Regular Channels

2.2.1.2.2　Eight Extraordinary Vessels

Eight extraordinary vessels are separate and different from the main channels, including *ren mai, du mai, chong mai, dai mai, yinwei mai, yangwei mai, yinqiao mai* and *yangqiao mai*. The eight extraordinary vessels are called "extraordinary" because they have no direct connection and pertaining relationships with *zang* and *fu* organs, and have no exterior-interior relationships. They have the actions to govern, communicate and regulate qi and blood within the twelve regular channels.

2.2.1.2.3　Twelve Divergent Channels

The twelve divergent channels are the channels branching out from the twelve regular channels. They originate respectively from the four limbs and run through the deeper parts of the body cavity and reach up the superficial parts of the neck. The divergent channels of the yang channels branch out from their channel-proper and still return to the channel-proper after running through the body internally; while the divergent channels of the yin channels branch out from their channel-proper, after running through the interior of the body, however, they join their external-internally related yang channels. The functions of the twelve divergent channels are mainly to strengthen the communication between the two external-internally related channels in the twelve regular channels. They also supplement certain weakness of the regular channels since they can reach some organs and components where the regular channels do not reach.

2.2.1.2.4　Fifteen Main Collaterals

The fifteen main collaterals are the larger and major collaterals. Each of the twelve channels,

Ren Mai and *Du Mai* has one and there is the other large collateral of the spleen channel. All these are collectively called the "fifteen main collaterals". The major functions of the fifteen main collaterals are to strengthen the communication in the exterior of the body between the two external-internally related channels, to supplement the regular channels by reaching some parts where the regular channels do not reach, and also to command all the yin and yang collaterals of the whole body.

The superficial collaterals are those collaterals running superficially and often appear in the surface. They are distributed widely without fixed region, playing roles of communication among the channels and transporting qi and blood onto the body surface. The minute collaterals are the tiniest and smallest collaterals distributed all over the body and numerous in the number. They are the sub-branches of the collaterals.

2.2.1.2.5 Twelve Channel Sinews

The twelve channel sinews are the system of tendons, muscles and joints where the qi of the twelve regular channels "concentrate, accumulate, distribute and connect". Their distribution is similar to the twelve regular channels. Muscles and tendons of the whole body can be divided into three yin and three yang of the hand and foot according to their distribution. In general, channel sinews originate at the extremities and converge at the bones and joints. Some of them enter the chest or abdominal cavity. However, they do not connect with *zang-fu* organs like the regular channels. The twelve channel sinews maintain the integrity of the body by connecting the limbs and the bones of the body, govern the movement of the joints and allow movement of the body. They are the affiliated portions of the twelve channels, with the actions of linking up the four limbs and bones, and dominating the motion of the joints.

2.2.1.2.6 Twelve Cutaneous Regions

The twelve cutaneous regions are the segments of the skin that are under the influence of a particular channel. They reflect the functional activities of the twelve regular channels, and also are the locations where the channel qi distributes. The cutaneous regions protect the body against invasion of exterior pathogenic factors. They are also very important in diagnosis as they represent the areas on the skin where the qi of the internal organs and channels manifest outwardly.

2.2.2 Acupuncture Points

2.2.2.1 Concept of the Acupuncture Point

Acupuncture points, "*shu xue*" in Chinese, refer to specific sites where qi and blood of *zang-fu* organs as well as channels are transported to the surface of the body. "*Shu*" means to transport while "*xue*" means hole or valley.

Acupuncture points are not only the sites where qi and blood are transported to the body surface, but they are also the reflecting places of disorders, and the sites to receive the stimulation by acupuncture, acupressure, cupping and moxibustion. There is a close relation between acupuncture points, channels and internal organs. Therefore stimulating these points may help promote flow of qi and blood in *zang-fu* organs, and regulate the balance between yin and yang so as to achieve the purpose of disease prevention and treatment.

2.2.2.2 Classification of the Points

Points are generally classified into three groups, namely: channel points, extra points and Ashi-points.

2.2.2.2.1 Channel Points

Channel points, which are collectively known as "points of the fourteen channels", refer to the points that are distributed along the course of the twelve regular channels as well as *Ren Mai* and *Du Mai*. There are 361 of them in total. Each channel point has its definite name, fixed location and specific indications.

2.2.2.2.2 Extra Points

Extra points refer to the points that have definite name, fixed location and specific indications but are not recognized as points of the fourteen channels. They are also known as "extra points outside the channels". Extra points have relatively fixed indications and most of them are very effective for some specific disorders.

2.2.2.2.3 Ashi-points

Ashi-points refer to the points that have neither the definite name nor fixed location, but are used for acupuncture and moxibustion by means of the tender spots, affected areas, or other sensitive spots reflecting the condition of disease. Ashi-points are usually located near to the affected areas. Acupuncture of these points may serve to dredge the channel for treatment of diseases.

2.2.2.3 Effects of the Points

Since they are the sites where qi and blood are transported, and the place where pathogenic factors invade, as well as the stimulation spots for acupuncture and moxibustion used for prevention and treatment of diseases, acupuncture points have the function of receiving stimulation, preventing and treating diseases. The stimulation of points by acupuncture and moxibustion may dredge the channel, regulate the flow of qi and blood, restore balance between yin and yang, harmonize *zang* and *fu* organs so as to achieve the purpose of strengthening the vital qi and eliminating the pathogenic qi. The effects of points can be classified into the following three aspects.

2.2.2.3.1 Local Therapeutic Effect

This means that all points can treat the disorders of adjacent locations. Local therapeutic effect is a characteristic property shared by all three groups of points. For example, *Jing ming* (BL1), *cheng qi* (ST1) and *si bai* (ST2) located around the eyes can be used for treatment of ophthalmic diseases.

2.2.2.3.2 Remote Therapeutic Effect

This means that some points are effective not only for disorders of adjacent location, but also effective for disorders of remote locations on the course of their pertaining channels. The remote therapeutic effect is a property of the channel points and especially those points of the twelve regular channels located distally to the elbow and knee joints. For example, *He gu* (LI4) not only serves to treat diseases of the upper limbs, but also diseases of the neck, head and face.

2.2.2.3.3 Special Therapeutic Effect

In addition to the local and remote therapeutic effects, points are also of some other special effects, namely: bi-directional regulation, general regulation and other relatively specific effects.

(1) The bi-directional regulation effect means that some points have the bi-directional regulation function. For example, *Tian shu* (ST25) may be used to relieve constipation for treatment of constipation, and relieve diarrhea for treatment of diarrhea.

(2) The general regulation effect means that some points may serve to treat general disorders. These points are usually located along the course of *yangming* channels, and *ren mai* and *du mai*.

(3) The relatively specific effect means that some points may be specifically effective for treatment of certain diseases. For example, *Lan wei* (EX-LE7) is effective in treating appendicitis.

2.2.2.4 Methods of Locating Points

The methods of locating points refer to the basic methods of determining the locations of points. Commonly used methods include the following three: measurement with anatomic landmarks, measurement with bone-length proportional units, and measurement with fingers.

2.2.2.4.1 Measurement with Anatomic Landmarks

This is a method for locating points by referring to the anatomic landmarks on the body surface. Anatomic landmarks may be divided into two types of fixed and moving ones.

(1) Measurement with Fixed Anatomic Landmarks

Fixed anatomic landmarks include the five sensory organs, hair, nails, nipples, umbilicus, and prominences and depressions of bones and muscles. These obviously found landmarks can be used directly to locate points. For example, *Yin tang* (EX-HN3) is the point located in the center of the two eyebrows.

(2) Measurement with Moving Landmarks

The points can be located according to moving landmarks like wrinkles, muscle crease, tendons and joint depressions appeared when the body or limbs are moving or in particular positions. For example, *Ting gong* (TE19) and *ting hui* (GB2) are located where the mouth opens. *Qu chi* (LI11) is located on the lateral side of the transverse crease when the elbow is bent.

2.2.2.4.2 Bone-Length Proportional Measurement

This is a method by taking the bones and joints of the body as major markers to measure the length and size of certain body parts and then converting their length or size into proportional units based on the measuring criteria for locating points. The proportional measurements of different parts of the body are introduced in the following table (Please see Table 2-5, Figure 2-5).

2.2.2.4.3 Finger Measurement

This is a measurement by using the length and width of the patient's finger (s) as a standard to locate points. There are usually three methods: middle finger measurement, thumb measurement and four-finger measurement.

(1) Middle finger measurement: This means that when the patient's middle finger is bent, the distance between the two medial ends of the creases of two interphalangeal joints is taken as one cun (Please see Figure 2-6).

Table 2-5 Standards for Bone-Length Proportional Measurement

Portion of the body	Distance	Proportional measurement	Method	Notes
Head	Anterior hairline to posterior hairline	12 cun	Longitudinal measurement	If the anterior and posterior hairlines are indistinguishable, the distance from the glabella to *da zhui* (GV14) is measured as 18 cun. The distance from the glabella to the anterior hairline is taken as 3 cun, and the distance from GV14 to the posterior hairline is 3 cun
	Between the two frontal angles along hairline	9 cun	Transverse measurement	For locating points on the head by transverse measurement
	Between the two mastoid processes	9 cun		
Chest and abdomen	*Tian tu* (CV22) to Xiphosternal symphysis	9 cun	Longitudinal measurement	The longitudinal measurement of the chest and hypochondriac region is generally based on the intercostal spaces. Each intercostal space is taken as 1.6 cun (the distance between CV22 and CV21 as 1 cun is an exception)
	Xiphosternal symphysis to center of umbilicus	8 cun		
	Between the center of the umbilicus and the upper border of the symphysis pubis	5 cun		
	Between the two nipples	8 cun	Transverse measurement	For females, the distance between two mid-clavicular lines can be taken as the substitute of the transverse measurement of the two nipples
Back	*Da zhui* (GV14) to sacrum	21 vertebra	Longitudinal measurement	The longitudinal measurement of the back is based on the spinous processes of the vertebral column
	Between the two medial borders of the scapula	6 cun	Transverse measurement	Usually, the lower angle of the scapula is about at the same level of the 7th thoracic spinous process, and the iliac spine is about at the same level as the 4th lumbar spinous process
Lateral side of the trunk	Tip of the axillary fossa on the lateral side of the chest to tip of the 11th rib	12 cun	Longitudinal measurement	
	Tip of the 11th rib to prominence of the greater trochanter of femur	9 cun	Longitudinal measurement	

Continue

Portion of the body	Distance	Proportional measurement	Method	Notes
Upper limbs	End of the axillary anterior fold to transverse cubital crease	9 cun	Longitudinal measurement	For locating points of three yin and three yang channels of the hand
	Transverse cubital crease to transverse wrist crease	12 cun		
Lower limbs	Upper border of symphysis pubis to medial condyle of femur	18 cun	Longitudinal measurement	
	Lower border of medial condyle of the tibia to tip of medial malleolus	13 cun		
	Prominence of the greater trochanter of the femur to popliteal transverse crease	19 cun	Longitudinal measurement	The distance between the transverse crease of the hip to the middle of the patella is measured as 14 cun
	Popliteal transverse crease to the tip of lateral malleolus	16 cun		
	Tip of lateral malleolus to sole	3 cun		

(2) Thumb finger measurement: This means that the width of the interphalangeal joint of the patient's thumb is taken as one cun (Please see Figure 2-7).

(3) Four-finger measurement: This means that when the patient's four fingers (index, middle, ring and little fingers) extend and touch closely together, the width of the four fingers at the level of the crease of the proximal interphalangeal joint of the middle finger is taken as three cun (Please see Figure 2-8).

2.2.2.5 Frequently Used Points

Each point is of its own relatively extensive indications. The location, indications and manipulations of frequently used points are listed in the following table (See Table 2-6).

Table 2-6 Location, Indications and Manipulations of Frequently Used Acupuncture Points

Channel	Point	Location	Indications	Manipulations
Hand *taiyin* Lung Channel	*chi ze* (LU5)	On the cubital crease, at the lateral side of the tendon of biceps brachii	Spasmodic pain in the elbow and arm, cough, asthma, distending pain of the chest and rib-side, infantile convulsion	Pressing, kneading, grasping, pointing
	kong zui (LU6)	7 cun above the wrist crease, on the line joining *tai yuan* (LU9) and *chi ze* (LU5)	Cough, hemoptysis, hoarseness, sore-throat and pain in the elbow and arm	Pressing, kneading, grasping, pointing
	lie que (LU7)	1.5 cun above the transverse crease of the wrist, above the styloid process of the radius	Cough, shortness of breath, rigid neck and headache, toothache	One-finger pushing, pressing, kneading

Continue

Channel	Point	Location	Indications	Manipulations
Hand *taiyin* Lung Channel	*tai yuan* (LU9)	At the radial end of the transverse crease of the wrist and in the depression on the radial side of the radial artery	Cough, asthma, distension of breast, sore-throat and pain of the wrist	Pressing, kneading, nipping
	yu ji (LU10)	On the midpoint of the 1st metacarpal bone, at the junction of the white and red skin	Pain in the chest and back, headache, dizziness, sore-throat, fever and aversion to cold	Pressing, kneading, nipping
	shao shang (LU11)	On the radial side of the thumb, 0.1 cun posterior to the corner of the nail	Faint due to apoplexy, spasmodic pain in the fingers and infantile convulsion	Nipping
Hand *yangming* Large Intestine Channel	*he gu* (LI4)	Between the 1st and 2nd metacarpal bones, on the midpoint of the 2nd metacarpal bone	Headache, toothache, fever, sore-throat, spasmodic pain of fingers; pain of arm and distorted face	Grasping, pressing, pointing, kneading
	shou san li (LI10)	2 cun below *qu chi* (LI11)	Spasm of elbow, difficulty in stretching and bending the arm, numbness and aching pain of the arm	Grasping, pressing, pointing, one-finger pushing
	qu chi (LI11)	In the depression lateral to the elbow crease when the elbow is bent	Fever, hypertension, swelling and pain of the arm and paralysis of the upper limbs	Grasping, pressing, kneading
	jian yu (LI15)	In the depression below the acromion when the arm is raised	Pain of the shoulder, dysfunction of the shoulder joints and paralysis	Pressing, kneading
	ying xiang (LI20)	0.5 cun lateral to the nose and in the naso-labial groove	Rhinitis, nasal obstruction and distorted face	Scrubbing, pressing, kneading
Foot *yangming* Stomach Channel	*si bai* (ST2)	Directly below the pupil and in the depression at the infraorbital foramen when looking straight forward	Distorted face, redness and itching of eyes	Pressing, kneading, pointing
	di cang (ST4)	0.4 cun lateral to the corner of mouth	Drooling and distorted face	Pressing, kneading, pointing
	xia guan (ST7)	In the depression between the zygomatic arch with mandibular notch which is visible when the mouth is open and invisible when the mouth is closed	Facial paralysis and toothache	Pressing, kneading
	tou wei (ST8)	0.5 cun directly above the anterior hairline at the corner of the forehead	Headache	Rubbing, pressing, kneading, scattering

Continue

Channel	Point	Location	Indications	Manipulations
Foot *yangming* Stomach Channel	*tian shu* (ST25)	2 cun lateral to the navel	Diarrhea, constipation, abdominal pain, irregular menstruation	Kneading, rubbing, one-finger pushing
	zu san li (ST36)	3 cun below *du bi* (ST35) and one finer-breadth lateral to the anterior border of the tibia	Abdominal pain, diarrhea, constipation, cold numbness of the lower limbs and hypertension	Pressing, kneading, pointing, one-finger pushing
	feng long (ST40)	On the middle of the line between the lateral part of the knee and the external ankle	Headache, cough, swollen limbs, constipation, mania and epilepsy, and paralysis of the lower limbs	Pressing, kneading
Foot *taiyin* Spleen Channel	*san yin jiao* (SP6)	3 cun above the tip of the medial malleolus, posterior to the center of the tibial border	Insomnia, abdominal distension, anorexia, enuresis, unsmooth urination, women diseases	Pressing, pointing, kneading, grasping
	di ji (SP8)	3 cun below *yin ling quan* (SP9)	Abdominal pain, diarrhea, edema, unsmooth urination, seminal emission	Grasping, pressing, pointing, kneading,
	yin ling quan (SP9)	In the depression posterior and inferior to the medial condyle of the tibia	Aching pain of the knee joints, unsmooth urination	Grasping, pressing, pointing, kneading,
	xue hai (SP10)	2 cun above the medio-superior border of the patella	Irregular menstruation, aching knees	Grasping, pressing, pointing, kneading,
	da heng (SP15)	4 cun lateral to the navel	Diarrhea and dysentery due to deficiency- cold, constipation, lower abdominal pain	Rubbing, kneading, pressing
Hand *shaoyin* Heart Channel	*ji quan* (HT1)	In the center of armpit	Chest oppression and hypochondriac pain, coldness and numbness of the arm and elbow	Grasping, plucking
	shao hai (HT3)	In the depression at the ulnar side of the elbow crease when the elbow is bent	Pain of the elbow joint, tremor and spasm of elbow	Grasping, plucking
	tong li (HT5)	1 cun above *shen men* (HT7)	Palpitation, severe palpitation, vertigo, sore-throat, sudden loss of voice, difficulty to speak due to stiffness of the tongue, pain of wrist and arm	Nipping, pressing, kneading
	shen men (HT7)	On the radial side of the tendon of the flexor carpi ulnaris and at the transverse crease of the wrist	Palpitation, insomnia and amnesia	Nipping, pressing, kneading

Continue

Channel	Point	Location	Indications	Manipulations
Hand *taiyang* Small Intestine Channel	shao ze (SI1)	At the lateral to the ulnar side of the small finger, about 0.1 cun posterior to the corner of the nail	Fever, unconsciousness in apoplexy, lack of lactation and sore-throat	Nipping
	hou xi (SI3)	In the depression proximal to the 5th metacarpophalangeal joint, on the junction of the red and white skin	Stiffness and pain in the head and neck, deafness, sore-throat, toothache, cataract and spasmodic pain in the arm and elbow	Nipping
	jian zhen (SI9)	1 cun posterior to the crease of armpit	Aching pain in the shoulder joint, difficulty in movement, and paralysis of the upper limbs	Grasping, pressing, kneading, rolling
	tian zong (SI11)	In the centre of the depression of the subscapular fossa	Aching pain of the shoulder and back, difficult movement of the shoulder joint, and stiffness of the neck	Pressing, pointing, kneading, rolling
Foot *taiyang* Bladder Channel	jing ming (BL1)	0.1 cun lateral to the inner canthus	Eye disorders	Pointing, kneading
	cuan zhu (BL2)	In the depression proximal to the eyebrow	Headache, insomnia, pain in the orbital bone and redness of eyes	Pointing, kneading
	tian zhu (BL10)	1.3 cun lateral to the *ya men* (GV15) and in the depression on the lateral side of the trapezius	Headache, stiff neck, stuffed nose, and pain in the shoulder and back	Grasping, kneading, pointing, pressing
	da zhu (BL11)	1.5 cun inferior to and lateral to the 1st thoracic vertebra	Fever, cough, stiff neck, aching pain in the scapula	Pointing, pressing, kneading, rolling
	feng men (BL12)	1.5 cun lateral to the 2nd thoracic vertebra	Common cold, cough, stiff neck and pain in the waist and back	Rolling, pressing, pointing, kneading, one-finger pushing, plucking
	fei shu (BL13)	1.5 cun inferior to and lateral to the 3rd thoracic vertebra	Cough, panting, chest oppression, muscular overstrain it the back	Rolling, pressing, pointing, kneading, one-finger pushing, plucking
	xin shu (BL15)	1.5 cun interior to and lateral to the 5th thoracic vertebra	Insomnia, palpitation	Rolling, pressing, pointing, kneading, one-finger pushing, plucking
	ge shu (BL17)	1.5 cun inferior to and lateral to the 7th thoracic vertebra	Vomiting, dysphagia, panting, cough and night sweating	Rolling, pressing, pointing, kneading, one-finger pushing, plucking
	gan shu (BL18)	1.5 cun inferior to and lateral to the 9th thoracic vertebra	Hypochondriac pain, hepatitis and blurred vision	Rolling, pressing, pointing, kneading, one-finger pushing, plucking

Continue

Channel	Point	Location	Indications	Manipulations
Foot *taiyang* Bladder Channel	*da shu* (BL19)	1.5 cun inferior to and lateral to the 10th thoracic vertebra	Hypochondriac pain, bitter taste in the mouth and jaundice	Rolling, pressing, pointing, kneading, one-finger pushing, plucking
	pi shu (BL20)	1.5 cun inferior to and lateral to the 11th thoracic vertebra	Distending pain in the stomach, dyspepsia and chronic infantile convulsion due to fright	Rolling, pressing, pointing, kneading, one-finger pushing, plucking
	(BL21)	1.5 cun inferior to and lateral to the 12th thoracic vertebra	Stomach disease, infantile vomiting of milk and indigestion	Rolling, pressing, pointing, kneading, one-finger pushing, plucking
	san jiao shu (BL22)	1.5 cun inferior to and lateral to the 1st lumbar vertebra	Borborygmus, abdominal distension, vomiting, and stiffness and pain in the waist and back	Rolling, pressing, pointing, kneading, one-finger pushing, plucking
	shen shu (BL23)	1.5 cun inferior to and lateral to the 2nd lumbar vertebra	Kidney asthenia, lumbago, seminal emission, irregular menstruation	Rolling, pressing, pointing, kneading, one-finger pushing, plucking
	(BL24)	1.5 cun inferior to and lateral to the 3rd lumbar vertebra	Lumbago	Rolling, pressing, pointing, kneading, one-finger pushing, plucking
	da chang shu (BL25)	1.5 cun inferior to and lateral to the 4th lumbar vertebra	Pain in the waist and leg, lumbar muscular sprain, intestinal inflammation	Rolling, pressing, pointing, kneading, one-finger pushing, plucking
	guan yuan shu (BL26)	1.5 cun inferior to and lateral to the 5th lumbar vertebra	Lumbago and diarrhea	Rolling, pressing, pointing, kneading, one-finger pushing, plucking
	ba liao (BL31-34)	In the first, second; third and forth sacral foramina	Pain in the waist and leg, disorders of the urinary and reproductive systems	Pressing, pointing, kneading, scrubbing
	zhi bian (BL54)	3 cun lateral to and inferior to the 4th sacral foramina	Pain in the waist and thigh, flaccidity of the lower limbs, unsmooth urination, constipation	Rolling, pressing, pointing, kneading
	yin men (BL37)	6 cun inferior to the centre of gluteal groove	Sciatica, paralysis of the lower limbs and pain in the waist and back	Rolling, pressing, pointing, kneading, patting

Continue

Channel	Point	Location	Indications	Manipulations
Foot *taiyang* Bladder Channel	kun lun (BL60)	In the depression between internal malleolus and the tendo calcaneus	Headache, stiff neck, lumbago and sprain of ankle	Pressing, grasping, pointing
	shen mai (BL62)	In depression at the lower border of the lateral malleolus	Mania and epilepsy, aching pain in the waist and leg	Nipping, pointing, pressing
Foot *shaoyin* Kidney Channel	yong quan (KI1)	In the depression of the sole	Migraine, hypertension and infantile fever	Scrubbing, pressing, kneading, pointing
	tai xi (KI3)	In the depression between internal malleolus and the tendo calcaneus	Sore-throat, toothache, insomnia, seminal emission, impotence and irregular menstruation	Grasping, pressing, kneading, pointing
	zhao hai (KI6)	In the depression below the medial malleolus	Irregular menstruation	Pressing, kneading, pointing
Hand *jueyin* Pericardium Channel	nei guan (PC6)	2 cun above the wrist crease and between tendon palmaris longus and tendon of flexor carpi radialis	Stomachache, vomiting, palpitation, mental derangement	Pressing, pointing, kneading, grasping
	da ling (PC7)	In the middle of the wrist crease and between tendon palmaris longus and tendon of flexor carpi radialis	Stomachache, palpitation, stomachache, vomiting, epilepsy and pain in the chest and hypochondrium	Pressing, pointing, kneading, grasping
	lao gong (PC8)	In the palmar crease and between the second and third metacarpal bone	Palpitation and tremor	Pressing, pointing, kneading, scrubbing
Hand *shaoyang sanjiao* Channel	zhong zhu (TE3)	In the depression at the lower border of the fourth and fifth between the metacarpal bone	Migraine, inflexibility of the fingers, and pain of the elbow and arm	Pointing, pressing, kneading
	yang chi (TE4)	On the transverse crease of the dorsum of wrist and on the ulnar side of the tendon of the extensor digitorum communis	Pain of the shoulder and wrist, malaria, consumptive disease and deafness	Pointing, pressing, kneading
	wai guan (TE5)	2 cun above the dorsal crease of the wrist and between the radius and ulna	Headache, pain and inflexibility of the elbow, arm and fingers	Pointing, pressing, kneading
	jian liao (TE14)	Inferior to the acromion and in the depression about 1 cun posterior to *jian yu* (LI15)	Aching pain of the shoulder and arm, difficult movement of the shoulder joint	Rolling, pointing, pressing, kneading
Foot *shaoyang* Gallbladder Channel	feng chi (GB20)	Between musculi sternocleidomastoideus and trapezius muscle, parallel to *feng fu* (GV16)	Migraine, headache, common cold and stiff neck	Pressing, kneading, grasping, one-finger pushing
	jian jing (GB21)	On the middle of the line between *da zhui* (GV14) and acromion	Stiff neck, pain of shoulder and back, difficulty to raise hands	Grasping, rolling, one-finger pushing, pressing, kneading

Continue

Channel	Point	Location	Indications	Manipulations
Foot *shaoyang* Gallbladder Channel	*huan tiao* (GB30)	On the point 1/3 lateral and 2/3 median of the line between the Greater trochanter of femur and sacral hiatus	Lumbago, leg pain and paralysis	Rolling, pointing, pressing, kneading
	feng shi (GB31)	On the middle point lateral to the high and 7 cun above the popliteal crease	Paralysis, aching pain of the knee joints	Rolling, pointing, pressing, kneading
	yang ling quan (GB34)	In the depression anterior and inferior to capitulum fibulae	Aching pain of the knee joints and hypochondriac pain	Plucking, pointing, pressing, kneading
	guang ming (GB37)	5 cun above the external ankle and on the posterior border of the fibula	Aching knees, pain of the lower limbs, pain of eyes, night blindness and breast distension	Plucking, pointing, pressing, kneading
	qiu xu (GB40)	Anterior and inferior to the external ankle, in the depression lateral to the tendon of long extensor muscle of toe	Pain of the ankle joint, chest and hypochondrium	Pressing, kneading
	zu lin qi (GB41)	On the dorsum of foot and 1.5 cun above the crease of the fourth and fifth toes	Scrofula, hypochondriac pain, foot swelling, pain and spasm	Nipping, pressing, kneading
Foot *jueyin* Liver Channel	*tai chong* (LR3)	On the dorsum of foot, in the depression between the first and the second metatarsal bone	Headache, vertigo, hypertension and infantile convulsion	Nipping, pressing, kneading
	li gou (LR5)	5 cun above the internal ankle and on middle of the median side of the tibia	Unsmooth urination, irregular menstruation, flaccidity of tibia	Pressing, kneading, one-finger pushing
	zhang men (LR13)	At the end of the 11th rib	Pain of chest and hypochondrium, chest oppression	Rubbing, pressing, kneading
	qi men (LR14)	Directly below the nipple and the sixth costal space	Chest and hypochondriac pain	Rubbing, pressing, kneading
Ren Mai	*guan yuan* (CV4)	3 cun below the navel	Abdominal pain, dysmenorrheal and enuresis	One-finger pushing, rubbing, pressing, kneading
	qi hai (CV6)	1.5 cun below the navel	Abdominal pain, irregular menstruation, enuresis	One-finger pushing, rubbing, pressing, kneading
	zhong wan (CV12)	4 cun above the navel	Stomachache, abdominal distension, vomiting, and indigestion	One-finger pushing, rubbing, pressing, kneading
	tan zhong (CV17)	On the front midline and parallel to the 4th costal space	Cough, asthma, chest oppression and pain	One-finger pushing, rubbing, pressing, kneading

Continue

Channel	Point	Location	Indications	Manipulations
Du Mai	*chang qiang* (GV1)	0.5 cun below the point of sacrum	Diarrhea, constipation and proctoptosis	Pressing, kneading
	ming men (GV4)	Below the second lumbar vertebral spinous process	Pain of the waist and spine	Pressing, kneading, one-finger pushing
	da zhui (GV14)	Below the 7th vertebral spinous process	Common cold, fever and stiff neck	Pressing, kneading, rolling, one-finger pushing
	feng fu (GV16)	1 cun directly above the middle of the posterior hairline	Headache and stiff neck	Pressing, kneading, one-finger pushing
	Baihui (GV20)	7 cun directly above the middle of the posterior hairline	Headache, vertigo, coma, hypertension and prolapse of anus	Pressing, kneading, one-finger pushing
	ren zhong (GV26)	On the middle point 1/3 above and 2/3 below the nasolabial groove	Convulsion and distorted face	Nipping
Extra Points	*yin tang* (EX-HN3)	On the middle of the line between the brows	Headache, rhinitis and insomnia	Rubbing, one-finger pushing, pressing, kneading
	tai yang (EX-HN5)	In the depression 1 cun posterior to the point between the brow and the outer canthus	Headache, common cold and eye problems	Rubbing, one-finger pushing, pressing, kneading
	yu yao (EX-HN4)	Middle of the brows	Pain of the orbital bone, redness and pain of eyes, tremor of the eyelids	Rubbing, one-finger pushing, pressing, kneading
Extra Points	*yao yan* (EX-B7)	In the depression 3.3 cun lateral and below the fourth lumbar vertebral spinous process	Lumbar sprain and ache of the waist and back	Rolling, pressing, kneading, scrubbing,
	jia ji (EX-B2)	0.5 cun below the first to the 5th thoracic and vertebral spinous process	Painful and stiff spine, visceral disease	Rolling, pressing, kneading, scrubbing, plucking
	shi xuan (EX-UE11)	Tips of the ten fingers, 0.1 cun to the nails	Coma	nipping
	he ding (EX-LE2)	In the depression on the middle of the upper border of patella	Swelling and pain of knee joint	Pressing, kneading, pointing
	lan wei (EX-LE7)	2 cun below *zu san li* (ST36)	Appendicitis and abdominal pain	Pressing, kneading, pointing
	dan nang (EX-LE6)	1 cun directly below *yang ling quan* (GB34)	Colic of gallbladder	Pressing, kneading, pointing

(Ma Liangxiao)

2.3 Basic Characteristics of TCM Nursing Medicine

TCM Nursing shares its cardinal characteristics of concept of holism and treatment based on pattern differentiation. In the long-term health care and nursing practice, nursing professionals further develop TCM nursing into a discipline which is also characterized by concept of holism and nursing based on pattern differentiation.

2.3.1 Concept of Holism

Holism refers to the concept that the human body is an organic whole, and emphasizes the unity of man and nature and society.

2.3.1.1 Human Body as an Organic Whole

TCM points out that the integral unity is formed by taking the five viscera as its center, combining with the six bowels to link the such tissues and organs of the whole body as five body constituents, sensory organs, orifices, four limbs and the skeleton to be an organic whole through the connection of channels and collaterals system; and to maintain harmonious physiological functions through the actions of essence, qi, blood and body fluids.

Different parts of the body would affect each other in pathological conditions as well. For example, as the kidney opens into the ears, and is external-internally related with the bladder. In patients with kidney deficiency, not only the function of the kidney will decline, but also the function of the ears and bladder will be affected. The clinical manifestations could be hearing loss, tinnitus, deafness, frequent urination, enuresis, etc. As the kidney is associated with the bone in constituent and could affect the bones, fragile and weak bone subjected to fracture are often seen in old patients with kidney deficiency.

Therefore, in nursing practice, internal pathological changes of the viscera and bowels and qi-blood in the patients can be understood through the external changes of sensory organs, orifices, body constituents, complexion, and pulse conditions.

2.3.1.2 Close Relation between Man and Nature

2.3.1.2.1 Unity of Man and Nature

Human are living in the natural world and the natural world provides them with the necessary conditions for existence. When the natural changes directly or indirectly influence the human body, they will result in corresponding physiological and pathological reactions. For example, different changes of seasons, the day and night, geographical environment may influence the human body.

Effects of season on human body are very obvious. During one year, with climatic changes of warm-spring, hot-summer, damp-late-summer, dry-autumn and cold-winter, human body must adapt itself to the season. For example, in spring and summer, yang qi goes outward and flourishes, qi and blood of the body trends to go and circulate superficially, marked by relaxation of the skin, more sweating and less urine. But in autumn and winter, yang qi goes inward and astringes, qi and blood of the body trends to go internally, manifested as compaction of the skin, less sweating and more urine. The pulse manifestation may also have an adaptable change following the changes of the season. For example, during the spring and summer, the pulse is often floating and large; and during autumn and winter, it is usually deep and small.

The changes of day and night can also influence human body. The alternation of day and night is the waning and waxing of yin and yang in nature. The qi-blood and yin-yang of the body can also conduct an adaptable change following the changes of day and night. For example, along with the rise of the sun in the morning, human's yang qi rises. At the noon, yang qi gets to peak, the function increases. At night yang qi astringes internally so as to facilitate rest and recover energy.

In addition, the geographical difference in living environment is also an important factor directly influencing the physiological function of human body. For instance, in the south of China, it is low-lying and the weather is usually damp and hot, the striae and interstices of most people there are porous. But in the north of China, it is high and the weather is cold and dry, the striae and interstices of most people there are compact.

2.3.1.2.2   Close Relation of Man and the Society

People are fundamental elements of society. People can influence society and the changes of society also can bring the corresponding effect on people's physiological, psychological function and pathological changes. There are many factors influencing mentality of the human body in social environment. Mental activity and physiological activity interact mutually. For example, great anger damages the liver; excessive joy damages the heart; over thinking damages the spleen. TCM nursing emphasizes coexistence, interdependence and interaction between body and spirit, and stresses mutual harmony between man and social environment.

2.3.1.3   The Holistic TCM Nursing

The concept of holism permeates all respects in TCM, especially in nursing practices. The holistic TCM nursing links local illness with general disorders during observation of patients and provision of nursing care. The holistic TCM nursing emphasizes the influences of external environment changes on people. Appropriate nursing plans should be made according to the changes of seasons, geographical environment, timing of the day and social factors.

2.3.2   Pattern Differentiation and Nursing

Pattern differentiation and nursing is composed of two processes that are respectively pattern differentiation and nursing.

Pattern differentiation is to synthetically analyze the patients' history, signs and symptoms collected by the four examinations (inspection, listening and smelling, inquiry, palpation), to clearly differentiate the cause of disease, nature of disease, location of disease, and relationship between pathogenic qi and healthy qi, to differentiate and recognize pattern of disease.

Nursing is to consider and formulate the corresponding nursing principle and method, make the nursing plan and interventions according to the result of pattern differentiation. Pattern differentiation is the prerequisite and basis for nursing, and nursing is the means and method for care of disease. The results of nursing are also a check for making sure whether the conclusion from pattern differentiation is sound or not.

The nurses should view the relationship between symptom and pattern properly in clinical practice. Symptom means a discomfort feeling subjected by patients, such as headache, aversion to cold, cough, flushed face, red tongue. Pattern is a group of symptoms at a given stage of disease, which reveals the cause, location, nature of disease, and relationship between pathogenic qi and healthy qi. The nurses should clearly differentiate the pattern.

Take common cold as an example, there are two different patterns: wind-cold and wind-heat. Only by clearly differentiating wind-cold or wind-heat pattern can one decide the method of nursing. For the wind-cold patients, nurses should tell them to avoid wind-cold and keep warm. The temperature in the ward should be warm enough for them. Food with the action of releasing the exterior with acrid-warm medicinals should be provided, such as Douchi soup, ginger, brown sugar and so on. For the wind-heat patients, the temperature in the ward should be cool for them. Food with the action of clearing heat and promoting fluid production should be provided, such as mung bean soup, watermelon, bitter gourd and so on.

The relationship between disease and pattern should be properly understood. Different patterns can be seen in one disease, while one pattern may appear in different diseases. Thus different nursing methods could be used for one disease while the same nursing method may be used for different diseases.

The so-called that the same disease can be nursed in many different ways means that the nursing method for one same disease can be different because of different time and geographic area of the attack, and different reaction of different patients, or because of different stage of development of disease. Also take common cold as an example, there are two different patterns, wind-cold and summer-heat-damp. Releasing the exterior with acrid-warm is different from dispelling summer heat and removing dampness.

The so-called that many different diseases can be nursed in the same way means that the same or similar nursing method can be taken to different diseases which have the same pattern in their course of development. For instance, gastroptosis, proctoptosis in a long standing diarrhea, and hysteroptosis are different diseases, however if they belong to the pattern of sinking of center qi, they can all be cared with the method of raising center qi. For example, the patient can be advised to have sufficient rest and avoid over exertion for cultivating center qi. Some food for fortifying the spleen and boosting qi can be recommended, such as *fu ling* (Poria cocos) porridge, *yi ren* (Coix Seed) porridge. Acupuncture *bai hui* (GV20), *guan yuan* (CV4) in order to supplement the center and boost qi.

It is quite evident that TCM nursing pays attention to disease differentiation, but pays more attention to pattern differentiation. If the pathomechanism and pattern are the same, the nursing method will be basically the same. Otherwise, the nursing method should be different. This principle that contradictions of different natures occurring in the course of disease are resolved by different nursing measures sufficiently reflects the essence of pattern differentiation and nursing.

2.4 Principles of TCM Nursing

The principles of TCM nursing are rules that the nurses must comply in clinical care, and they are extensions of therapeutic principles of TCM in nursing. They are also based on pattern differentiation. According to the results of pattern differentiation, the correct principles of nursing shall be determined and specific nursing methods shall be made. They are often universal guiding principles for caring all kinds of diseases.

2.4.1 Reinforcing Healthy Qi and Dispelling Pathogenic Qi

The course of disease is the process of the struggle between the two contradictory aspects of healthy qi and pathogenic qi. When healthy qi gains the upper hand, the disease will subdue; when the pathogenic qi gains the upper hand, the disease will progress. Thus the basic principle of treatment and nursing is that reinforcing healthy qi and dispelling pathogenic qi should be carried out to change the ratio in strength of the two sides in order to promote the patient to recover as soon as possible.

Reinforcing healthy qi means to build up a good physique and boost the resistance of the body against pathogenic qi by applying therapies of medicament, diet therapies, physical exercises, acupuncture and massage so as to gain the goal of dispelling pathogenic qi and resuming health. It is suitable for cases whose healthy qi is deficient.

Dispelling pathogenic qi means to eliminate pathogenic qi of disease by applying therapies of medicament, acupuncture and cupping to attain the goal of resuming healthy qi. It is suitable when there is an excess of pathogenic qi with no deficiency of healthy qi.

In nursing practice, proper methods such as reinforcing healthy qi, dispelling pathogenic qi or reinforcing healthy qi first and then dispelling pathogenic qi or dispelling pathogenic qi first and then reinforcing healthy qi or reinforcing healthy qi and dispelling pathogenic qi simultaneously should be chosen according to relative exuberance and debilitation of pathogenic qi or healthy qi. Generally speaking, reinforcing healthy qi is only suitable for cases whose healthy qi is deficient but pathogenic qi is not excessive. Dispelling pathogenic qi is only suitable when there is an excess of pathogenic qi with no deficiency of healthy qi. Reinforcing healthy qi before dispelling pathogenic qi is mainly suitable for a case with excess pathogens in which healthy qi is too weak to stand the attack. Dispelling pathogenic qi before reinforcing healthy qi is mainly suitable for the case with rampancy of a pathogen that needs urgently for dispelling pathogenic qi in which healthy qi is deficient, but is not so serious and still can stand the reduction. Reinforcing healthy qi and dispelling pathogenic qi simultaneously is mainly suitable for cases of both deficient healthy qi and excessive pathogenic qi.

2.4.2 Nursing Aiming at Seeking the Root of a Disease

Patient's condition is changeable in the course of disease. In the majority of cases the manifestations of a disease are consistent with its nature. In some cases the manifestations and nature of a disease are not consistent. Therefore, nurses must see through the phenomena into the nature of disease so as to resolve the disease by taking appropriate nursing intervention.

Nursing aiming at seeking the root of a disease means that the root of cause must be sought out in order to provide appropriate nursing methods. This is a cardinal principle for nursing based on pattern differentiation.

2.4.2.1 Straight Nursing

Straight nursing is used for a case whose signs and symptoms are consistent with its nature, which is also named "allopathic nursing" because it goes against the nature of disease.

This means to differentiate cold, heat, deficiency, and excess by analyzing clinical symptoms and signs, and then to apply respectively the different methods of treating cold with heat, treating heat with cold, treating deficiency with supplementation and treating excess with drainage.

For example, warm and hot medicine and approaches can be applied to care the cold pattern caused by cold pathogen. The temperature in the ward should be high in order to make the patients feel warm and comfortable. The patients should take decoction and food while it is warm. Cold food or drink should not be served for the patients. For the patients with heat pattern caused by heat pathogen, opposite nursing methods should be used.

2.4.2.2 Paradoxical Nursing

The so-called "paradoxical nursing", also named "consistent nursing", is used for cases whose manifestations are opposite to the nature of disease. This means to provide nursing methods that seem to follow the false manifestations of disease.

Manifestations of some complicated and serious diseases are often not consistent with the nature of diseases. Therefore nurses should see through the false appearances to determine the nature and provide care. Commonly-used methods are as follows:

2.4.2.2.1 **Treating Heat with Heat** It is a method to treat the pattern with false heat signs by applying various warm and heat medicines. It is indicated for patients with true cold with false heat caused by exuberant yin repelling yang. Some patients appear the true cold signs of reversal counterflow cold of the four limbs and faint pulse with the false heat signs, such as fever and red complexion. So the warm and heat medicine and other approaches should be taken for nursing. For instance, the patients should take food and decoction with warm property, and take it while they are warm, and the nurses should keep the temperature in the ward high to keep the patients warm.

2.4.2.2.2 **Treating Cold with Cold** It is a method to treat the pattern with false cold signs by applying various cold and cool medicines. It is indicated for patients with true heat with false cold due to exuberant yang repelling yin. For example, some patients with fever from external contraction appear the true heat signs of high fever, thirst with a desire for cold drink, deep urine scanty in volume, at the meantime appear the false cold signs, such as reversal cold of four limbs and deep pulse. So it still needs cold-cool medicine and other approaches for nursing. For instance, the patients should take drink and decoction with cool or cold property, and take it while they are cool, and the nurses should keep the temperature in the ward low.

2.4.2.2.3 **Treating the Blocked by Blocking** It is a method to treat deficiency pattern with false obstruction signs by applying various supplementing medicines. It is indicated for patients with true deficiency with false excess. For example, some patients with spleen qi deficiency appear the true deficiency signs of abdominal distention and fullness, poor appetite and digestion caused by failure of the spleen to transport and transform, but there is no stagnation of either water-dampness or indigested food, therefore those should be cared by fortifying the spleen and boosting qi, or treating the blocked by supplementation. The patients should take common yam rhizome porridge, Chinese date porridge, acupuncture and massage in order to reinforce the effect of the decoction and replenish spleen qi.

2.4.2.2.4   Treating the Flowing by Promoting its flowing   It is a method to treat excess pattern with diarrhea signs by applying various evacuant medicines. It is indicated for patients with true excess with false deficiency. For example, for a diarrhea resulting from food stagnation or functional disorder of spleen and stomach, antidiarrheal agents are banned; on the contrary, agents of digestant and evacuant need to be given to remove the food accumulation. The symptom of diarrhea will be relieved if the pathogenic qi of the disease is removed.

2.4.3   Emergency or Chronicity and Root or Branch

The root and the branch are relative concepts with multiple meanings in TCM. "The branch" is the phenomena of disease; "the root" is the nature of disease. For instance, healthy qi is the root and pathogenic qi is the branch; the cause of a disease is the root and the symptom is the branch; the old or primary disease is the root while the new or secondary one is the branch. In terms of location of disease, the viscera are the roots, the tendons, muscles, joins and skin are the branches. If the nurses master the branch and the root of disease, they could determine the priority and select the suitable nursing method. Because the process of disease is changeable and complicated and is different between the branch and the root, nursing method in the clinical practice is planned depending on the emergency or chronicity of the root and the branch of disease.

2.4.3.1   In Urgent Conditions, Nursing the Branch

When the branch condition is very serious and becomes the principal aspect of disease, it will endanger the life of the patient or influence the treatment and nursing of the root condition, if not cared promptly, then measures of "nursing the branch in urgent conditions" should be taken first. For example, when the patient of ulcer disease with severe symptoms, such as vomiting blood, having blood in the stool, no matter what kind of disease it is, emergency measures should be taken first to stop bleeding for the branch. Then after the bleeding stops, the root condition is cared.

2.4.3.2   In Moderate Conditions, Nursing the Root

When the branch condition is not serious, the nature of disease should be differentiated and the root cause of disease be cared. For example, in the case of fever due to yin deficiency, fever is the branch and yin deficiency is the root, so nursing method should be enriching yin for caring the root when the symptom of fever is not serious. When yin deficiency is solved, the symptom of fever can be relieved.

2.4.3.3   Nursing the Branch and the Root Simultaneously

When both the branch and the root conditions are acute, the branch and the root should be cared at the same time. For example, a patient with qi deficiency gets contraction of external pathogen and has a cold. Healthy qi is too weak to defeat external pathogen. So qi deficiency is the root and external pathogen is the branch. If only dispelling pathogenic qi is used, healthy qi will be injured further. For this case the principle of reinforcing healthy qi and dispelling pathogenic qi should be carried out simultaneously in nursing.

2.4.4 Balancing Yin and Yang

The relative balance of yin and yang maintains healthy life activity. When their relative balance is destructed, signs of the abnormal exuberance and debilitation of yin or yang will appear. Therefore, yin and yang should be coordinated to remedy and restore their relative balance in clinical nursing.

Balancing yin and yang is to rectify excess or deficiency of yin and yang by eliminating the surplus and supplementing the deficient in order to restore and reconstruct the relative balance of yin and yang.

2.4.4.1 Eliminating the Surplus

Eliminating the surplus is clinically indicated for an excess pattern of yin or yang by treating excess with drainage in nursing. For example, treating heat with cold is used for an excess-heat pattern due to exuberance of yang heat, and nursing methods include keeping the room ventilating, taking decoction when it is cool, avoiding excessive mood swings, providing food with the action of clearing heat and promoting fluid production, such as watermelon juice, pear juice, mung bean and so on.

2.4.4.2 Supplementing the Deficient

Supplementing the deficient is clinically indicated for a case with a deficiency of yin or yang by treating deficiency with supplementation in nursing. If yin fails to restrict yang due to its deficiency, which is often manifested by yin deficiency with yang hyperactivity, it should be cared with methods of enriching yin and subduing yang, and the corresponding nursing measures may include keeping the room cool and ventilating, providing food with the action of enriching yin and clearing heat, such as tremella, lily bulb, soft-shelled turtle and so on. If yang fails to restrict yin due to its deficiency, which usually presents with yang deficiency and yin hyperactivity, it should be cared with methods of supplementing yang and subduing yin, and the corresponding nursing measures may include keeping the room warm, providing food with the action of supplementing yang and subduing yin. In case of yin and yang deficiency, supplementing both yin and yang is needed. According to the theory of interdependence of yin and yang, the cases of either yin or yang deficiency may involve the other. Therefore, in nursing deficiency of either yin or yang, one should also pay attention to "seeking yin within yang" or "seeking yang within yin". That is, when enriching yin, supplementing yang should be appropriately considered; and when supplementing yang, enriching yin also should be appropriately considered.

2.4.5 The Three Considerations of Time, Place and Person in Nursing

This is to determine different nursing measures for disease according to different season, region, and individual. The occurrence, development and transformation of the disease can be affected by many factors, such as season, climate, geographic environment, especially the patient's sex, age, individual constitution, customs and so on. So in nursing of disease, analyze the concrete conditions, and thus provide different nursing care accordingly. Only in this way will the appropriate nursing plan be established.

2.4.5.1   Administering Treatment at the Most Optimal Time

A nursing principle established on the basis of characteristics of different seasons is "administering treatment at the most optimal time". Climatic changes of four seasons may exert a certain impact on physiological functions and pathological changes. Abnormal climatic change is a key factor of inducing diseases. For example, in spring and summer, yang qi rises and the interstitial space of people open and discharge. The patients should not lie on the bed covered with quilts or have hot drinking to avoid injuring body fluids with too much dispersion after take releasing the exterior decoction. In autumn and winter, the interstitial space of people is compact and yang qi stays internally. If a patient is suffering from contraction of wind-cold, he should take hot exterior-releasing decoction and drink in order to reinforce the effect of the decoction and keep warm to prevent cold. In addition, pay attention to some seasonal disease, such as *bì* syndrome, asthma and stroke, and take preventive nursing.

2.4.5.2   Administering Treatment according to Geographical Location

A principle in nursing determination based on geographic characteristics is known as "administering treatment according to geographical location". Different geographic environments and people's customs directly affect physiological functions and pathological changes. Nursing methods should differ as well. For example, it is cold and dry with little rainfall in northwestern China, people there often suffer from invasion by wind-cold. Warm and heat herbs should be used, but cold and cool herbs should be used with caution. In the coastal areas of southeastern China, it is damp and hot, people there often suffer from invasion by warm and damp heat, and nursing care should therefore be provided to remove dampness and clear heat with cool-cold herbs, warm and heat herbs should be used with caution.

2.4.5.3   Administering Individualized Treatment for Each Patient

A principle in nursing determination based on characteristics of the patient's age, sex and constitution is known as "administering individualized treatment for each patient". The physiological states and abundance or deficiency of qi and blood differ in people of different ages. For example, aged people, whose vitality is in the decline with deficient qi and blood, often suffer from deficiency pattern. In nursing, supplementing methods should be used. Children are full of vitality, but their qi and blood are not abundant enough and their viscera and bowels are delicate. They are likely to suffer from cold, heat, deficiency or excess pattern with changeable conditions of illness. Therefore supplementation should be carefully prescribed for children, and the dosage of herbs should be smaller. In addition, women differ from men physiologically. Women have their special conditions such as menstruation, leucorrhea, pregnancy and delivery, which all need to be considered when nursing measures are taken. Some drug taboo should be considered seriously. Because of the differences in innate endowment and health care after birth, individuals have different types of constitution such as cold or heat. For example, a person with a constitution of yang deficiency should keep warm and have warm and hot natured and supplementing food, and avoid cold and cool food. A person with a constitution of yin deficiency should stay in a cool and well-ventilated room and be given food with action of promoting fluid production and enriching yin.

In summary, the principles of the three considerations of time, place and person fully embody the concept of holism of TCM nursing, and the principle and adaptability in clinical practice. Only by comprehensively observing the conditions, concretely analyzing the idiographic instance, can gain the better curative effect.

2.4.6 Preventive Nursing

It has always been focused on illness prevention in TCM. Preventive care is an important part in the theoretical system of TCM. Preventive nursing means taking a certain measure in advance to prevent the occurrence, development, transmission and recurrence of disease under the guidance of the basic theory of TCM. Preventive nursing is also called "nursing disease before it arises" in TCM nursing, which includes preventing disease before it arises and controlling the development of existing disease.

2.4.6.1 Preventing Disease Before it Arises

This implies that before a disease occurs, various measures should be taken to prevent its occurrence. The onset of a disease has close relationship with healthy qi and pathogenic qi. The invasion of pathogenic qi is the external factor and a deficiency of vital qi is the internal factor for the onset of disease. For prevention of disease, on one hand, the invasion of pathogenic qi should be avoided, on the other hand, healthy qi should be enhanced to increase resistance against disease.

2.4.6.1.1 Protecting Healthy Qi to Increase Resistance against Disease

If healthy qi is abundant, the qi-blood and yin-yang of the body is vigorous, the function of viscera and bowels is strong, the resistance of the body against disease is strengthened. Protecting healthy qi is the key to increase resistance against disease.

(1) Having regular lifestyle, taking moderate work and rest

According to climate changes of four seasons, people should arrange work and rest time reasonably and have regular living habits to improve the ability of adapting to the environment change of nature. People can maintain spirit and qi, keep vigorous energy and strong vitality if they have moderate work and rest. Otherwise, people will be lack of energy, their vitality will decline and be easy to sick if they have abnormal living or over work and rest for a long time.

(2) Taking care of diet, protecting the spleen and stomach

The spleen is the foundation of acquired constitution and the source of qi and blood production. The spleen qi has the actions to promote the digestion of food taken in and the absorption of the foodstuff essence and further to distribute the essence. Foodstuff essence coming from diet is the substantial foundation for production of qi and blood. If the qi-blood is vigorous, healthy qi is abundant, the body is not easy to be invaded. Having proper diet emphasized in

TCM nursing means that the diet should be appropriate and regular. One should pay attention to the nature and flavor of food to make heat and cold harmonized, and the five flavors balanced. One should cultivate a good dietetic habit, has his diet at relatively fixed time and in relatively fixed quantity, neither starve nor overeat. In addition, one should also pay attention to dietetic sanitation to avoid "disease from the mouth". Improper diet, such as over drinking and eating, will lead to the occurrence of disease.

(3) Cultivating mental health, training the body

Spirit and mind activities take essence, qi, blood and body fluid as their substantial foundation, and they are closely related to visceral function and qi-blood movement. For example, joy may make flow of qi and blood smooth, the visceral function coordinative and the vital qi abundant. So the resistance against disease is enhanced to prevent its occurrence. While depression may lead to qi stagnation and blood stasis, dysfunction, decrease of resistance. So in TCM nursing, mental training is emphasized, one must keep "a peaceful and happy mood with humility and few desires to have vigorous healthy qi internally", so that he can attain the aim of "securing emotion balance and never suffering from a disease". A healthy physique often results from unremitting physical exercises. Many famous Chinese doctors have created series of classical exercises, such as the *Tai Ji Quan* (shadowboxing), *Wu Qin Xi* (five mimic-animal exercise), *Ba Duan Jin* (the Eight Pieces of Brocade). By doing proper physical exercises, one can both improve blood circulation to make the joints flexible, and make qi dynamic and free, strengthen the resistance against diseases, and prevent and reduce the occurrence of disease. The body will be healthy because of the unity of spirit and form.

(4) Medicinal prevention, protecting essential qi for anti-aging

By applying artificial immunization, the immunity will be enhanced to prevent and reduce the occurrence of disease. The "human variolation" was created in ancient China to prevent smallpox. It is our contribution to the world preventive medicine. In recent years, more and more attention has been paid to application of herbs in disease prevention. For instance, *ban lan gen* (Radix Isatidis), *guan zhong* (Cyrtomium Rhizome) or *da qing ye* (Folium Isatidis) are used to prevent flu; *ma chi xian* (Herba Portulacae) is used to prevent dysentery, and *yi chen* (Capillary Wormwood Herb), *zhi zi* (Fructus Gardeniae) are used to prevent hepatitis with good effects. Furthermore, rise and fall of essential qi in kidney is directly related to growth, development and the degree of aging. If essential qi in kidney is abundant, the body will be energetic, healthy, and longevity. Protecting kidney to keep essential qi is helpful for strengthening the resistance against diseases by reducing desire, using dietetic therapy, Chinese medicine, massage, and doing physical exercises.

2.4.6.1.2 Avoiding Invasion by Pathogenic Qi to Protect Healthy Qi

Pathogenic qi and pestilent qi are an important condition in onset of disease. Therefore prevention before occurrence of a disease includes protecting healthy qi and avoiding invasion by pathogenic qi. People should keep away from pathogenic qi and comply with the changes of four seasons for nourishing yang in spring and summer while nourishing yin in autumn and winter so that the interstitial space of people is compact and defense qi (*wei* qi) is dense for preventing invasion by pathogenic qi. When the weather is abnormal or epidemic disease is prevalent, people should avoid pathogenic qi, and do a good job in isolation to prevent the environment, water and food from contamination. In addition, people should avoid trauma and insect animal bites.

2.4.6.2 Controlling the Development of Existing Disease

Once a disease already occurs, one should strive for an early diagnosis and treatment to control the development of existing disease. Therefore, clinical nurses should watch out for changing state of disease and offer effective care.

2.4.6.2.1 Watching out for Changing State of the Disease in Order to Strive for an Early Diagnosis and Treatment

At early stages, disease is often mild, and its location is superficial and healthy qi is not deficient. If effective treatment and care is delivered timely, the disease is easier to cure. If external pathogenic qi has invaded the human body and proper treatment hasn't been provided yet, pathogenic qi will go inside to invade the viscera and the disease will progress. According to watching out for changing state of the disease and synthetically analyzing, the nurses differentiate and recognize the pattern of the disease to provide a reliable basis for an early diagnosis and effective treatment to stop the disease from further development and transmission.

2.4.6.2.2 Effective Nursing to Prevent Transmission

In clinical treatment of a liver disease, the method of strengthening the spleen is often taken as an auxiliary method, which means that not only treatment and nursing of liver disease but also strengthening the spleen should be provided to prevent transmission of liver disease, when liver disease hasn't affected the spleen yet. Therefore, clinical nurses should understand the development and transformation of disease, watch out for changes of the disease and take preventive treatment and nursing to prevent the progress of the disease. The part that has not been invaded by the pathogenic qi must be treated first to stop the disease from further development and transmission.

(Yang Xiaowei)

3

Commonly Used Techniques of Traditional Chinese Nursing

3.1 Auricular Seeds Taping Therapy

Auricular seeds taping therapy is taping small, round, hard and smooth objects such as vaccaria seed (Semen Vaccariae) and small magnetic beads to particular auricular points. The taped objects are then pressed in order to stimulate the auricular points and attain therapeutic results. This method has been widely used because of its wide range of indications, convenient for use, safety, and lack of side effects.

3.1.1 Anatomical Nomenclature of the Surfaces of the Auricle

The anatomical nomenclature of the surfaces of the auricle (Please see Figure 3-1).

Helix: It is the curved free rim of the auricle.

Helix tubercle: The tubercle is located on the posterior-superior portion of the helix.

Helix cauda: The inferior part of the helix is at the junction of the helix and the lobe.

Helix crus: It is the transverse ridge of the helix that continues backward into the concha of the ear.

Antihelix: It refers to the "Y" shaped prominence that is roughly parallel to the helix, including the body of the antihelix, superior antihelix crus and inferior antihelix crus.

Body of the antihelix: It refers to the main part of the antihelix that extends in a vertical direction.

Superior antihelix crus: It is the superior branch of the bifurcation of the antihelix.

Inferior antihelix crus: It is the inferior branch of the bifurcation of the antihelix.

Triangular fossa: This refers to the triangular depression formed by superior and inferior antihelix crus and the corresponding helix.

Scapha: This refers to the depression between the helix and the antihelix.

Tragus: It is the flap-shaped tubercle in front of the auricle.

Supertragic notch: This is the depression between the tragus and helix.

Antitragus: This refers to the flap-shaped tubercle opposite of the tragus and superior to the ear lobe.

Intertragic notch: This refers to the depression between the tragus and antitragus.

Helix notch: This refers to the depression between the antihelix and antitragus.

Ear lobe: This is the lowest part of the auricle devoid of cartilage.

Concha: This is the hollow area formed by parts of the helix and antihelix, tragus, antitragus and the orifice of the external auditory meatus.

Cavum concha: This is the concha inferior to the helix crus.

Cymba concha: This is the concha superior to the helix crus.

Orifice of the external auditory meatus: It is the opening in front of the cavum concha.

3.1.2 Distribution Rules of Auricular Points

Auricular points are the specific areas distributed over the ear. When there is an illness in the body, it may manifest on the ear as tenderness, deformities, discoloration, and disturbances in the skin electrical properties. All these changes and manifestations can be used for diagnosis as well as for treatment.

There exists some regularity in the distribution of auricular points. They are based on the upside down fetus distribution theory, which is explained below. Points related to the portions of the head are located on the ear lobe. Points related to the upper limbs are located on the scapha. Points related to the lower limbs are located on the superior and inferior antihelix crus. Points related to the organs in the chest are located on the cavum concha. Points related to the organs in the abdomen are located on the cymba concha. Points related to the spine and trunk are located on the antihelix. Points related to the pelvic cavity are located in the triangular fossa. Points related to the digestive tract are distributed around the helix crus. Points related to the urinary tract are located at the junction of the inferior antihelix crus and the cymba concha (Please see Figure 3-2).

3.1.3 Locations and Indications of Auricular Points

For the locations of auricular points [Please see Figure 3-3 (a) and (b)].

3.1.3.1 Points on the Helix (12 areas, HX1-HX12)

The whole helix is divided into 12 areas. The helix crus is HX1. The part of the helix from the helix notch to the upper edge of the inferior antihelix crus is divided into 3 equal areas, which are HX2, HX3, and HX4 counting from below to above. The helix between the two crura of the antihelix is HX5. HX6 extends from the anterior edge of the superior crus of the antihelix to the apex of ear. HX7 extends from the apex of ear to the upper edge of the helix tubercle. The area from upper edge to the lower edge of the helix tubercle is HX8. The part from the lower edge of the helix tubercle to the notch of helix-lobe is equally divided into 4 areas, which from above to below are HX9, HX10, HX11, and HX12 respectively (see Table 3-1).

Table 3-1   Locations and Indications of Points on the Helix

Name	Location	Indications
Ear Center (HX1)	On the helix crus; on HX1	Hiccups, urticaria, pruritus, infantile enuresis, hemorrhagic diseases
Rectum (HX2)	On the helix close to the notch superior to the tragus, on HX2	Constipation, diarrhea, prolapse of the anus, haemorrhoids
Urethra (HX3)	On the helix superior to Rectum, on HX3	Frequent, painful, or dripping urination; retention of urine

Continue

Name	Location	Indications
External Genitals (HX4)	On the helix superior to Urethra, on HX4	Testitis, epididymitis, vulvar or scrotal pruritus
Anus (HX5)	On the helix anterior to the triangular fossa, on HX5	Haemorrhoids, anal fissure
Ear Apex (HX6, 7 i)	On the apex where the ear is folded forward at the juncture of HX6 and HX7	Fever, hypertension, ocular sty, acute conjunctivitis, toothache
Node (HX8)	On the tubercle of the helix, on HX8	Dizziness, headache, hypertension
Helix1 (HX9)	Inferior to the helix tubercle, on HX9	Tonsillitis, upper respiratory tract infection, fever
Helix2 (HX10)	Inferior to the helix1, on HX10	Tonsillitis, upper respiratory tract infection, fever
Helix3 (HX11)	Inferior to the helix2, on HX11	Tonsillitis, upper respiratory tract infection, fever
Helix4 (HX12)	Inferior to the helix3, on HX12	Tonsillitis, upper respiratory tract infection, fever

3.1.3.2 Points on the Scapha (6 areas, SF1-SF6)

The scaphoid fossa is separated horizontally into 6 equal sections, which from upper to lower part of the scapha are SF1, SF2, SF3, SF4, SF5, and SF6 respectively (see Table 3-2).

Table 3-2　Locations and Indications of Points on the Scapha

Name	Location	Indications
Finger (SF1)	On the uppermost section of the scaphoid fossa, on SF1	Paronychia, pain and numbness of the fingers
Wrist (SF2)	On the section inferior to SF1, on SF2	Pain in the wrist
Wind Stream (SF1, 2 i)	Between the sections of Fingers and Wrist, midpoint between SF1 and SF2	Urticaria, pruritus, allergic rhinitis
Elbow (SF3)	On the third section from the top of the scaphoid fossa, on SF3	External humeral epicondylitis, pain in elbows
Shoulder (SF4, 5i)	On the fourth and fifth sections from the top of the scaphoid fossa, on SF4 and SF5	Periarthritis of the shoulder, pain of the shoulder
Clavicle (SF6)	On the lowermost section of the scaphoid fossa, on SF6	Periarthritis of the shoulder

3.1.3.3 Points on the Antihelix (13 areas, AH1-AH13)

Both the superior and inferior crus of antihelix are separated into 3 equal sections. The lower 1/3 of the superior crus of the antihelix is AH5. The middle 1/3 is AH4. The upper 1/3 is divided horizontally into 2 equal subparts, of which the lower half is AH3. The upper half is once again divided perpendicularly into 2 subparts, the posterior half is AH2 and the anterior half of which is AH1. The front and middle 2/3 of the inferior crus are AH6, and back 1/3 of which is AH7. The body of the antihelix is separated horizontally into 5 equal sections. Then it is also divided vertically into 2 sections, the medial side taking 1/4, the lateral side taking 3/4. Thus the body of antihelix is divided into 12 areas. The anterior superior 2/5 are AH8, while the posterior superior 2/5 are AH9; the front intermediate 2/5 are AH10 while the back intermediate 2/5 are AH11; the front inferior 1/5 is AH12 while the back inferior 1/5 is AH13 (see Table 3-3).

Table 3-3   Locations and Indications of Points on the Antihelix

Name	Location	Indications
Heel (AH1)	On the anterosuperior portion of the superior antihelix crus, on AH1	Heel pain
Toe (AH2)	On the posterosuperior portion of the superior antihelix curs inferior to the apex, on AH2	Paronychia, toe pain
Ankle (AH3)	At the part inferior to heel and toe, on AH3	Sprained ankle
Knee (AH4)	At the middle 1/3 of the superior antihelix crus, on AH4	Pain of the knee joint, sciatica
Hip (AH5)	At the lower 1/3 of the superior antihelix crus, on AH5	Hip joint pain or sprain, pain in lumbosacral area, sciatica
Sciatic Nerve (AH6)	At the inferior 2/3 of the inferior antihelix crus, on AH6	Sciatica, lower limb paralysis
Sympathesis (AH6a)	On the juncture between the terminus of the inferior antihelix crus and the helix	Spasms of the stomach and intestines, angina, biliary colic, ureterolith, functional disorders of autonomic nerves
Buttock (AH7)	On the posterior 1/3 of the inferior antihelix crus, on AH7	Sciatica, gluteal fascitis
Abdomen (AH8)	On the upper 2/5 of the front part of the body of the antihelix, on AH8	Abdominal pain or distension, diarrhea, acute lumbar muscle sprain, dysmenorrhea, labor pain
Lumbosacral Vertebrae (AH9)	Posterior to AH8, on AH9	Pain in the lumbosacral region
Chest (AH10)	On the central 2/5 of the front part of the body of the antihelix, on AH10	Pain and fullness in the chest or ribsides, intercostal neuralgia, oppression of the chest, mastitis
Thoracic Vertebrae (AH11)	Posterior to AH10, on AH11	Chest pain, premenstrual spargosis, mastitis, postpartum hypogalactia
Neck (AH12)	On the lower 1/5 of the front part of the body of the antihelix, on AH12	Stiff neck, pain of the neck
Cervical Vertebrae (AH13)	Posterior to AH12, on AH13	Stiff neck, cervical spondylopathy

3.1.3.4 Points on the Triangular Fossa (5 areas, TF1-TF5)

The triangular fossa is separated into 3 equal sections. The middle 1/3 is TF3. The uppermost 1/3 is separated into 3 equal sections again. The upper 1/3 is TF1 and the middle and lower 2/3 are TF2. The lowest 1/3 section is separated into 2 equal sections, the upper half of which is TF4 and lower half of which is TF5 (see Table 3-4).

Table 3-4 Locations and Indications of Points on the Triangular Fossa

Name	Location	Indications
Superior triangular fossa (TF1)	On the upper part of the superior 1/3 of the triangular fossa, on TF1	Hypertension
Internal Genitals (TF2)	At the lower 2/3 part of the superior 1/3 of the triangular fossa, on TF2	Dysmenorrhea, irregular menstruation, leukorrhagia, dysfunctional uterine bleeding, impotence, seminal emission, premature ejaculation
Middle triangular fossa (TF3)	In the middle 1/3 of the triangular fossa, on TF3	Asthma
Shenmen (TF4)	On the upper part of the posterior 1/3 of the triangular fossa, on TF4	Insomnia, profuse dreaming, withdrawal syndrome, epilepsy, pain disorders
Pelvis (TF5)	On the lower part of the posterior 1/3 of the triangular fossa, on TF5	Pelvic inflammation, adnexitis

3.1.3.5 Points on the Tragus (4 areas, TG1-TG4)

The external surface of the tragus is divided into 2 equal parts from above to below, the upper 1/2 is TG1 and lower 1/2 is TG2. The internal surface of the tragus is separated into 2 equal sections too, the upper part of which is TG3 and the lower part of which is TG4 (see Table 3-5).

Table 3-5 Locations and Indications of Points on the Tragus

Name	Location	Indications
Upper tragus (TG1)	On the upper 1/2 of the external surface of the tragus, on TG1	Laryngitis, rhinitis, simple obesity
Lower tragus (TG2)	On the lower 1/2 of the external surface of the tragus, on TG2	rhinitis, nasal obstruction, simple obesity
External Ear (TG1u)	Anterior to the superior tragic notch nearby the helix, on the upper edge of TG1	Otitis externa, otitis media, tinnitus
Apex of Tragus (TG1p)	On the center of the upper eminence of the tragus, posterior to the edge of TG1	Fever, toothache, squint
External Nose (TG1, 2)	At the middle part of lateral side of the tragus, the junction of upper and lower tragus	Nasal vestibulitis, rhinitis
Adrenal Gland (TG2p)	On the center of the lower eminence of the tragus, on the posterior edge of TG2	Hypotension, rheumatic arthritis, mumps, dizziness, asthma, shock, allergic diseases
Pharynx and larynx (TG3)	On the upper 1/2 of the internal side of the tragus, on the TG3	Loss of voice, pharyngitis, tonsillitis
Internal nose (TG4)	On the lower 1/2 of the internal side of the tragus, on the TG4	Rhinitis, maxillary sinuitis, nose bleeding
Anterior intertragic notch (TG2b)	At the lowest part of the front of the intertragic notch, the lower edge of the area of lower tragus	Pharyngitis, stomatitis, eye disorders

3.1.3.6 Points on the Antitragus (4 areas, AT1-AT4)

Draw a vertical line from the apex of antitragus down to upper line of ear lobe. Draw another line from the midpoint between the apex of antitragus and antihelix-antitragus notch down to upper line of ear lobe. Therefore, the antitragus is separated into 3 sections on its external surface. The anterior area is AT1, the intermediate area of which is AT2 and posterior area of which is AT3. The internal surface of the antitragus is AT4 (see Table 3-6).

Table 3-6 Locations and Indications of Points on the Antitragus

Name	Location	Indications
Forehead (AT1)	On the anterior part of the outer side of the antitragus, on the AT1	Frontal headache, insomnia, profuse dreaming
Posterior intertragus (AT1b)	On the anteroinferior part of the antitragus, posterior to intertragus and the lower edge of forehead	Prosopantritis, eye disorders
Temple (AT2)	On the middle part of the lateral side of the antitragus, on the AT2	Migraine, dizziness
Occiput (AT3)	On the posterior part of the lateral side of the antitragus, on the AT3	Dizziness, headache, epilepsy, asthma, neurasthenia
Subcortex (AT4)	On the medial side of the antitragus, on AT4	Pain, neurasthenia, pseudomyopia, insomnia
Apex of the antitragus (AT1, 2, 4 i)	At the free end of the apex of the antitragus, at the junction of AT1, AT2 and AT4	Asthma, mumps, testitis, epididymitis, neurodermatitis
Central rim of the antitragus (AT2, 3, 4 i)	On the free rim of the antitragus, at the midpoint of the apex of the antitragus and antihelix-antitragus notch at the juncture of AT2, AT3, and AT4	Enuresis, aural vertigo, diabetes insipidus, functional uterine bleeding
Brain Stem (AT3, 4 i)	On the antihelix-antitragus notch at the junction of AT3 and AT4	Dizziness, occipital headache, pseudomyopia

3.1.3.7 Points on the Concha (18 areas, CO1-CO18)

It is necessary to know the marker points and lines on the auricle firstly. The concha is separated into 18 areas by those marker points and lines. Point A is located at the medial edge of the helix, at the junction between the middle and upper 1/3 of the line from the notch of helix crus and the inferior edge of the inferior antihelix crus. In the concha, draw a level line from the end of the helix crus to the concha edge of the helix. Point D is located at the cross point of the line with the edge of the antihelix. Point B is located at the junction of the middle and posterior 1/3 of the line extending from the end of the helix crus to Point D. Point C is located at the junction of the upper 1/4 and lower 3/4 of the posterior edge of the orifice of the external auditory meatus. Draw a curved line similar to the concha edge of the antihelix from Point A to B. Draw a curved line similar to the inferior edge of the helix crus from Point B to C (Please see Figure 3-4).

Divide the part, formed by the inferior edge of the helix crus and its opposite BC line (the front part), into 3 equal areas. There are area 1, 2 and 3 counting from front to back. The fan-shaped area at the end of the helix crus is area 4. Divide the part, formed by the superior edge of the helix crus and its opposite AB line (the front part), into 3 equal areas. They are from the back to the front area 5, 6 and 7 respectively. Connect Point A with the junction of the anterior 1/3 and the posterior 2/3 of the lower edge of the inferior crus of the antihelix. The concha anterior to this line is area 8. Divide the part posterior to area 8 and superior to area 6 and 7 into two areas. The anterior area is area 9 and posterior area id area 10. Divide the part posterior to area 10 and superior to line BD into 2 areas. The superior area is area 11 and the inferior area is area 12. Draw a line from the helix notch to point B. The area between this line and BD line is area 13. Take the middle point of cavum concha as the center of a circle. The circle with a radius of half the distance from the center to line BC is area 15. Make two tangents from the highest and lowest points to the office of the external auditory meatus, the area with the lines is area 16. The area external to area 15 and 16 is area 14. Draw a line from the lowest point of the orifice of the external auditory meatus to the middle point of the concha edge of the antitragus, and then divide the part inferior to the line is divided into 2 areas. The upper area is area 17 and lower is area 18 (see Table 3-7).

Table 3-7　Locations and Indications of Points on the Concha

Name	Location	Indications
Mouth (CO1)	On the anterior 1/3 of the area inferior to the crus of helix, on CO1	Facial paralysis, stomatitis, cholecystitis, cholelithiasis, withdrawal syndrome, periodontitis, glossitis
Esophagus (CO2)	On the middle 1/3 of the area inferior to the crus of the helix, on CO2	Esophagitis, esophagospasm
Cardia (CO3)	On the posterior 1/3 of the area inferior to the crus of the helix, on CO3	Cardiospasm, nervous vomiting
Stomach (CO4)	On the terminus of the helix crus, on CO4	Gastrospasm, gastritis, gastric ulcer, nausea and vomiting, insomnia, toothache, indigestion
Duodenum (CO5)	On the posterior 1/3 of the area superior to the helix crus, on CO5	Duodenal ulcer, cholecystitis, cholelithiasis, pylorospasm, abdominal distension and pain, diarrhea
Small Intestine (CO6)	On the middle 1/3 of the area superior to the helix crus, on CO6	Indigestion, abdominal pain and distension, tachycardia
Large Intestine (CO7)	On the anterior 1/3 of the area superior to the helix crus, on CO7	Diarrhea, constipation, cough, toothache, acne
Appendix (CO6, 7 i)	At the junction of CO6 and CO7	Appendicitis, diarrhea
Angle of superior concha (CO8)	At the anterior part under the inferior antihelix crus, on CO8	Prostatitis, urethritis
Bladder (CO9)	At the intermediate part under the inferior crus of antihelix, on CO9	Cystitis, enuresis, retention of urine, lower back pain, sciatica, occipital headache
Kidney (CO10)	At the posterior part under the inferior crus of antihelix, on CO10	Lower back pain, tinnitus, neurasthenia, pyelitis, asthma, nocturnal enuresis, irregular menstruation, seminal emission, premature ejaculation

Continue

Name	Location	Indications
Ureter (CO9, 10 i)	At the junction of Kidney (CO9) and Bladder (CO10)	Urethral colic
Pancreas and gallbladder (CO11)	At the posterior part of the cymba concha, on CO11	Cholecystitis, cholelithiasis, biliary ascariasis, migraine, herpes zoster, otitis media, tinnitus, acute pancreatitis
Liver (CO12)	On the posteroinferior area of the superior cymba concha, on CO12	Pain in the chest and rib-sides, dizziness, premenstrual syndrome, irregular menstruation, menopause syndrome, hypertension, myopia, simple glucoma
Center of superior concha (CO6, 10 i)	In the center of the superior concha, at the junction of Small Intestine (CO6) and kidney (CO10)	Abdominal pain or distension, biliary ascariasis
Spleen (CO13)	At the part inferior to BD line, posterosuperior part of the cavum concha, on CO13	Abdominal pain or distension, diarrhea, constipation, poor appetite, dysfunctional uterine bleeding, leukorrhagia, Meniere's disease
Heart (CO15)	In the depression at the center of the cavum concha, on CO15	Rapid or slow heart beating, angina pectoris, aortic arch syndrome, neurasthenia, hysteria, oral ulcers
Trachea (CO16)	At the part between the Heart (CO15) and the orifice of the external auditory meatus, on CO 16	Asthma, bronchitis
Lung (CO14)	In the cavum concha around Heart (CO15) and Trachea (CO16), on CO14	Cough, asthma, pain or fullness in the chest, loss of voice, acne, pruritus, urticaria, constipation, withdrawal syndrome
San Jiao (CO17)	At the part posteroinferior to the orifice of the external auditory meatus and between the Lung (CO14) and Endocrine (CO18), on CO17	Constipation, abdominal distension, pain on the lateral side of the upper limb
Endocrine (CO18)	At the inside of the notch of the intertragus and anteroinferior part of cavum concha, on CO18	Dysmenorrhea, irregular menstruation, menopausal syndrome, acne, hyperthyroidism or hypothyroidism

3.1.3.8   Points on the Earlobe (9 areas, LO1-LO9)

A grid of 9 sections is delineated on the frontal surface of the earlobe by drawing three equidistant horizontal lines below the lower border of the cartilage of the notch between the tragus and the antitragus, and two equidistant vertical lines. From front to back, the upper 3 areas are LO1, LO2 and LO3; the middle areas are LO4, LO5 and LO6; and the lower areas are LO7, LO8 and LO9 (see Table 3-8).

Table 3-8   Locations and Indications of Points on the Earlobe

Name	Location	Indications
Teeth (LO1)	On the anterosuperior area of the front surface of the earlobe, on LO1	Toothache, periodontitis, hypotension
Tongue (LO2)	On the central superior area of the front surface of the earlobe, on LO2	Glossitis, stomatitis
Jaw (LO3)	On the posterosuperior area of the front surface of the earlobe, on LO3	Toothache, dysfunction of the temporomandibular joint
Anterior Ear Lobe (LO4)	On the anterior central area of the front surface of the earlobe, on LO4	Neurasthenia, toothache
Eye (LO5)	On the center of the front surface of the earlobe, on LO5	Acute conjunctivitis, electric opthalmitis, stye, myopia
Internal Ear (LO6)	On the central posterior part of the front surface of the earlobe, on LO6	Tinnitus, hearing impairment, otitis media, Meniere's disease
Cheek (LO5, 6 i)	On the central posterior part of the front surface of the earlobe, at the junction between LO5 and LO6	Facial paralysis or spasm, trigeminal neuralgia, acne, verruca plana, mumps
Tonsil (LO7, 8, 9)	On the inferior part of the front surface of the earlobe, including LO7, 8, 9	Tonsillitis, pharyngitis

3.1.3.9   Points on the Posterior Surface of the Ear (5 areas, P1-P5)

The dorsal side of the ear is separated into 5 areas. Draw 2 horizontal lines passing through the back corresponding points of the bifurcation of the antihelix crura and helix notch, thus the posterior surface is thereby divided into 3 parts. The upper part is P1, the lower part is P5. The middle part, once again, is divided equally into 3 equal areas. The medial area is P2, the middle area is P3 and the lateral area is P4 (see Table 3-9).

Table 3-9   Locations and Indications of Points on the Posterior Surface of the Ear

Name	Location	Indications
Heart of Posterior Surface (P1)	On the upper portion of the posterior surface of the auricle, on P1	Palpitation, insomnia, dream-disturbed sleep
Lung of Posterior Surface (P2)	On the centromedial portion of the posterior surface of the auricle, on P2	Cough, asthma, pruritus
Spleen of Posterior Surface (P3)	On the posterior surface of the auricle close to the terminus of the crus of the helix, on P3	Gastric pain, indigestion, poor appetite
Liver of Posterior Surface (P4)	On the centrolateral portion of the posterior surface of the auricle, on P4	Cholecystitis, cholelithiasis, pain in rib sides
Kidney of Posterior Surface (P5)	On the lower portion of the posterior surface of the auricle, on P5	Dizziness, headache, neurasthenia
Groove of posterior Surface (GPS)	On the posteromedial surface of the ear formed by the superior and inferior antihelix crura	Hypertension, pruritus

3.1.3.10   Points on the Root of the Ear

Table 3-10   Locations and Indications of Points on the Root of the Ear

Name	Location	Indications
Upper Ear Root (R1)	At the top of the root of the ear	Epistaxis
Root of Ear Vagus (R2)	At the ear root on the posterior groove of the helix crus	Cholecystitis, cholelithiasis, abdominal pain, diarrhea, nasal congestion, tachycardia
Lower Ear Root (R1)	On the lowest part of the ear	Hypotension, paralysis of the lower limbs, sequelae of infantile paralysis

3.1.4   Clinical Application of Auricular Seeds Taping Therapy

3.1.4.1   Indications of Auricular Seeds Taping Therapy

Auricular seeds taping therapy can be used to treat painful disorders such as sprains, headaches, and neuropathic pains.

This can be indicated for inflammatory and infectious diseases like acute and chronic colitis, periodontitis, laryngopharyngitis, tonsillitis, cholecystitis, influenza, whooping cough, bacillary dysentery and mumps, etc.

This can be used to treat functional disorders and allergic diseases such as dizziness, hypertension, arrhythmia, neurasthenia, hives, asthma, rhinitis and purpura, etc.

It may be adopted to treat endocrinal and metabolic disorders such as hyperthyroidism, hypothyroidism, diabetes, obesity and menopausal symptoms, etc.

It can also be applied for conditions such as anaphylactic reactions to transfusion and infusion, for beauty therapy, smoking and drug addictions, anti-aging and disease prevention as well.

3.1.4.2   Principles for Selecting Auricular Points

Choosing the corresponding points to the location of the diseased or affected part of the body is important. There will be one or more sensitive points on the ear when a disease is present. For example, choose the stomach (CO4) for the treatment of stomachache.

Choose points based on the visceral manifestation theory. For instance, choose the kidney (CO10) for alopecia or the lung (CO7) and large intestine (CO14) for skin disorders.

Furthermore, choose points based on the channel pattern identification. For example, choose the bladder (CO9) or pancreas and gallbladder (CO11) for sciatica. Choose the large intestine (CO7) for toothache.

Overall, choose points as instructed by biomedical principles. For example, choose the adrenal gland (TG2p) for inflammatory diseases such as asthma. Choose Shen men (TF4) and subcortex (AT4) points for painful conditions and inflammations. Finally, choose the endocrine (CO18) for irregular periods.

Choosing points is based on clinical experience. There are some effective points discovered in clinical practice, but they do not meet the criteria of the above principles. For example, choose the external genital (HX4) for pain in the lower back and legs, the ear apex (HX6, 7 i) for bloodletting and for red, swollen and painful eyes.

3.1.4.3 Procedures and Methods of Auricular Seeds Taping Therapy

3.1.4.3.1 Auricular Diagnostic Methods

Inspection: Auricular inspection is to check for abnormal changes on the ear in order to diagnose diseases or disorders. The most commonly seen positive changes include deformities, discoloration, pimples, desquamation, nodules, congestion, depression, blisters and so on.

Detection of the tender spot: This method searches for the tender spots on the ears with a probe, the head of an acupuncture needle handle, or the end of a matchstick by pressing and moving on the surface of the ear gently and smoothly.

Measurement of electrical resistance: This technique detects decreased electrical resistance in points with an electrical detector that has an indicator lamp or special sound.

3.1.4.3.2 Selecting auricular points

After making clear diagnosis, proper auricular points are selected according to above principles or positive reaction spots detected by above diagnostic methods can be used.

3.1.4.3.3 Disinfection

The auricular points should be disinfected with 75% alcohol.

3.1.4.3.4 Manipulation

The vaccaria seed (Semen Vaccariae) and small magnetic beads are mainly used for auricular seeds taping. Holding the auricle with one hand, use a detection probe to press the auricular points hard enough to leave depressions with the other hand. Tape the seeds to the auricular points with a piece of adhesive tape sized in 0.5 cm square and press it for several minutes until a feeling of local heat, or distending pain is achieved. Mainly tape the auricular points of the affected side. Bilateral auriculae may be taped simultaneously or during alternate treatment sessions. The patient is asked to press the selected points 2 to 4 times a day. The seeds can be kept in place for 3 to 5 days. Remove the tape and seeds before the next treatment and modify the points according to the condition of the disease.

3.1.4.3.5 Precautions

Avoid exposure of the adhesive tape to moisture. Use other stimulating methods for patients with adhesive allergies.

In order to prevent injury to the auricle, do not rub in a sideways or circular motion while pressing the taped auricular points.

Auricular seeds taping is contraindicated in case of inflamed or frostbitten auricular.

Auricular seeds taping is contraindicated for pregnant women with a history of repeated miscarriage and patients with severe cardiac disease.

When treating a sprain or other soft tissue injuries, encourage the patient to move the affected part in order to increase the therapeutic outcome.

3.2 Tuina

Manipulations of Tuina are the standard techniques performed by the operator with hands or other parts of the body to stimulate the treated areas and activate the limbs. There are different types of manipulations with different operation methods of stimulation, intensity and time, such as pushing manipulation, pressing manipulation, and kneading manipulation and so on. They are essential contents of manipulations of Tuina. The combination of two more basic manipulations is called compound manipulation, such as pressing and kneading manipulation, pushing and rubbing manipulation and so on. These manipulations have effects of dredging channels, promoting qi and blood circulation, lubricating joints and regulating *zang-fu* organs etc.

3.2.1 Indications

Tuina manipulations for adults are indicated for disorders of orthopaedics and traumatism, such as stiff neck, cervical spondylopathy, acute lumbar sprain, chronic lumbar muscle strain, scapulohumeral periarthritis, prolapse of lumbar intervertebral disc, chronic strain of soft tissues, acute soft tissue injury, etc.; diseases of internal medicine, such as constipation, diarrhea, hypertension, headache etc.; diseases of gynaecology such as dysmenorrheal, irregular menstruation; diseases of otolaryngology such as toothache, deafness. Tuina manipulations for infants are indicated for cough, fever, asthma, vomiting, anorexia, constipation, etc.

3.2.2 Basic Requirements of Manipulations

The basic requirements of manipulation are being persistent, forceful, even speed rhythm, soft and deep penetration. "Persistent" means that the manipulation should be performed for a continuous period of time without any deformation. "Forceful" means the manipulation must be performed with moderate force which should be adjusted according to the patient's constitution, state of illness and the difference of treated areas, avoid performing with clumsy strength and by force. "Even speed rhythm" means that the manipulation is performed with rhythm, constant speed and pressure. "Soft" means that the manipulation is operated gently and carefully, not violently. "Deep penetration" is that the stimulation must be penetrated deeply into the deep tissues. Only when the manipulation is operated persistently, forcefully, evenly and softly can the purpose of deep penetration be achieved. The successful manipulation should take softness as the first and relaxation as prized.

3.2.3 Commonly Used Manipulations for Adults

3.2.3.1 One-Finger Pushing

Exert force by swinging the forearm and direct it to the treated areas or points continuously with the tip or the whorled surface of the thumb. This is the so-called one-finger pushing manipulation.

3.2.3.1.1 Operation Method

The operator grasps a hollow fist with suspended and flexed wrist and palm, and stretch the thumb straight naturally to cover the fist hole. Exert force on the body surface with the tip or whorled surface of the thumb. Lower the shoulder, drop the elbow and suspend the wrist. Swing the forearm initiatively to drive the wrist swinging transversely while flexing and extending the thumb joint to make the force on the channels and points continuously with the light and heavy force alternately. The frequency is 120 to 160 times per minute.

3.2.3.1.2   Essentials for Operation

(1) Lowering shoulders: Relax the shoulder joints with the scapulas dropping naturally. Keep the armpit free with the space of a fist. Avoid shrugging shoulders to exert strength.

(2) Dropping the elbow: Drop the elbow joint naturally and be a little lower than the wrist. Don't extend the elbow outwards or adduct excessively.

(3) Suspending the wrist: Flex the wrist joint and naturally suspend it. Get the wrist relax and try best to flex to 90°.

(4) Exerting force to the thumb: Fix the tip or the whorled surface of the thumb on the treated area or points, avoid pressing forcefully.

(5) Emptying the palm: Keep the palm and other four fingers except the thumb relaxed and grasp an empty fist. Accumulate the strength in the palm and send it from the fingers.

(6) Pushing fast and shifting slowly: Pushing fast refers to swing quickly, 120 to 160 times per minute; shifting slowly refers to fix on the surface of the skin with the tip or the whorled surface of the thumb and shift slowly along the channels or a special path. Don't slip or rub.

3.2.3.1.3   Precautions

(1) It is favorable to calm down, keep the heart and spirit in peace, concentrate on the operation. Only when the posture is correct and the essentials are complied with can the manipulation be performed effectively.

(2) There are two methods in performing one-finger pushing manipulation with, to be performed either with the thumb joint flexed or not flexed. If the operator's interphalangeal joint of thumb is stiff with the small activity range or soft stimulation is needed in the treatment, the manipulation can be done with the thumb joint flexed and extended. If the operator's interphalangeal joint of thumb is flexible, it is favorable to do the manipulation with straight thumb joint.

(3) When one-finger pushing manipulation is operated on the body surface, it should follow the principle of "pushing along the channels and pressing on the points" to select points along the channels.

3.2.3.2   Rolling

Take the ulnar side of opisthenar as the contact surface, swing the forearm to drive the wrist to flex and extend and roll the opisthenar on the treated areas. This is the so-called rolling manipulation.

3.2.3.2.1   Operation Method

The operator keeps the thumb straight naturally, grasps an empty fist, naturally flex the metacarpophalangeal joints of the little finger and the ring finger to about 90°, the flexed angles of the metacarpophalangeal joints of other fingers reduce gradually to make the palm round along the palm surface. Press the treated area with the dorsum of the hand close to the little finger. Swing the forearm initiatively to flex and extend the wrist in large amplitude and rotate the forearm as well. Roll the ulnar side of the opisthenar on the treated areas continuously. The swinging frequency is about 120 times per minute.

3.2.3.2.2 Essentials for Operation

(1) Lower the shoulders and drop the elbow with the elbow joint flexed naturally to 140° to keep a space of a fist to the chest. Relax the wrist and grasp an empty fist. The angle of the metacarpophalangeal joints from the little finger to the ring finger becomes small one by one, enable the back of hand to be an arch and fix on the treated area.

(2) The wrist joint flexes and extends about 120°, that is to say, flex the wrist about 80° when the arm swings outward while extending the wrist about 40° when the arm swings backward. Enable the half area of the opisthenar to touch the treated area successively. The forearm rotates outward while swaying externally and inwards while swaying backward.

(3) The stimulation should be changed with light and heavy force in turn, the ratio of heaviness and lightness for rolling forth and rolling back is 3:1, that is "rolling forward three times and rolling back once".

(4) The frequency should be fixed when applying the rolling manipulation. The shifting speed can't be too fast.

(5) The rolling manipulation is often used together with the passive limb movement of the patient in clinic. As one hand is doing the rolling manipulation, the other hand can help the patient to do the passive movement. The two hands should be harmonious and the passive movement should be "soft, short, and causal".

3.2.3.2.3 Precautions

(1) To perform the rolling manipulation, the flexing-extending movement of the wrist joint should be maximized. Avoid rotating the forearm mainly and flexing and extending the wrist joints insufficiently.

(2) It is favorable to fix on for performing the rolling manipulation; dragging, jumping or rotating-swinging is not allowed. Bumping between the opisthenar and body surface should be avoided.

(3) Avoid operating on the apophysial points of vertebral spinous process and other joints because it may cause discomfort.

3.2.3.3 Kneading

Fix on the body surface with the certain part of finger and palm and knead in circles to rotate gently and softly the subcutaneous tissues. This is the so-called kneading manipulation, one of the commonly used manipulations of Tuina. According to the different contacting surface during the operation, it can be divided into the palm base kneading manipulation, major thenar kneading manipulation and finger kneading manipulation.

3.2.3.3.1 Operation Method

(1) Palm-base kneading manipulation: Exert force with the palm base. Flex the fingers naturally and extend the wrist joint slightly backwards. Crook the elbow joint slightly as a fulcrum, swing the forearm initiatively to drive the palm base to knead on the treated area with the frequency of about 120 to 160 times every minute.

(2) Major thenar kneading manipulation: Exert force with the major thenar and crook the wrist joint slightly to 120° to 140°. Use the elbow joint as a pivot and swing the forearm

initiatively to knead with the major thenar on the treated area with the frequency of about 120 to 160 times every minute.

(3) Thumb kneading manipulation: Exert force with the whorled surface of the thumb while the other four fingers supporting on a suitable position. Flex the wrist joint slightly or straighten. Swing the forearm in small amplitude and drive the thumb to rotate on the treated area. The frequency is 120 to 160 time every minute.

(4) Middle finger kneading manipulation: Exert force with the whorled surface of the middle finger, extend straight the interphalangeal joint of the middle finger and slightly bend the metacarpophalangeal joints. Take the elbow joint as a fulcrum, swing the forearm initiatively in small amplitude and drive the whorled surface of the middle finger to rotate on the treated area. The frequency is 120 to 160 times every minute.

Kneading with the index finger or the juxtaposed index finger, middle finger and ring finger are called index finger kneading manipulation and three fingers kneading manipulation respectively. The operation essentials are the same as those of middle finger kneading manipulation.

3.2.3.3.2 Essentials for Operation

(1) In performing, the operator should lower the shoulders, drop the elbow and relax the wrist joint. Swing the forearm in small amplitude to rotate the contacting parts with force from the wrist joint.

(2) The subcutaneous tissues should be activated to move together. The movement should be flexible and rhythmic.

(3) The pressure should be moderate, making the patient feel comfortable.

3.2.3.3.3 Precautions

Avoid rubbing or slipping between the treated part and the body surface during the manipulation.

The force should be passed through the relaxed wrist joint. When performing this manipulation, the wrist joint should be kept in certain intensity, excessive stiffness of the wrist joint should be avoided.

3.2.3.4 Rubbing

Use the finger or palm surface as the touching part to make rhythmic and circular rubbing movement. This is the so-called rubbing manipulation, which is the gentlest Tuina manipulation.

3.2.3.4.1 Operation Method

(1) Palm-rubbing manipulation: Press on the body surface with the fingers juxtaposed, the palm straightened naturally, the wrist joint stretched slightly. Use the elbow joint as a fulcrum. Then move the forearm actively to rub in circles with the palm on the treated areas. It can be performed either clockwise or counter-clockwise with the frequency of 100 to 120 times every minute.

(2) Finger-rubbing manipulation: Take the surface of the index finger, middle finger, ring finger and little finger as the contacting surface with the fingers juxtaposed, the palm straightened naturally and the wrist joint flexed slightly. Use the elbow as a pivot and move the forearm actively to drive the surface of the four fingers to rub in circles on the treated area. It can be

performed either clockwise or counter-clockwise with the frequency of 100 to 120 times every minute.

3.2.3.4.2 Essentials for Operation

(1) Relax the shoulder joints, actively swing the forearm to drive the relaxed wrist joint to do the circular movement. When operating the finger-rubbing manipulation, the wrist joints should be kept in certain intensity, but avoid being stiff.

(2) The force should be moderate and the speed should be even. Finger-rubbing manipulation should be performed with lighter force and faster speed while palm-rubbing manipulation is performed with heavier force and slower speed.

3.2.3.4.3 Precautions

(1) It is suitable to perform the rubbing manipulation lightly and slowly, avoid operating fast and heavily.

(2) The direction of the manipulation should be chosen according to the deficiency and excess syndrome of the illness. Traditional Chinese medicine thinks that clockwise circular-rubbing manipulation is suitable for deficiency syndrome while counter-clockwise circular-rubbing manipulation is indicated for excess syndrome. In clinic, different directions of the rubbing manipulation are selected according to the anatomical structure of the treated areas and pathological conditions.

(3) When performing the rubbing manipulation, ointments with different kinds of function can be smeared according to the disease condition. Scallion and ginger juice, as well as turpentine can also be smeared to enhance the effect.

(4) Pay attention to the difference between rolling manipulation and circular rubbing manipulation: When performing rolling manipulation, fix the fingers and palm on a certain part of the body surface to drive the subcutaneous tissues to move with a relatively stronger force without rubbing movement with the body surface; when performing circular rubbing manipulation, the fingers and palm make circular rubbing with a relatively lighter force on the body surface without moving the subcutaneous tissues. The two manipulations are often used together in clinic.

3.2.3.5 Scrubbing

Exert force on the treated areas with the major thenar, the palm base and the hypothenar to do the linear rubbing movements back and forth, the heat generated by the rubbing can penetrate the body surface into the deeper layer. This is the so-called scrubbing manipulation. It can be divided into scrubbing with palm, scrubbing with major thenar and scrubbing with hypothenar.

3.2.3.5.1 Operation Method

(1) Scrubbing with the palm: Exert force on the body with the surface of the palm and extend the wrist joint straight. Take the shoulder joint as the fulcrum and move the upper arm actively with the surface of the palm scrubbing the body surface along a straight line back and forth. The frequency is 100 to 120 times every minute and it is mostly used in the chest and hypochondrium as well as in the abdomen.

(2) Scrubbing with the major thenar: Exert force on the body surface with the major thenar and extend the wrist joint straight. Take the shoulder joint as the fulcrum and move the upper arm

actively with the major thenar scrubbing on the body surface along a straight line back and forth. The frequency is 100 to 120 times every minute and it is mostly used in the chest and abdomen, waist and back and four limbs.

(3) Scrubbing with the hypothenar: Exert force on the body surface with the hyothenar, keep the palm vertical to the body surface and extend the wrist joint straight. Take the shoulder joint as the fulcrum and move the upper arm actively with the hyothenar scrubbing on the body surface along a straight line back and forth. The frequency is 100 to 120 times every minute and it is mostly used on the shoulder and back, waist and buttocks and lower limbs.

3.2.3.5.2　Essentials for Operation

The scrubbing route should be straight and long. No matter whether the scrubbing is from top to down or from left to right, the route should be kept straight. Moreover, the distance of moving back and forth should be long and continuous without pause.

The palm should be kept close to the treated area. The pressing force should be kept even. It is favorable not to make the skin fold during scrubbing. The frequency should also be even.

3.2.3.5.3　Precautions

(1) The operator should breathe naturally and not hold breath in the operation.

(2) Scrubbing manipulation can generate soft and warm stimulation. Scrubbing with the palm produces mild warm stimulation. Scrubbing with the hypothenar produces higher warm stimulation. Scrubbing with the major thenar produces moderate warm stimulation. It is operated until the patient feels warm.

(3) When operating scrubbing, smear some lubricant on the treated areas, which not only protects the skin, but also is good for the heat to permeate into the body.

(4) Since scrubbing is operated directly on the body surface, pay attention to keeping the operating room warm.

(5) After operating scrubbing, generally it is inadvisable to use other manipulations on the treated areas to avoid injuring the skin.

3.2.3.6　Pushing

Exert force on certain parts or points of the human body with fingers and palm or other parts of the body to make linear or arc movement in one direction, which is called pushing manipulation. It can be divided into flat pushing manipulation, straight pushing manipulation, spiral pushing manipulation, separate pushing manipulation and coalescent pushing manipulation.

3.2.3.6.1　Operation Method

(1) Flat pushing manipulation: According to the difference of force exerting parts, there are flat pushing manipulations with the thumb, with the palm and with the elbow. Exert force on the body surface with the thumb, palm and elbow. Push heavily and slowly in a one way direction along the channels or the direction of muscle fibers. Press and knead on the important treated areas or points.

(2) Straight pushing manipulation: Exert force on certain parts or points of the body with the radial surface of the thumb or the whorled surfaces of the index finger and middle finger. Push straightly in one way direction.

(3) Spiral pushing manipulation: Push spirally on the points by the whorled surface of the thumb. The frequency is about 200 to 240 times every minute.

(4) Separate pushing manipulation: Keep the whorled surfaces of the thumb or the palm of both hands close to the body surface. Push from the center part to the left or right side separately in a one way direction. The frequency is 120 times per minute.

(5) Coalescent pushing manipulation: Keep the whorled surfaces of the thumb or the palm of both hands close to the body surface. Push from either side of the points to the center of the points.

3.2.3.6.2 Essentials for Operation

(1) Flat pushing manipulation can exert comparatively stronger force among pushing manipulations. When operating, it is better to push with steady force, slow speed and along straight line in one way direction.

(2) To operate the straight pushing manipulation, the wrist, palm and fingers move straightly forwards in one direction with the elbow joint flexed and extended. The pressure used is lighter than that of the flat pushing manipulation. The movements should be light and continuous. It is better not to make the skin of the treated area red after the manipulation.

(3) When operating the spiral pushing manipulation, relax the elbow joint and wrist joint. Make the spiral movement in small amplitude by the thumb without the subcutaneous tissue movement. It is similar to the finger-rubbing manipulation.

(4) During the operation of separate pushing manipulation, it requires the strength of the two hands be even, the movement be soft and consonant. The pushing movement to both sides can be operated in a straight line or in a curved line.

(5) The operation essentials of coalescent pushing manipulation are the same as that of the separate pushing manipulation. But the operation should be done in the opposite direction.

3.2.3.6.3 Precautions

(1) Pushing manipulation should be performed along a straight line or a curved line in one direction and rubbing back and forth should be avoided.

(2) During the operation, the operating part should stick tightly on the body surface, the strength should be stable, even and moderate, the speed of pushing is not suitable to be fast.

(3) When pushing manipulation is operated on the body surface, talcum powder or the scallion and ginger juice can be smeared on the treated areas.

3.2.3.7 Wiping

The whorled surface of thumb is tightly close to the skin of treated area. Push up and down or left to right or along a curved path, which is called the wiping manipulation. It can be divided into wiping manipulation with fingers and wiping manipulation with the palm.

3.2.3.7.1 Operation Method

(1) Wiping manipulation with fingers: Exert force on the body surface with the whorled surface of one thumb or two thumbs and support with the other four fingers. Slightly exert force with the thumb and slowly shift up to down or left to right or along a curved line.

(2) Wiping manipulation with the palm: Exert force with one or two palms on the body

surface and relax the wrist joint. The forearm and upper arm exert force cooperatively to drive the palm to move up and down, or left to right, or along a curved line.

3.2.3.7.2 Essentials for Operation

(1) In the operation of wiping manipulation, the whorled surface of thumb or the palm should stick tightly on the body surface.

(2) In operating the wiping manipulation, the strength should be even, the movement should be soft and mild, and the distance of wiping back and forth in the treated area should be long as far as possible.

3.2.3.7.3 Precautions

(1) The stimulation of wiping manipulation is superficial and it is inadvisable to affect the subcutaneous tissues in deep layer.

(2) It is easy to confuse wiping manipulation with pushing manipulation. Pushing manipulation is linear movement in one direction while wiping manipulation can be done up and down, or in a straight line, or in a curved line, it is more flexible.

(3) When finger wiping manipulation is done on the head, the operating procedure is more fixed.

3.2.3.8 Scattering Manipulation

Push and rub back and forth along the channel of *shaoyang* over the temporal region with the radial surface of thumb and the tips of the other four fingers, which is called scattering manipulation.

3.2.3.8.1 Operation Method

The operator holds the patient's head with one hand and keeps close to the temple of the head with the radial surface of thumb and the tips of the other four fingers. Push and rub back and forth behind the ear along the *shaoyang* channel with slight force. The frequency is about 250 times every minute.

3.2.3.8.2 Essentials for Operation

The operator should lower the shoulder, drop the elbow and bend the elbow joint to 90° to 120°, keep the wrist joint relaxed.

Take the elbow joint as the fulcrum, actively swing the forearm to drive the wrist joint to swing, and push and rub on the temple back and forth with the operating hand.

3.2.3.8.3 Precautions

(1) During the operation, the exerting parts of the fingers should stick tightly on the scalp with slight strength. When pushing and rubbing forward, the strength should be heavier; while pushing and rubbing backward, the strength should be lighter.

(2) When operating this manipulation, the holding hand should fix the patient's head to avoid shaking and generating discomfort.

(3) The scattering manipulation should be operated along the channel forward and backward, the distance of movement should not be too long.

3.2.3.9 Foulage

Clip a certain part of the body or limbs with both palms, twist alternatively or quickly back and forth, which is called foulage manipulation.

3.2.3.9.1 Operation Method

(1) Foulage on the shoulders and upper limbs: The patient takes a sitting position with shoulders and arms relaxed and dropped naturally. The operator stands by the patient, the upper body slightly inclines forward, clips the front and back of the patient's shoulder with both palms. The foulage is done from upper limb to the wrist for 3 to 5 times.

(2) Foulage on the hypochondria: The patient takes a sitting position and slightly extends the two arms outside. The operator stands behind the patient and clamps the two hypochondriac regions of the patient with the two palms. Do foulage from armpits to waist for several times in the two sides.

(3) Foulage on the lower limbs: The patient takes the supine position and bends knees to about 60°. The operator stands beside the bed, clamps the two sides of the patient's thigh with two palms, do foulage from the upper down to the crus.

3.2.3.9.2 Essentials for Operation

The operator should exert force symmetrically with the palms and the patient should relax the limbs.

It is better to twist quickly and shift up and down slowly.

3.2.3.9.3 Precautions

The strength used should not be too heavy in the foulage.

Being a supplementary manipulation, this is often used on the shoulders and in the upper limbs and mainly used when the Tuina treatment goes to a close.

3.2.3.10 Shaking

Hold the distal end of the treated limbs with both hands or one hand to shake continuously up and down or from left to right in a small amplitude, which is called shaking manipulation.

3.2.3.10.1 Operation Method

The operator holds the distal end of the patient's upper or lower limbs (wrist or ankle) by hand, lifts the treated limbs to a certain angle (the upper limbs extend about 60° outside in the sitting position, the lower limbs lift to form about 30° angle between the extremity and the bed in the supine position). When pulling with slight strength, continuously shake up and down in small amplitude to make the parenchyma of the treated limbs of the patient generate the vibration and convey to the proximal end of the limbs.

3.2.3.10.2 Essentials for Operation

(1) The shaken limbs of the patient should naturally extend straight and relax. The operator should breathe naturally and can't hold breath.

(2) The amplitude of shaking should be small, and the frequency should be fast.

3.2.3.10.3 Precautions

(1) To shake the lower limbs, the amplitude of shaking can be larger than that of the upper limbs and the frequency should be lower because the lower limbs are heavier.

(2) The shaking is usually used as an ending of manipulation, the shaking manipulation of the upper extremities is commonly used.

3.2.3.11 Pressing

Exert force on the particular point or part of the body surface with the fingers or the palm and press down gradually, which is called pressing manipulation.

3.2.3.11.1 Operation Method

(1) Pressing manipulation with fingers: Extend the thumb straight, press on the channels and points of the body surface with the tip or the whorled surface of the thumb supported by the other extended four fingers. If the strength is not enough for one hand, overlap the other thumb on it to press down heavily with the surface of the thumb.

(2) Pressing manipulation with the palm: Press on the body surface with the palm root, thenar or the whole palm. If the strength is not enough for one hand, overlap the two hands to press.

3.2.3.11.2 Essentials for Operation

(1) The direction of pressing should be vertical. The strength used should be from light to heavy, stable and lasting to make the stimulation fully penetrate into the deep layer of the body tissue, and then decrease the pressure gradually. The principle "light-heavy-light" should be followed.

(2) If the bigger stimulation is needed in the pressing manipulation, the operator can slightly incline his upper body forward to increase the stimulation by his own gravity.

3.2.3.11.3 Precautions

Avoid using the sudden violent force to prevent the side effect.

The force should be changed rhythmically in operation. Pay attention to the difference between the lasting-pressing manipulation and pressing manipulation. In clinic, it is commonly used together with the kneading manipulation to form the compound manipulation of pressing and kneading manipulation.

3.2.3.12 Continuous Pressing Manipulation

Exert force on the special point or part of the body surface with the thumb, palm or the olecranon of the elbow and press downwards continuously, which is called continuous pressing manipulation.

3.2.3.12.1 Operation Method

The operator presses the body surface vertically with the whorled surface of the thumb, palm or the upper part of the forearm of the flexed elbow. Gradual slipping on the body surface can also be done during the pressing. Pressing with the upper part of the forearm is also called continuous pressing manipulation with elbow.

3.2.3.12.2 Essentials for Operation

Pressing manipulation is similar to continuous pressing manipulation, so they are always collectively called "pressure manipulation". If distinguished strictly, the former is more dynamic while the latter is more static; the lasting time of pressing manipulation is short while the continuous pressing manipulation is long; the force of pressing manipulation is small and the stimulation is light while the force of continuous pressing manipulation is great and the stimulation is strong.

3.2.3.12.3 Precautions

(1) When it is used on the back and waist, control the force to prevent side effect.

(2) The stimulation of the continuous pressing manipulation with elbow is stronger, so it is mostly used on the waist and buttocks of the strong people where there are thick muscles.

3.2.3.13 Pointing

Press on the certain point or part of the body with the tip of finger or the articular protrusion, which is called pointing manipulation. It can be divided into pointing with fingers and pointing with elbow in clinic.

3.2.3.13.1 Operation Method

(1) Pointing manipulation with fingers: The operator makes an empty fist, extends the thumb straight and makes it close to the middle interphalangeal joint of the middle finger. Exert force with the tip of the thumb or the interphalangeal joint of the thumb, or the tip of the middle finger supported by overlapping the index finger on the back of the middle finger. Press on a certain point or part with a steady force.

(2) Pointing manipulation with the elbow: The operator bends the elbow and exerts force with the olecranon, slightly inclines his body and presses continuously with the elbow. The pressure from the operator's own gravity is transmitted through the shoulder joint and upper arm to the elbow.

3.2.3.13.2 Essentials for Operation

The pointing manipulation is developed from the pressing manipulation, the essentials are basically the same, but the touching area is smaller and the stimulation is stronger.

3.2.3.13.3 Precautions

(1) In operating the pointing manipulation, the touching area is small, the stimulation intensity is big and the stimulation time is short. It is often used to relieve pain, also called "finger needle". After the pointing manipulation, kneading manipulation can be used to smooth qi and blood and prevent the lesion of parenchyma of the treated area as well.

(2) It should be carefully applied to people who are old, weak and frail.

(3) The part for exerting force in pointing manipulation with the elbow and pressing manipulation with the elbow is different. The former exerts force with the sharp olecroanon while the latter exerts force with the blunt upper part of the forearm.

3.2.3.14 Pinching

Exert force symmetrically with the thumb and other fingers and extrude the treated area, which is called pinching manipulation. The manipulation used to treat the spine is called spine pinching manipulation, which is usually used in children.

3.2.3.14.1 Operation Method

Clamp the treated area with the thumb, index finger and middle finger, or the thumb and the other four fingers and extrude symmetrically and loosen at once. Repeat the manipulation mentioned above and shift gradually.

3.2.3.14.2 Essentials for Operation

The force should be exerted with the thumb and other four fingers, symmetrically, evenly and softly. The movement should be consecutive and rhythmic.

3.2.3.14.3 Precautions

(1) The force should be exerted with the palm, not the tip of the finger.

(2) The force of the fingers is highly required, especially the combined force of thumb and other four fingers. People can adopt the relative exercise for basic training to improve the finger force.

3.2.3.15 Grasping

Exert force symmetrically with the thumb and the other four fingers to lift and pinch or clamp the limbs or skin, which is called grasping manipulation.

3.2.3.15.1 Operation Method

The operator relaxes the wrist joint, clamps the treated area symmetrically with the whorled surface of thumb and index finger, middle finger or other fingers to lift the skin and continuously do the kneading and pinching movement alternately with light and heavy strength.

3.2.3.15.2 Essentials for Operation

(1) Relax the wrist joint, extend the fingers straightly, exert force with the flat finger pulp to clamp the treated area, bend the metacarpophalangeal joints that is opposite to the thumb, lift and pinch the skin and the subcutaneous parenchyma symmetrically, which seems to be a scissor type.

(2) The strength should be slow, gentle and even, from light to heavy then from heavy to light, the kneading and pinching movement should be continuous.

3.2.3.15.3 Precautions

(1) In the operation of grasping manipulation, avoid bending the interphalangeal joint of the fingers to form the action of pinching the skin by the tip of fingers or nipping with the fingernails.

(2) During the operation of grasping manipulation, pinch the subcutaneous parenchyma as much as possible according to the clinical needs and avoid the fingers slipping on the body surface.

(3) After the grasping manipulation, kneading and rubbing manipulation can be used to smooth qi and blood.

3.2.3.16 Twiddling

Clamp the treated area with the thumb and index finger and twiddle while kneading and pinching symmetrically, which is called twiddling manipulation.

3.2.3.16.1 Operation Method

Exert force symmetrically and clamp the treated area with the whorled surface of thumb and the radial surface of the index finger, and make a quicker twisting with slight force like twiddling a thread. Twiddling is a supplementary manipulation and it is mostly used for the joints of fingers and toes.

3.2.3.16.2 Essentials for Operation

(1) Twiddling manipulation requires the movement be continuous and flexible, soft and powerful.

(2) The speed of the twiddling is quick, but the shift speed on the treated area should be slow.

3.2.3.17   Plucking

Press on the treated area with the thumb and pluck back and forth along the direction vertical to the direction of the tendons and muscles, which is called plucking manipulation.

3.2.3.17.1   Operation Method

Straighten the thumb and exert strength with the tip or the whorled surface of the thumb supported by the other four fingers. Press deeply with the thumb until the patient feels aching and distending. Then pluck back and forth along the direction vertical to the direction of the muscle fiber and tendon. If the force of one finger is not enough, it can be operated by two thumbs overlapped.

3.2.3.17.2   Essentials for Operation

(1) In operating plucking manipulation, the thumb should not rub and move on the body skin but should pluck with the subcutaneous muscle fiber or tendon and ligament together.

(2) In operating plucking manipulation, the strength used should be increased gradually according to the patient's endurance.

3.2.3.17.3   Precautions

(1) Plucking manipulation is usually operated on the tenderness.

(2) The stimulation of plucking manipulation is stronger, so it is better to use kneading and rubbing manipulation to smooth qi and blood after operating this manipulation.

3.2.3.18   Patting Manipulation

Patting in rhythm on the body surface with the empty palm is called patting manipulation.

3.2.3.18.1   Operation Method

The operator juxtaposes the fingers and thumb together, flexes the metacarpophalangeal joints slightly so as to form an empty palm. Then pat the treated parts in rhythm at a frequency of 100 to 120 times per minute.

3.2.3.18.2   Essentials for Operation

(1) The shoulder joint and wrist should be relaxed and dropped. The wrist joint should be relaxed. The patting should be light and steady. The palm should rise up as soon as patting the treated area. Pat in rhythm until the skin turns to reddish with congestion.

(2) The manipulation can be operated by one hand or both hands.

3.2.3.18.3   Precautions

(1) The palm patting on the body surface should be steady, avoid dragging on the body surface.

(2) Avoid using this manipulation in the patient who suffers from tuberculosis, serious osteoporosis, bone tumor, and coronary heart disease.

3.2.3.19   Striking Manipulation

Strike the treated parts in rhythm with the palm base, the hypothenar, the back of a fist, finger tip or the stick made of mulberry twigs, which is called striking manipulation.

3.2.3.19.1   Operation Method

(1) Striking manipulation with the palm root: Fingers stretch naturally, the wrist joint stretches slightly backward and tap the body surface with the palm root.

(2) Striking manipulation with the hypothenar: Fingers stretch naturally, the wrist joint

stretches slightly backward and then strike the body surface with the hypothenars of both hands alternately.

(3) Striking manipulation with fist: Hold a fist and keep the wrist joint straight and strike the body surface with the back of fist. The frequency is 3 to 5 times per time.

(4) Striking manipulation with the finger tips: Strike the treated parts lightly and quickly with the five finger tips juxtaposed together.

(5) Striking manipulation with a stick: Strike the body surface with the upper 1/2 of the stick made of mulberry twigs.

3.2.3.19.2 Essentials for Operation

(1) The force used should be quick with a short duration. Strike vertically to the body surface with an even and rhythm frequency.

(2) When operating striking manipulation with palm root, take the palm root as the force origin, strike with the strength from the forearm. The arms can flirt in great amplitude. The frequency is 3 to 5 times per time.

(3) Striking manipulation with the hypothenar can be operated with one hand or both hands. Take the elbow joint as the supporting point and make the forearm move actively. When operating, the hypothenar should be perpendicular to the direction of the muscle fiber and the movement should be rhythmic and rapid.

(4) When operating striking manipulation with the fist, take the elbow joint as the supporting point and strike with the force from the flexion and extension of the elbow joint and the forearm. The force should be steady.

(5) When operating striking manipulation with finger tips, relax the wrist joint and flex and extend the elbow joint in a small amplitude. Strike the body surface with the finger tips lightly at a rapid speed just like rain drops.

(6) When operating striking manipulation with stick, hold the 1/3 part of the lower part of the mulberry stick, move the forearm actively and strike the treated part with the upper part of the stick in rhythm.

3.2.3.19.3 Precautions

(1) When operating striking manipulation, pay attention to the rebounding. The stick should bounce up at one after it touches the treated parts. Do not pause or drag on the body surface.

(2) Strictly grasp the treated parts and indications of different striking manipulations, avoid striking violently.

(3) Striking manipulation with the palm root in mainly indicated for *da zhui* (GV14), lumbosacral region. Striking manipulation with a stick can be used on *bai hui* (GV20), *huan tiao* (GB30). Striking manipulation with the finger tips is usually used on the head. In operating with a stick, the body of the stick, not the tip should be used. The ordinate axis of the stick body should parallel with the direction of the muscle fiber except the lumbosacral parts.

3.2.3.20 Flicking

Press the back side of the index finger tightly with the middle finger and spring swiftly to flick the part or point of the body, which is called flicking manipulation.

3.2.3.20.1   Operation Method

Flex the forefinger, press the back side of the forefinger with the whorled surface of middle finger and then flick the treated parts rapidly. The frequency is about 120 to 160 times per minute. The manipulation is usually used as a supplementary manipulation on the head and in the face.

3.2.3.20.2   Essentials for Operation

This manipulation should be operated evenly and continuously. The intensity of flicking should be controlled to avoid inducing pain.

3.2.3.21   Vibrating

Vibrating is a kind of continuous rapid vibration done by fingers or palm on certain acupuncture points or areas of the human body.

3.2.3.21.1   Operation Method

(1) Finger-vibrating manipulation: Drop the elbow and put the tips of fingers on the performed area. Straighten the fingers and flex the elbow slightly. The muscles of the forearm and hands exert intensive motionless power to make rapid vibration of the arm. The vibration is transported to the body of the patient through the tips of fingers, producing easy and warm feeling in the performed area.

(2) Palm-vibrating manipulation: Stretch the wrist joint slightly backwards and extend fingers naturally. Press the performed area of the patient gently with the palm and flex the elbow slightly. The muscles of the forearm and hands exert intensive motionless power to make rapid vibration of the arm. The vibration is transported to the body of the patient through the center of the palm, producing easy and warm feeling in the performed area.

3.2.3.21.2   Essentials for Operation

(1) Relax the shoulder and the upper arm. Slightly flex the elbow joint.

(2) The muscles of the forearm and palm should exert intensive motionless power which is to tighten the muscles of the hand and the forearm without doing active movements.

(3) The mind should be concentrated on the fingertips and the center of the palm with natural and easy breath.

(4) The movement should be continuous and constant with high frequency of 300 to 400 times per minute.

3.2.3.21.3   Precautions

(1) Except the motionless power from the muscles of the forearm and hand, other parts of the body should be relaxed during the operation. Don't hold the breath.

(2) Do not press downward too much during the operation.

(3) Vibrating needs long time practice. The practice of *Shao Lin* internal exercise (*Shao Lin Nei Gong*) can improve the quality of the manipulation efficiently.

3.2.3.22   Nipping

Nipping is done by the finger nails to irritate the acupuncture points forcefully without injury of the skin.

3.2.3.22.1   Operation Method

Nip the points by nails of thumb or index finger forcefully without injury of the skin.

3.2.3.22.2 Essentials for Operation

(1) The nipping direction should be perpendicular. The strength should be started from gentle to strong. Do not dig with the finger to avoid damage the skin of the performed points.

(2) Kneading with the belly of thumb gently can be performed to the points after nipping to relieve the pain.

3.2.4 Self-Massage for Healthcare

3.2.4.1 Effect and Requirement of Self-Massage

Self-massage for healthcare based upon the theories of traditional Chinese medicine, means that people may use some basic manipulations to work on certain parts or acupoints of the body in order to regulate the channels, activate and promote transportation and circulation of qi and blood so as to achieve the purpose of strengthening body constitution, preventing and treating diseases, preserving health and prolonging life.

3.2.4.1.1 Effect of Self-Massage

(1) Regulating Yin and Yang

The balance between yin and yang is the key to heath. The imbalance between yin and yang can lead to various diseases and pathological changes. Self-massage functions to dredge the channels, invigorate qi and blood, soothe the limbs and skeleton, and nourish the viscera. It also has the capability of regulating the excess or deficiency of yin and yang in order to restore the balance between them and keep the normal physiological functions of the body.

(2) Dredging the Channels and Collaterals

When the physiological activities of channels are normal, qi and blood within the channels flow freely so that the *zangfu* organs are well nourished and they can communicate with the surface of the body effectively. When the channels fail to work normally, the flow of qi and blood will be blocked, normal body functions will be disturbed and the person will become ill. Properly stimulating the channels and points with Tuina methods can adjust the function of vital organs, dredge the channels, promote the flow of qi and blood, improve body metabolism and enhance the natural ability of the body to prevent diseases.

(3) Strengthening Body Constitution

To apply manipulations of self-massage to one specific part of the body may exert effect of activating healthy qi, consequently promoting production, transportation and circulation of qi and blood, and improving body immunity. It has a double directional function of adjusting the viscera so as to normalize the dysfunction, and regulate the active function of qi to release the fatigue of the mentality and body; improve local circulation of blood and nutrition support for hairdressing or loss of weight, thereby, to achieve the purpose of strengthening body constitution and keeping good health.

3.2.4.1.2 Requirement of Self-Massage

(1) Self-massage or family-massage should be done through definite diagnosis, please go to see the doctor in time if one feels uncomfortable.

(2) Keep moderate temperature and humidity to prevent cold. To give comfortable position

and lay some skin lubricant such as massage paste on the exposed skin.

(3) Manipulations of self-massage should be harmonious and tender, energize moderately, from gently to strongly, from shallowly to deeply. It can last 20 to 30 minutes every time according to different conditions. Self-massage should be done step by step, the time, frequency and intensity of application should be carefully monitored for permanent impact.

(4) Do not choose parts in the lower abdominal and lumbar region for pregnant women or some acupoints such as *he gu* (LI4), *san yin jiao* (SP6). Do not do massage when one exercises excessively, is too full or famished, feels fatigue, is drunken, feels nervous or is during menstruation period. Do not apply self-massage if one is seriously ill, or suffers from trauma and infectious disease.

(5) Self-massage can be easily applied with sure security and efficiency, and it is suitable for people of different age to preserve health, prevent and treat diseases.

3.2.4.2 Practical Manipulations of Self-Massage

3.2.4.2.1 General Self-Massage

Self-massage is a common therapy of health cultivation and health care. People can use manipulations to work on the skin or acupoints of their own body in order to prevent and treat diseases, improve and strengthen body constitution. It should be operated flexibly step by step according to individual conditions and in accordance with the passage of the channels and collaterals of the five viscera. One can also do the general self-massage for healthcare from the head to foot. Good effects will be obtained if self-massage is done properly as follows:

Tapping the teeth → cleaning the mouth → wiping the face → kneading the eyes → press *jing ming* (BL1) points → brushing the *ying xiang* (LI20) points → pressing the temples → *Ming Tian Gu* (auricular drilling) → combing the hair → kneading the neck → pinching the shoulder → swing the hands → broadening the chest → kneading the abdomen → beating the back → rubbing the waist → pressing the *huan tiao* (GB30) points → rubbing the thigh → kneading the calf → rubbing the *yong quan* (KI1) points.

3.2.4.2.2 Broadening the Chest

The normal physiological function of the lung is to ensure normal respiration, nutrition and water metabolism. If the function of the lung is abnormal, it will lead to difficulty in breath stuffiness in the chest, cough, asthmatic breath, and even edema. Thus, the manipulation of broadening the chest may effectively prevent and treat diseases of the lung.

(1) Kneading the breast: Use the middle finger to press and knead below the collarbone and between the ribs from inside to outside, from upper to lower, from one side to another until aching or bulging feeling is present.

(2) Vibrating the chest: Hold greater pectoral muscle of the left side and grasp with the right hand for 9 times, repeat the same manipulation on the right side with the left hand. Then, cross the fingers, hold the nape with the elbow flexed horizontally. Try to extend the elbow backward as much as possible when breathing out. Repeat the same procedure for 9 times, and relax it from inner to forth.

(3) Tapping the chest: Put the right hollow palm over the right breast, pat with proper force

and move to the left horizontally, back and forth for 9 times until warm feeling at the local area is felt.

(4) Rubbing the chest: Cross the hands with fingers and put them on the chest, transversely rub back and forth forcefully for 36 times until warm feeling at the local area is felt.

(5) Pushing the *dan zhong* (CV17): Put the hands one over the other at CV17 between the nipples, rub up and down for 36 times.

(6) Kneading *zhong fu* (LU1): Cross the hands in front of the chest. Put the tips of middle fingers at LU1 on both sides. Knead the point with slightly forceful strength clockwise and counterclockwise for 36 times respectively.

(7) Hooking *tian tu* (CV22): Hook CV22 with the tip of the index finger and knead for 1 minute.

(8) Removing obstruction from the lung channel: Take a sitting or standing position, put the right hand above the left breast and rub in circles till it is warm in the local area. Then rub backward and forward along the front of the shoulder, anterior border of medial aspect of the arm, and radial side of the wrist and dorsum of the index finger (the course of the lung channel) for 36 times. Then repeat the same procedure with the left hand on the right side.

3.2.4.2.3 Strengthening the Spleen

When the spleen functions well in transportation and transformation, the food nutrient is absorbed continuously, qi and blood are constantly produced, the body is well nourished, the lips are red and lustrous. If the spleen does not function well, it will cause emaciation, muscular atrophy and weakness, tastelessness or abnormal taste in the mouth, and pale lips without luster. The manipulation for strengthening the spleen and regulating the stomach can effectively prevent and treat disorders of the spleen and stomach.

(1) Rubbing *zhong wan* (CV12): Put the left or the right hand on CV12. Rub the epigastric region counterclockwise in circles for 36 times from small to large circles. Then perform the same rubbing movement clockwise for 36 times from big to small circles.

(2) Kneading *tian shu* (ST25): Take a sitting position, or lie down on the back. Press and knead ST25 with the index and middle fingers simultaneously clockwise and counterclockwise for 36 times respectively.

(3) Pressing epigastric region: Juxtapose the four fingers of the left or the right hand and put them on CV12. Take abdominal respiration, press downward when breathing in and knead in circles when breathing out. Repeat the whole procedure for 36 times.

(4) Separating yin and yang: Put the hands on the xiphoid process with fingers pointing to each other. Perform pulling manipulation from the front midline to the hypochondriac regions along the rib arcs and shift to the lower abdomen. Repeat the whole procedure for 9 times.

(5) Rubbing the navel: Put the palm center of one hand on the navel, press the back of the hand with another hand, clockwise for 3 to 5 minutes.

(6) Pressing *zu san li* (ST36): Put the thumbs, index or middle finger on ST36, press and knead with slight strength for about 3 minutes until aching and distending feeling in the local area is felt.

(7) Kneading *xue hai* (SP10): Take a sitting position, knead SP10 with the thumbs clockwise and counterclockwise for 36 times respectively.

(8) Pinching *he gu* (LI4): Press LI4 with the thumb and index finger of the right hand for about 1 minute. Then perform the same procedure with the left hand on the other side.

3.2.4.2.4　Calming the Mind

The normal function of the heart is manifested as vigorous spirit, sound mental activities, agile movement, moderate and forceful pulse as well as light reddish tongue with moist coating. Insufficient heart qi may cause low spirit, slow reaction, irregular pulse, and dark purple or pale tongue property. Thus, the manipulation for tranquilizing the heart and calming the mind can effectively prevent and cure diseases of the heart.

(1) Rubbing the chest: Put the right hand on the area between the breasts with fingers pointing downward to the side of the abdomen. Push first downward to the area below the left breast and rub the heart area, and then return in the initial position. Then withdraw the hand to the area below the right breast to repeat rubbing in circles. Push and rub in this way to form a figure of "∞" (horizontal 8) for 36 times.

(2) Patting the calvaria: Use the palm to pat the calvaria with rhythm. It should be gently done at the beginning. Then strengthen gradually when there is no bad reaction, tap about 10 times each procedure.

(3) Grasping the heart channel: Put the thumb of the right hand under the left armpit and the rest other four fingers on the medial aspect of the upper arm, grasp, press and knead simultaneously. Then shift the hands bit by bit to *shen men* (HT7). Repeat the same procedure up and down for 9 times. Then change the hand to perform the same procedure on the right arm.

(4) Kneading *shen men* (HT7): Take a sitting position, put the middle finger over the index finger of the right hand to knead HT7 on the left hand for about 1 minute. Then change the hand and repeat the same procedure on the opposite side.

(5) Squeezing *nei guan* (PC6): Take a sitting position, press PC6 on the left side with the thumb of the right hand, the other four fingers assist to squeeze the point from the back of the wrist. Press and squeeze for 9 times. Then change the hand and perform the same manipulation the right side.

(6) Beating heaven drum: Press the hands on the ears with the bottom of the palms pointing to the front with the five fingers pointing to the back. Hit the occiput region with the index, middle and ring fingers for 3 times, and then move the hands away suddenly. Repeat the same procedure for 9 times.

(7) Stirring the sea: Rotate the tongue to rub the outside and inside of the gums, from the right to the left and the left to the right for 9 times respectively. Swallow the saliva excreted in 3 times.

3.2.4.2.5　Soothing the Liver

If liver qi is sufficient, the tendons will be strong, the nails will be firm and the eyes will be bright. Deficiency of liver qi will result in soft and weak tendons and blurred vision. Thus, frequently application of the manipulations for soothing the liver and smoothing the gallbladder is an effective way to prevent and treat diseases of the liver.

(1) Kneading *dan zhong* (CV17): Take a sitting position, juxtapose the four fingers and put them on CV17, knead clockwise and counterclockwise for 36 times respectively with relatively forceful strength.

(2) Rubbing the hypochondriac region: Take a sitting position, put the hands over the chest at the sides of the nipples with the left hand over the right hand, rub horizontally along the ribs and gradually shifting downward to the floating ribs, then put the right hand over the left side and perform the same movement again. Repeat the same process until warm feeling in the hypochondriac region is felt.

(3) Rubbing the lower abdomen: Take a sitting or supine position, put the hands below the hypochondriac regions, rub forcefully along an oblique line to the lower abdomen and pubis for 36 times.

(4) Pointing and pressing *zhang men* (LR13): Put the tips of the middle fingers on LR13, press the point for about 1 minute with slightly strong force till aching and numb feeling is felt.

(5) Kneading *qi men* (LR14): Take a sitting or supine position, put the palm root of the left hand on the right LR14, knead it forcefully clockwise and counterclockwise for 36 times respectively, then change the other hand to repeat the same manipulation.

(6) Nailing *tai chong* (LR3): Take a sitting position, press LR3 with the tips of thumbs forcefully for about 1 minute till aching and numb feeling is felt, then knead the point gently with the whorl surface of the thumbs.

3.2.4.2.6 Strengthening the Kidney

The kidney is considered as "the foundation of congenital constitution" and is the energy source of life. The major function of the kidney is to store essence, control reproduction and development and regulate metabolism of body fluid. In addition, its role in accepting qi is of great importance to respiration. This manipulation can help strengthen and consolidate kidney function, prevent and cure disorders of the kidney system.

(1) Rubbing *guan yuan* (CV4): Take CV4 as the centre of a circle, rub in circles clockwise or counterclockwise with the left and right hands for 36 times respectively. Then press CV4 inward and downward for 3 minutes with the rhythm of respiration.

(2) Rubbing the lower abdomen: From the area below hypochondriac regions to the pubis, two hands push and rub repeatedly along an oblique course until it is warm in the local area.

(3) Rubbing the lumbosacral region: Lean the body forward slightly, flex the elbow, put two palms on the sides of the lower back. Then rub the sacral region up and down with the whole palm or hypothenar until it is warm in the local area.

(4) Rubbing kidney regions: Put the hands over *shen shu* (BL23), rub and turn for 36 times in circles with both hands simultaneously (Rubbing clockwise is reinforcing and counterclockwise is reducing. It is not advisable to apply reducing method on BL23). If one has the problems of kidney deficiency or lumbago, it is necessary to increase the times of turning activity.

(5) Kneading *ming men* (GV4): Put the index finger and middle finger on GV4 and knead the point in circles clockwise and counterclockwise for 36 times respectively.

(6) Rubbing *yong quan* (KI1): Take a sitting position with the legs crossed, rub both hands till they are hot, then rub back and forth from *san yin jiao* (SP6) to the toe until the skin is hot, then rub KI1 with both hands respectively until it is warm inside. The rubbing movement should be done in proper rhythm.

(7) Contracting the anus and perineum: Relax the body in a quiet environment, take abdominal respiration (breathe in with the abdomen protruded and breathe out with the abdomen contracted). During the expiration, slightly contract the anus and perineum. During inspiration, relax the abdomen. Repeat the whole procedure for 36 times.

(Ma Liangxiao)

3.3 Acupressure

Acupressure is a healing technique using fingers, palms, knuckles and elbows to apply pressure at acupuncture points to inspire qi of the channels, regulate yin and yang according to the basic theory of TCM. Acupressure is derived from acupuncture. Both of them use the same points and channels, but acupuncture employs needles, while acupressure uses the fingers or certain manual manipulations. Acupressure is one of the most frequently used techniques of TCM nursing due to its advantages of easy operation, low cost, safety, extensive indications and satisfied efficacy.

3.3.1 Indications of Acupressure

Acupressure has the effects of releasing tension, relaxing the sinews and alleviating pain, invigorating blood and dissolving stasis, and dredging the channels and collaterals. Therefore, acupressure has extensive indications and can be used for nursing various diseases involving internal medicine, gynecology, surgery, pediatric, and traumatology, especially for pain, injury of soft tissues, emotional tension, functional disorders of *zang-fu* organs.

3.3.1.1 Diseases of Traumatology
Fibromyalgia, lumbago, cervical spondylopathy, periarthritis of shoulder, chronic muscular strain, ankle and knee sprain, etc.

3.3.1.2 Internal Diseases
Common cold, headache, dizziness, insomnia, cough, asthma, stomachache, diarrhea, constipation, impotence, hypertension, coronary heart disease, sequelae of wind stroke, chronic fatigue syndrome, depression, etc.

3.3.1.3 Diseases of Surgery
Hyperplasia of the mammary gland, postoperative gastrointestinal dysfunction, adverse reactions of chemotherapy and radiotherapy, etc.

3.3.1.4 Gynecological Diseases
Irregular menstruation, dysmenorrhea, menopausal syndrome, etc.

3.3.1.5 Diseases of Five Sensory Organs
Myopia, tinnitus, rhinitis, etc.

3.3.2 Frequently Used Manipulations and Points of Acupressure

The majority of Tuina manipulations can be used in acupressure, especially those techniques using fingers and palms to apply certain pressure at acupuncture points. The essentials of acupressure techniques are steady, forceful, even speed rhythm, soft and penetration. In general, gradual, steady and penetrating pressure on each point for approximately three minutes is ideal. How much pressure to apply to any point depends on the physique of the patient and the location of the point. Each body and each area of the body requires a different amount of pressure. The area being pressed may result in aching, numbness, heavy, distention and pain sensations. If it hurts a great deal, then use light touch instead of pressure. The calves, the face, and genital areas are sensitive and need gentle pressure. The back, buttocks, and shoulders, especially if the musculature is developed, usually need deeper, firmer pressure.

The frequently used acupressure techniques include: one-finger pushing, kneading, rubbing, scrubbing, mopping, pressing, continuous pressing, pointing, grasping, plucking, nipping, etc. For the details of operation methods, essentials and precautions of those techniques, please refer to Section 1 "Tuina" of Chapter 3.

For the frequently used acupressure points and its techniques, please refer to Form 2-3 in Section 2 "Channels, Collaterals and Acupuncture Points" of Chapter 2.

3.3.3 Contraindications of Acupressure

3.3.3.1   Surgery diseases such as acute peritonitis, enterobrosis, acute appendicitis, fracture, etc.

3.3.3.2   Various acute and chronic infectious diseases such as typhoid, epidemic cerebrospinal meningitis, epidemic encephalitis B, hepatitis, tuberculosis, syphilis, gonorrhoea, AIDS, etc.

3.3.3.3   Various acute poisoning, such as food poisoning, gas poisoning, drug poisoning, alcoholism, venomous snake bites, etc.

3.3.3.4   Various severe hemorrhagic conditions, such as cerebral hemorrhage, gastrorrhagia, metrorrhagia, hematochezia, hematuria, traumatic bleeding, etc.

3.3.3.5   Various life-threatening diseases and serious medical problems, such as acute myocardial infection, renal failure, heart failure, etc.

3.3.4 Precautions for Acupressure

3.3.4.1   Maintain an appropriate room temperature and good ventilation prior to acupressure.

3.3.4.2   In order to make the patient comfortable and facilitate location of points, the patient should be placed in a posture according to the condition of disease, constitution, age and gender of the patient and suitable to the points selected.

3.3.4.3   Apply finger pressure in a slow, rhythmic manner to enable the layers of tissue and the internal organs to respond. Never press any area in an abrupt, forceful, or jarring way.

3.3.4.4   Do not do acupressure immediately when a patient is famished, tired, or extreme nervous. Avoid practicing acupressure right after a big meal or on a full stomach. Wait until at least an hour after eating a light meal.

3.3.4.5　Do not choose points in the lower abdominal region for pregnant women in the first trimester. For pregnant women over 3 months, acupuncturing points on the abdominal and lumbosacral areas should be avoided. Certain points including *san yin jiao* (SP6), *he gu* (LI4), *kun lun* (BL60) and *zhi yin* (BL67), which intensively promote blood circulation, are contraindicated during the entire pregnancy. Acupressure should not be applied to women during their menstrual periods, unless they are treated for irregular menstrual periods.

3.3.4.6　Acupressure should not be applied to the infected, ulcerated, or scarred skin or tumors.

3.3.4.7　Lymph areas, such as the groin, the area of the throat just below the ears, and the outer breast near the armpits, are very sensitive. These areas should be touched only lightly and not pressed.

3.4　Moxibustion

Moxibustion is a therapy that utilizes cauterization or heating with ignited flammable material and drug to stimulate the acupuncture points or certain areas of the body in order to treat and prevent diseases.

Moxibustion has effect of warming and dredging the channels, dispersing the wind and relieving the exterior syndrome, warming the middle *jiao* and dispersing the coldness, warming and strengthening the spleen and kidney, supporting yang to rescue collapse, removing blood stasis and stagnation, disease prevention and health maintenance.

Among the materials used in moxibustion, moxa-wool is the most common material which is made of dry mugwort leaves that are purified and formed into fine and soft fibers. Mugwort leaves are fragrant, warm pungent in nature, and bitter in flavor. They are combustible with mild firepower, which can be used in moxibustion to treat lots of illnesses.

3.4.1　Indications

Moxibustion is indicated for various diseases, especially for deficiency syndromes, cold syndromes and yin syndromes. It is used for conditions caused by cold-damp obstruction and blood stagnation, such as joint pain due to wind-cold-dampness pathogen, dysmenorrhea, amenorrhea and abdominal pain; for vomiting and diarrhea due to exterior cold syndromes or deficient cold syndrome of middle *jiao*; for prolonged diarrhea, rectocele, impotence, and enuresis caused by deficiency of spleen and kidney yang; for profuse sweating, cold limbs and feeble pulse due to collapse of yang qi; for prolapse of internal organs, rectum and uterus caused by sinking of middle *jiao* qi. Moxibustion also can be applied to the early stage of abscess and carbuncles, as well as chronic sores, to promote discharge of pus and fascinating the recovery.

3.4.2　Contraindications

3.4.2.1　Moxibustion is contraindicated for any conditions with swift and rapid pulse in both exterior heat syndrome and interior heat syndrome due to yin deficiency. Do not use moxibustion for high fever, convulsion, extreme exhaustion and emaciation. Avoid using moxibustion to treat the patient with excess-heat syndrome and fever due to yin deficiency.

3.4.2.2   Avoid using moxibustion in the cardiac apex area, areas with big arteries, abdominal and lumbosacral region of pregnant women, nipple and external genitals. Avoid using scarring moxibustion on the face, places with large vessels, and joints.

3.4.3   Classifications of Moxibustion

There are many kinds of moxibustion, with the most common ones listed in Figure 3-5.

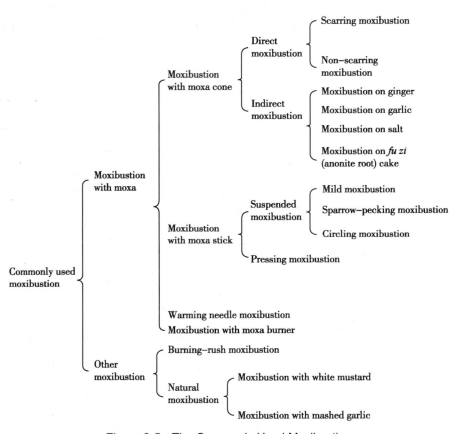

Figure 3-5   The Commonly Used Moxibustion

3.4.4   Commonly Used Operation of Moxibustion

3.4.4.1   Moxibustion with Moxa Cone

This is a method that moxa cone which is formed by shaping a small amount of moxa wool tightly into a cone is put on a selected area of the body and ignited to treat diseases. The size of a moxa varies depending on the conditions and the parts of the body to be treated. A small sized cone is of a wheat grain shape. A middle one is of half of the kernel of Chinese date, and a big one is of half of an olive. Every cone after burning is called one "zhuang". Moxibustion with moxa cone is divided into direct moxibustion and indirect moxibustion.

3.4.4.1.1 Direct Moxibustion

Direct moxibustion is a method that an ignited cone with appropriate size is put directly on the skin. It can be further divided into scarring moxibustion and non-scarring moxibustion according to whether there are scars on the skin after moxibustion. Because scarring moxibustion makes the patient feel great pain, it is rarely used in clinical practice, so only non-scarring moxibustion is introduced here.

Non-scarring moxibustion is also known as non-pustulating moxibustion. It is a method that there will not be a scar on the skin. It is indicated for pain syndrome caused by wind-cold pathogen, and abdominal pain, diarrhea and dysmenorrhea due to deficiency-cold. Smear a bit vaseline on the selected point. Put the moxa cone on the point and ignite it. When 3/5 of the cone is burnt and the patient feels a slight pain, take it off with a forceps and place a new one and ignite it again for the second cone or *zhuang*. Three to seven cones or *zhuang* are needed for each point until the local skin becomes congested and reddish without blister.

3.4.4.1.2 Indirect Moxibustion

It is also known as material isolated moxibustion, or namely a method that the ignited moxa cone is isolated with some materials from contacting the skin directly. Generally speaking, moxibustion on ginger, moxibustion on garlic, moxibustion on salt and moxibustion on *fu zi* (aconite root) cake are commonly used.

(1) Moxibustion on ginger: This method is indicated for deficiency-cold syndrome such as abdominal pain, diarrhea, vomiting and dysmenorrheal and so on. Cut ginger into a slice 2 to 3cm in diameter and 0.2 to 0.3cm in thickness, and puncture some holes in it. Smear a bit vaseline on the selected point. Put ginger slice on the point. Put the moxa cone on it. Ignite the cone and replace a new one and ignite it again for the second cone or *zhuang* when the first cone completely burns out and the ashes are removed. Five to ten cones or *zhuang* are needed for each point until the local skin becomes reddish without blister.

(2) Moxibustion on garlic: This method is mainly used to treat pulmonary tuberculosis and abscesses at the initial stage. Cut a slice of the garlic about 0.2 to 0.3cm thick, and puncture some holes in it. Smear a bit vaseline on the selected point. Put garlic slice on the point. Then put the moxa cone on it. Ignite the cone and replace a new one and ignite it again for the second cone or *zhuang* when the first cone completely burns out and the ashes are removed. Five to seven cones or *zhuang* are needed for each point until the local skin becomes reddish without blister.

(3) Moxibustion on salt: This method is used to treat acute abdominal pain due to cold pathogen, vomiting, diarrhea, dysentery and flaccid pattern of stroke. *Shen que* (CV8) is frequently used. Fill the umbilicus with salt, and put a piece of ginger with holes on the salt to prevent burning the patient. Then put the moxa cone on the ginger and ignite it. Replace a new one and ignite it again for the second cone or *zhuang* when the first cone completely burns out and the ashes are removed. The number of cones or *zhuang* is not limited.

(4) Moxibustion on *fu zi* (aconite root) cake: This method is used to treat diseases due to insufficiency of vital essence such as impotence, premature ejaculation and a ruptured abscess. Grind a piece of aconite root into a fine powder, mix the powder with yellow rice wine into the

paste and shape it into a cake 3 cm in diameter and 0.8 cm in thickness, and puncture some holes in it. Put a moxa cone on the aconite cake and ignite it. Replace a new one and ignite it again for the second cone or *zhuang* when the first cone completely burns out and the ashes are removed. Five to seven cones or *zhuang* are used per point.

3.4.4.2　Moxibustion with Moxa Stick

A moxa stick is prepared by wrapping moxa wool with a piece of Cortex Mori paper and shaping it into a cylinder. Ignite one end of the moxa stick and point it at the point or the diseased area. It can be divided into suspended moxibustion and pressing moxibustion.

3.4.4.2.1　Suspended Moxibustion

It can be further divided into mild moxibustion, sparrow-pecking moxibustion and circling moxibustion based on the way of operation. Materials used in the operation includes moxa-sticks, lighter, forceps and clean disc.

(1) Mild moxibustion: Prepare the materials used in mild moxibustion. Choose points based on the disease condition. Help the patient to select a comfortable posture, and expose the area needing treatment. Ignite one end of the moxa stick and keep it 2 to 3cm away from the skin to warm the area. Patient should feel warm but without causalgia. Each point should usually be heated for 10 to 15 minutes until the skin becomes reddish. The method is used to treat chronic diseases due to deficiency-cold, such as abdominal pain, dysmenorrhea and so on.

(2) Sparrow-pecking moxibustion: Prepare the materials used in sparrow-pecking moxibustion. Choose points based on the disease condition. Help the patient to select a comfortable posture, and expose the area needing treatment. Ignite one end of the moxa stick to warm the area. Move the ignited end upwards and downwards between 2 and 5cm as if a bird is pecking. Each point should usually be heated about 5 minutes. This method is often used to treat acute diseases because the patient will have a stronger feeling of warmth.

(3) Circling moxibustion: Prepare the materials used in circling moxibustion. Choose points based on the disease condition. Help the patient to select a comfortable posture, and expose the area needing treatment. Ignite one end of the moxa stick, keep it about 3cm away from the skin and move it left and right or in a circular motion to warm the area. Each point should usually be heated for 20 to 30 minutes. This method is often used to treat acute diseases.

The three methods mentioned above can be used solely or together.

3.4.4.2.2　Pressing Moxibustion

Place a piece of cloth or several layers of paper on the selected point, and then press the ignited end of the moxa stick onto the cloth or paper tightly until it is extinguished. Ignite and press it again. This method is indicated for dual syndrome of wind-cold-dampness and deficiency-cold.

3.4.4.3　Natural Moxibustion

It is also known as drug moxibustion or vesiculate moxibustion. In fact, it is an external application rather than normal moxibustion. Spread some irritant herbs on the selected point or the diseased part in order to induce blisters and congestion. Moxibustion with mashed garlic and white mustard seed are commonly used.

3.4.4.3.1   Moxibustion with Mashed Garlic

Take 3 to 5g of mashed garlic and apply it on the selected point for 1 to 3 hours until the local skin is itching, flushed and blistered. This moxibustion on *yong quan* (KI1) and *he gu* (LI4) can respectively treat hemoptysis and tonsillitis.

3.4.4.3.2   Moxibustion with White Mustard Seed

Grind a certain amount of white mustard seed into fine powder, mix it with water to make a paste, apply it on the selected point, cover it with oiled paper and then affix it with adhesive plaster. This method is usually used to treat arthralgia. It can be combined with other medication to treat asthma as well.

3.4.4.4   Precautions

3.4.4.4.1   Make explanation to the patient before treatment and help the patient to take a comfortable posture to prevent scalding due to change of posture during the treatment.

3.4.4.4.2   Follow the sequence of moxibustion. In general, moxibustion is applied first on the yang channels and then the yin channels; first on the upper part and then lower part; first with a smaller moxa cone and then a bigger one; first on a point or area with fewer moxa cones and then an area with more moxa cones.

3.4.4.4.3   Pay attention to asking how the patient feels during the treatment. When treating the elderly, infants and patients with sensation disorder, use hand to feel the temperature and adjust the distance between the burning moxa and the patient's skin in time in order to avoid scalding.

3.4.4.4.4   Remove the ashes in time to prevent scalding. Put the ash in the disc where there is some water to avoid burning again.

3.4.4.4.5   If the patient's skin appears to be red or the patient feels the area a little burnt, it is normal and it does not need to be managed. The liquid in small blister can be absorbed by the body. If the blister is large, the liquid can be suck out by a sterile syringe. The area needs to be covered with sterile gauze to prevent infection.

3.5   Cupping Therapy

Cupping is a therapy that a jar is attached to the skin surface using negative pressure brought by means of suction or inducing a flame into the cup so as to form a local congestion or blood stagnation to prevent or treat diseases. It is also called "horn" method, for the buffalo horn is most used as a cup in the ancient time.

3.5.1   Indications

Cupping therapy can free channels and collaterals, dispel wind and scatter cold, relieve swelling and pain, suck toxin and evacuate purulence. It is often used in clinical practice to treat headache due to wind and cold pathogen, arthralgia and ache of the waist and back due to wind-cold-dampness pathogen, cough and asthma due to deficiency cold and snakebite.

3.5.2 Contraindications

Don't apply cupping to the part which is uneven or hairy.

Don't apply cupping to the part where there is ulcer, swelling and where large blood vessels are distributed.

Don't do cupping in the abdominal and lumbosacral region of the pregnant women.

Don't do cupping for the patient with high fever, spasm or clotting disorder.

Don't do cupping for the patient with severe heart disease, heart failure and sever edema.

Don't do cupping for those with severe nervousness, after drunk, extreme tired, excessive eating and over-thirst.

3.5.3 Types of the Cup

At present, bamboo cup, pottery cup, glass cup and piston air-sucking cup are mainly used in clinical practice, of which glass cup is the most commonly used.

3.5.3.1 Bamboo Cup

It is a cup made of a jointed section of bamboo that is 3 to 5cm in diameter and 6 to 10cm in length. The rim of the cup should be smooth and polished. Its advantages are that it is easily-made, light, cheap and durable, suitable for boiling in a medicinal liquid. Its disadvantages are that it cracks and leaks the air out easily. It can be disinfected by boiling.

3.5.3.2 Pottery Cup

It is made of pottery. It can create a strong suction but it is heavier and easily broken. It can be disinfected by boiling or soaking in disinfector.

3.5.3.3 Glass Cup

Glass cup is the most commonly used in clinical practice. It's made of glass and looks like a ball. It comes in a variety of sizes such as large, medium and small. Its advantage is transparent so that the patient's reaction can be observed and the time during which the cup is retained can be controlled. Its disadvantages are fast heat conduction causing the possibility of scalding and easily broken. It can be disinfected by boiling or soaking in disinfector.

3.5.3.4 Sucking Cup

It is made of transparent plastic with a piston inside. The suction is created by moving the piston upwards to draw the air out. It is convenient and safe and is difficult to break. It can be disinfected by soaking in disinfector.

3.5.4 Cup-Sucking Methods

Cup-sucking method here means adopting a certain way to expel air in the cup to create negative pressure so that the cup is attached tightly to the skin. The commonly used methods to attach the cup onto the body are fire cupping, water cupping and sucking cupping.

3.5.4.1 Fire Cupping

Fire cupping is used to expel air in the cup by a flame to create suction and attach the cup to the skin. The most commonly used method is flash-fire cupping.

Hold a cup with appropriate size by one hand, ignite a 95% alcohol-soaked cotton ball held with forceps by the other hand. Put the flame quickly into the cup and take it out after circling it inside once or twice. Place the cup on the patient's skin quickly. This is a safe and the most commonly used method. Do not keep the flame at the opening of the cup to avoid causing scalding.

3.5.4.2 Water Cupping

Water cupping is used to expel air inside the cup by the water vapor with high temperature to create suction and attach the cup to the skin. It is also named cup-boiling method. Boil the bamboo cup in boiling water or medicinal water for 5 to 10 minutes. Take is out with a long forceps and pour the excess liquid out with the opening of the cup downward. Cover the opening with a cold wet towel and place the cup on the skin.

3.5.4.3 Sucking Cupping

Place the cup tightly on the skin, and draw out the air by pulling the piston to attach the cup onto the skin.

3.5.5 Method for Removing Cups

When local skin of cupping turns red or ecchymosis appears after certain time of cupping, the cups can be removed. The attached cup should be removed by holding it with one hand and pressing the skin around the cup with the thumb or other fingers of another hand to let air in. Do not remove the cup with force, this may cause pain or local skin injury.

3.5.6 Manipulation Procedures of Fire Cupping

Here, take flash-fire cupping as an example to introduce preparation and process of operation.

3.5.6.1 Preparation before Operation

Prepare glass cups, 95% ethanol immersed swab, lighter, forceps and clean disc. Prepare vaseline when planning using moving cupping.

3.5.6.2 Procedure of Operation

Explain the purpose and notice of the operation. Check medical order again.

Choose points due to patient condition. Help the patient to apply a comfortable position, and expose the area needing treatment.

Choose a suitable cup. Check whether the edge of the opening is smooth.

Choose the method to fire and attach the cup against the skin. Retain the cup for 10 to 15 minutes.

Pay attention to the condition of the skin while retaining the cup.

Remove cup, wipe off the dirty, help the patient put on and apply a comfortable position.

Tidy up, wash the hands, and take a record.

3.5.7 Clinical Application of Cupping Methods

3.5.7.1 Retaining Cupping

Attach the cup onto the skin and retain it for 5 to 15 minutes. Remove the cup when the local skin forms congestion and blood stagnation. If the cup is large and the suction is strong, the time of retaining cupping should be properly shortened to avoid forming blisters. This method can be applied to all kinds of diseases. A single-cup or multi-cup retaining can be used.

3.5.7.2   Moving Cupping

Smear some unguent or vaseline to the treated area, attach the cup onto the skin. Hold the body of the cup with one hand. Move it up and down or left and right. Remove the cup when the skin becomes reddish, congested and stagnated. This method is suitable for places with thick muscles in such large areas as the back, waist, buttocks and thighs. Select the cup whose opening is large, smooth and polished. Moving cupping is mainly used for acute heat syndromes, paralysis, numbness, *Bi* syndrome due to wind-cold-dampness, muscular atrophy, etc.

3.5.7.3   Flashing Cupping

It refers to attach and remove the cup quickly and repeatedly until the skin turns reddish, congested and stagnated. This method is usually indicated for local numbness and pain.

3.5.8   Precautions

3.5.8.1   Cupping should be applied to the areas with thick muscles. Help the patient to take a comfortable posture.

3.5.8.2   Select the proper sized cup depending on the treated area. Pay attention to examining whether the opening of the cup is smooth and whether there are cracks.

3.5.8.3   The operation should be done steadily, correctly and swiftly.

3.5.8.4   Pay attention to asking how the patient feels and observing the reaction of the local skin during the treatment. Remove and attach the cup again when the patient has feeling of heat, tightness, ache, pain in the treated area.

3.5.8.5   Help the patient to cover the cloth and quilt to keep warm during the retaining cupping.

3.5.8.6   The cupping procedure should be done with great care in order to avoid burning the skin. If a few small blisters appear due to excessive burning or prolonged cup retention, cover them with sterilized gauze to protect the area and avoid infection. If the blisters are large, they may be pricked and the liquid in them can be drawn out by syringe. Cover them with sterilized gauze to avoid infection.

3.5.8.7   Observe whether the patient has the reaction of cupping syncope. When the patient suddenly presents symptoms of dizziness, nausea, pale complexion, etc., stop cupping immediately, and remove all the cups. Help the patient to lie on supine posture and keep his or her body warm. In minor cases, ask the patient to have a rest, and give him or her some warm water or sugar water to drink. The symptoms will be removed shortly. For severe cases, inform the doctor and give remedy to the patient according to the symptoms.

3.6   Scraping Therapy

Scraping therapy is a method to scrape repeatedly on the skin of certain parts of the human body with the dull and smoothly edged instrument so as to form a local congestion or blood stagnation to prevent or treat diseases. Through scrapping, the evil qi of *zangfu* organs can be easily expelled from the skin and muscles, thereby, the blood and qi of the whole body can be quickly free-flowing. The aim of treatment is thus achieved.

3.6.1   Indications

It is indicated for high fever, headache, nausea, vomiting due to exogenous dampness pathogen and heatstroke, bellyache, diarrhea caused by exogenous summer-dampness pathogen.

3.6.2   Contraindications

3.6.2.1   Avoid using scraping for patients with severe or life-threatening diseases, such as acute infectious diseases and sever heart disease, etc.

3.6.2.2   Avoid using scraping for patients with bleeding tendency such as thrombopenia or dysfunction of coagulation, etc.

3.6.2.3   Avoid using scraping at areas with skin ulcers, sores, scalding, recent fracture, or skin masses due to unclear reason.

3.6.2.4   Avoid using scraping among the old, or people with weak constitution, and the excessively thin.

3.6.2.5   Avoid using scraping on the abdomen, lumbosacral region and certain acupuncture points of pregnant women, such as SP6, LI4, GB21, BL60, etc. Do not use scraping on the crown of the head of an infant since his or her fontanelle has not closed yet.

3.6.2.6   Avoid using scraping for people with excessive hunger, overeat, fatigue or nervousness.

3.6.3   Scraping Instruments

At present, scrapping board made by buffalo horn is the most commonly used instrument for scrapping. Coin or spoon with smooth edges and without breakage can also be selected.

3.6.4   Parts for Scraping

Head: Usually scrape the part between the eyebrows and temples.

Neck and nape: Scrape the neck part, the two sides of the nape part.

Chest: Scrape the intercostal spaces and the sternum. The nipples are forbidden to be scraped.

Shoulder and back: Shoulders and the two sides of vertebral column which are the most commonly used parts.

Upper and lower limbs: The medial side of the upper limb, elbow fossa, the medial side of the thigh, and the popliteal fossa are mainly used for scraping.

3.6.5   Manipulations

3.6.5.1   Preparation before Operation

This includes plate, scrapping instrument, lubricant in bowl such as clean water, sesame oil or blood-activating lubricant, a piece of cloth or paper.

3.6.5.2 Procedure of Operation

Prepare all the materials and take them to the ward. Make explanation to the patient to get his or her cooperation.

Help the patient to select a comfortable posture according to the disease and expose the selected parts. The body position of the sufferer: Normally choose the supine position, ventricumbent position and the position of leaning on one's back; it depends on the comfort of the sufferer.

Examine the edge of the instrument and make sure it is smooth and there is no breakage.

Hold the instrument with the hand and dip the lubricant to scrape gently on the selected parts. Keep the angle between the instrument and the skin at an angle of 45° to 90°. Scrap the neck and two sides of vertebral column up to down while scraping the chest and back inside to outside. Scrape along one direction. The strength should be even, moderate. Don't scrape by force. Keep the instrument wet during operation. Scrape until the skin appears red or mauve blood stagnation.

The strip number of scrapping should depend on the disease condition. Generally, 8 to 10 strips should be scrapped once, 6 to 15cm long every strip, 20 times per strip.

Wipe the oil or the water. Assist the patient to put on clothes, and make the bed.

3.6.6 Precautions

3.6.6.1 Keep the fresh air circulating in the room. Avoid the patient being blown directly.

3.6.6.2 The scrapping board should be cleaned after using and disinfected with 75% alcohol. It is recommended to fix the scrapping board for each person.

3.6.6.3 The force should be moderate and even during scrapping, which is decided by the tolerance of the patient. Scrape no more than 10 minutes in each area, or stop on the appearance of red spots under the skin. Red spots should not be importuned if there is no or little.

3.6.6.4 Pay attention to observing the color change of the local skin and asking how the patient feels. Stop scrapping immediately when the patient has the symptoms of abnormal pain, cold sweating, chest discomfort and dysphoria.

3.6.6.5 Tell the patient to take a rest, keep good mood, take light and digestive food, avoid eating cold and greasy food and avoid catching cold after the treatment.

3.6.6.6 The next scrapping is done until blood stagnation disappears, generally the interval is 3 to 6 days, and a treatment course consists of 3 to 5 sessions.

(Ma Liangxiao)

3.7 Hot Compress Therapy

Hot compress therapy is a method to put the heated medicine into a cloth bag and move the bag back and forth or circularly on the certain part or point of the human body. It includes hot medicinal compress, hot scallion compress, and hot salt compress.

3.7.1 Purpose

Hot compress therapy makes use of heat and medicine to warm the channels and unblock the collaterals, dissipate cold and relieve pain, move qi and invigorate blood, dispel stasis and disperse swelling.

3.7.2 Contraindications

Avoid using this method to treat the patients with excess-heat syndrome or unconsciousness patients. Don't use it in the abdomen where the patient has mass of uncertain character, or in the abdominal and lumbosacral region of pregnant women. Don't use it in the places with large vessels, on the injured skin and in the insentient parts.

3.7.3 Different Hot Compress Therapy

Hot medicinal compress therapy is a method to mix the herbs with white spirit or vinegar and heat up them, and put them into a bag, then move the bag back and forth or circularly on the certain part or point of the patient.

3.7.3.1 Hot Medicinal Compress Therapy

3.7.3.1.1 Indications

Gastric cavity pain, diarrhea due to deficiency-cold of the spleen and stomach, cold pain or numbness or soreness of joints caused by *bi* syndrome due to wind-damp.

3.7.3.1.2 Preparation before Operation

This includes treatment plate, medicine, white spirit or vinegar, treatment bowl, 2 double-layered gauze bags, cotton swab, vaseline, big towel, wok, induction cooker, bamboo spade or bamboo chopsticks.

3.7.3.1.3 Procedures of Operation

(1) The practitioner dresses clean and tidy. Wash hands and wear a mask. Put the medicine into the wok according to the doctor's advice, then add moderate white spirit or vinegar and mix them. Saute them to 60 or 70℃ by low flame and put them into the bag, wrapped by the big towel, and keep it warm.

(2) After the materials are prepared, take them to the ward and check again. Explain the purposes and ways of the operation to the patient in order to get his/her cooperation. Assist the patient to take a comfortable posture according to the disease condition and expose the body parts to be treated. Make sure the patient feel warm and private, pull the drapes if necessary.

(3) After smearing appropriate amount of vaseline on the selected skin or the corresponding point, move the medicine bag on the part or point back and forth with the even force. At the beginning, the force should be small but the speed could be relatively high. The force can be increased gradually but the speed can be slowed with the fall of the temperature. When the medicine bag's temperature is too low, change the medicine bag in time to keep warm and enhance the effects. During the compress, observe the appearance of the skin and ask patients if there is any burning pains in order to prevent burns.

(4) The operation usually lasts for 15 to 30 minutes every time, once or twice every day.

(5) After finishing the operation, clean the local skin, assist the patient to put on the clothes and take a comfortable lying posture.

(6) Clean up the materials, wash hands and make notes.

3.7.3.1.4 Precautions

(1) Pay attention to keeping safety during sauting the herbs. When adding the white spirit to the herbs, take the wok away from the fire to prevent danger.

(2) Before the operation, make a full explanation to the patient and tell him/her to empty the bladder.

(3) Pay attention to keeping warm in winter. The temperature in the room should be comfortable in order to prevent contraction of wind-cold.

(4) During the compress, pay attention to observing the skin to prevent burns. Keep the temperature of the medicinal bag at 50 to 60℃. The temperature of the medicinal bag should not be higher than 70℃. For the old, infants, children, the temperature of the medicine bag shouldn't be higher than 50℃.

(5) During the operation, keep the medicine bag warm, change or heat the bag timely. If the patient feels uncomfortable, the compress should be stopped.

3.7.3.2　Hot Scallion Compress

It is a kind of therapy applying hot scallion compress on the patient's abdomen using 200 to 250g fresh scallion stalk (cut into 2 to 3cm segments) that is sauted to heat and put 30ml white spirit, then put into the cloth bag, which achieves the effect of ascending the clear and descending the turbid. For the patient with urine retention, move the scallion bag up and down from the right side of peripheral umbilicus to the left side, right ascending and left descending, which can achieve the effect of discharging ascites and accumulation of qi, and promoting urination as well as stool. For the patient with flaccidity syndrome, paralysis, compress on the painful parts directly. The operation takes about 20 minutes, twice a day.

3.7.3.3　Hot Salt Compress

It is a kind of therapy applying heated sea salt (500-1000g) with the similar size into the cloth bag, and moves it on the affected parts or special parts repeatedly when the bag's temperature is appropriate. It is applied to the gastric or abdominal region of the patient with chronic stomachache and diarrhea due to deficiency cold. If the patient suffers from bì syndrome, flaccidity syndrome, paralysis or pain of muscles and bones, directly compress on the painful parts. For the patient with urinary retention, compress shen que (CV8) or the lower abdomen. The salt bag can be put under the head as a pillow if the patient has dizziness and tinnitus. It can be applied on the center of the thenar for the patient with kidney yang deficiency. This operation lasts for 20 to 30 minutes every time, twice a day.

3.8　Steaming and Washing Therapy

It is an external treatment to steam and fumigate local skin first, to bathe, soak local or whole body with the hot herbal decoction in appropriate temperature.

3.8.1 Purpose

This is an external approach to prevent or treat diseases by fumigating or steaming the body surface or deep tissues through direct action of the herbs and the vapor from the boiling herbs so as to open and discharge the striae and interstices, clear heat and resolve toxins, remove swelling and relieve pain, kill parasites and relieve itching, warm the channels and unblock the collaterals, invigorate blood and dissolve stasis, scatter wind and dissipate cold, dispel wind and eliminate dampness, regulate function of the viscera.

3.8.2 Indications

This method is widely used in many kinds of diseases of internal medicine, surgery, gynecology, pediatrics, orthopedics, otorhinolaryngology and dermatology. It is commonly used in common cold due to wind-cold, sore, carbuncle, perianal abscess, vulva itches, soreness of bones and muscles, *bì* syndrome due to wind-cold, stye, eczema, skin itchiness, tinea of feet and hands.

3.8.3 Contraindications

Steaming and washing therapy should be contraindicated for the patients with fever, coma, local part edema, psychotic, malignant tumor, jaundice, hemorrhagic tendency, qi and blood deficiency, severe heart diseases, asthma attack. Sitz bath and body bathing therapy is not allowed for female patients in menstrual period or pregnancy.

3.8.4 Preparation

3.8.4.1 Eyes Steaming and Washing Therapy
Prepare tray, treatment bowl (filled with herbal decoction), thermometer, gauze and tweezers.
3.8.4.2 Limb Steaming and Washing Therapy
Washbasin or cask, herbal decoction, thermometer, bath towel or middle-size sheet, oval forceps and small towels.
3.8.4.3 Sitz Bath
Prepare tray, small towels, herbal decoction, thermometer, bidet, chair and wood lid with hole.
3.8.4.4 Body Bathing Therapy
Bathtub, herbal decoction, hot water, thermometer, tressel, drop cloth, bath towel, soft towel, clothes and slippers.

3.8.5 Procedures of Operation

3.8.5.1 The practioner dresses clean and tidy. Wash hands and wear a mask. Prepare herbal decoction according to the doctor's advice.

3.8.5.2 After the materials are prepared, take them to the ward and check again. Explain the purposes and ways of the operation to the patient in order to get his/her cooperation. Assist the patient to take a comfortable posture according to the disease condition and expose the body parts to be treated. Pull the drapes when necessary. Adjust the temperature of the wards according to the disease condition.

3.8.5.3　Different parts of steaming and washing therapy

(1) Eyes steaming and washing therapy

Pour the herbal decoction into the treatment bowl. Put the gauze with the hole on the treatment bowl. Assist the patient to take a sitting posture. Aim the hole at the sick eye to steam. When the temperature of herbal decoction is 40℃, wash the sick eye with the soaked sterile gauze with tweezers. The treatment duration usually lasts for 15 to 30 minutes each time.

(2) Limb steaming and washing therapy

Pour the herbal decoction into the wash basin or cask. Put the patient's sick limb on the wash basin or cask. Drape the bath towel or middle-size sheet over the patient's sick limb and the wash basin or cask in order to stream the sick limb. When the temperature of herbal decoction is 38~41℃, soak the patient's sick limb in the herbal decoction. The treatment duration lasts from 10 to 20 minutes each time.

(3) Sitz bath

Pour the herbal decoction into the bidet. Put the bidet on the chair and cover the wood lid with hole. Ask the patient to expose the buttocks and sit above the bidet to steam. When the temperature of herbal decoction is reduced to 40℃, remove the wood lid and soak the buttocks in herbal decoction. 20 to 30 minutes for each time is appropriate.

(4) Body bathing therapy

Pour the herbal decoction into the bathtub. When the temperature of herbal decoction is reduced to 50℃, put the tressel into the bathtub in order to ensure the safety of the patient. Ask the patient to take off clothes and sit on the tressel for steaming. Drape the drop cloth over the patient's body in order to stream the body. When the temperature of herbal decoction is at 38 to 41℃, soak the patient's body and four limbs in the herbal decoction. 10 to 20 minutes for each time is appropriate. Help the patient to soak with the soft towel and move all joints of four limbs. 20 to 40 minutes for each time.

3.8.5.4　During the operation, keep an eye on the response of patients. If the patient feels uncomfortable, stop the operation at once and offer anti-symptomatic treatment.

3.8.5.5　After finishing the operation, clean the local skin, assist the patient to put on the clothes and take a comfortable lying posture to rest.

3.8.5.6　Clean up the materials, wash hands and make notes.

3.8.6　Precautions

3.8.6.1　Pay attention to keeping warm in winter in order to prevent contraction of wind-cold.

3.8.6.2　The temperature of the herbal decoction should not be too high. Keep the temperature at 50 to 70℃. The temperature of the herbal decoction for washing should be at 40℃ to prevent scalding.

3.8.6.3　Generally once every day. 20 to 30 minutes for each time. According to the disease condition, twice every day where necessary.

3.8.6.4   Don't do the operation when the patient is on an empty stomach. Don't do the operation within half an hour before and after meal. The old and the weak patients should not do the operation by themselves. The operation shouldn't be lasted too long to prevent patients from collapse.

3.8.6.5   Sterile operation is necessary for the wound when it is receiving the steaming and washing therapy.

(Yang Xiaowei)

4

General Nursing

General nursing means recuperation and maintenance. In broad sense, it is to prevent disease and enrich well-being with theories and methods of TCM. In narrow sense, it refers to TCM nursing, which consists of daily life nursing, dietary nursing, emotional nursing, exercise nursing, etc.

4.1 Daily Life Nursing

As for daily life, it refers to the basic activities in people's daily life including life style, habits and customs, work style, etc. Daily life nursing means that people should comply with the changes in nature and live regularly. Daily life is closely related to health. People should follow the changes in nature, adapt to the seasonal changes, keep normal dietary and regular daily life in order to maintain health and prolong life. Conversely, people will fall to diseases if they eat improperly and live irregularly.

4.1.1 Complying with the Four Seasons to Regulate the Body and Spirit

4.1.1.1 Significance of Complying with the Four Seasons to Regulate the Body and Spirit

The changes of yin and yang in the four seasons dictate the changes in the world. In terms of changes in four seasons, yang qi works as the commander to generate and cultivate things in spring and summer because yang qi is in charge of generation while yin qi is for nourishing; in autumn and winter all things are under the control of yin qi when yang qi tends to wither up all things and yin qi to store them, and then, all things are sheltered for storage. In *Su Wen* (*Basic Questions*), it is said that the function of the human body is corresponded to *Tian qi* (qi of nature), which means human can communicate with natural rules on the basis of changes of yin-yang in nature. Basically, health preservation in four seasons is to adjust yin-yang in human body according to rise and fall of yin-yang in nature thereafter the vital activities within body can correspond to changes of nature.

It is recorded in the *Su Wen* (*Basic Questions*) that people should "cultivate yang in spring and summer, and nourish yin in autumn and winter", which is put forward according to the time, characteristics, states of the waxing and waning of yin and yang, qi's ascent and descent, viscera function's rise and fall. In spring and summer, everything recovers from dormant winter, grows to prosperity. This vitality growing from weak to strong is a symbol of yang qi of the natural world in spring and summer. Likewise, the function of yang qi prevails in human vital activities at that time. Therefore, people should adapt their vital activities to the natural changes for preserving yang. From autumn to winter, everything goes from fruition to hiding and storing, because the natural world is dominated by yin qi at that time, so is human body. Therefore, it is time to store yang qi and nourish yin essence to adapt to natural changes. This is the basic principle of yin-yang changes in four seasons. If this basic principle is gone against yin-yang balance within human body, many diseases will occur. Therefore, people should follow the basic principle of "cultivating yang in spring and summer, and nourishing yin in autumn and winter" in seasonal health preservation.

4.1.1.2 Daily Life Nursing in the Four Seasons
4.1.1.2.1 Daily Life Nursing in Spring

In spring, yang qi has gradually been more and more prosperous and works predominantly in nature after being stored in winter, it governs the growth and everything is about to boom. There is a vigorous picture in nature. People should comply with the vital qi and adjust daily life.

(1) The principle of daily life nursing in spring

The principle of daily life nursing in spring is to follow the upward trend of yang qi in nature, be consistent with growing trend and the vitality of everything in nature, support yang qi within the human body, regulate the functions of the liver and gallbladder, keep away from evil qi in nature in order to maintain exuberance of qi of the *shaoyang* meridian in the body and lay a solid foundation for health preservation in summer.

(2) Maintenance of daily activities

All the daily activities should function to stretched, smooth, dispersing and unobstructed state in spring, sleeping a little later at night, getting up as early as possible in the morning, doing some outdoor exercises, wearing loose and comfortable clothes, leaving one's hair loose and relaxing the body as comfortable as possible. If unrestrained, yang qi will be generated and enriched. Doing exercises in the daytime can relieve fatigue and having entertainment after a hard day at work in the evening would be helpful to relieve physical and mental stress. But, people should follow certain basic rules, that is, people should choose different exercises according to the individual constitutions and inclinations. Activities or exercises should not be too strong in case of too much physical exertion, so that the human body can be kept in a stretched and relaxed condition. All the activities or exercises should not be too strong so that the human body is kept in a stretched and relaxed condition instead of being tired. Sitting, watching and sleeping for a long continuous time will be disadvantageous to relaxation of muscles and tendons and will block qi and blood circulation in the channels and collaterals and cause dysfunction of the liver and gallbladder. Less staying sedentary indoors and choose an outdoor venue, such as carry on outdoor activities in the park or grass field to communicate with nature and breathe the fresh air. Thus yang qi in the human body will rise gradually in spring by doing these sports.

(3) "*Chun Wu*" (keep warm in spring) fosters yang qi

"Keep warm in spring" means that people should take off the winter clothing as late as possible and keep warm energy in the body to foster inner condition for the generation of yang qi. In spring, yang qi begins to rise but is not strong enough and cold qi fades away gradually. This is the reason why the weather is cold one minute and hot the next minute in early spring. It is very difficult for the body to adapt to the changeable weather. Therefore, if people take off winter clothing too early, the cold pathogen will attack the human body easily and cause diseases ultimately, because yang qi is still insufficient to resist the spring cold at this time. If the principle of "keep warm in spring" is followed properly, yang qi will be prosperous. This also means that the healthy qi is strong enough so the deficiency-type pathogen and abnormal weather will have no opportunities to attack the body. Clothes in spring should be loose, soft and warm, and add or take off clothes according to the climatic changes. Don't take off winter clothing too early. Cold usually comes in from the foot, so traditional health preservation suggests dressing in spring should be thicker in feet and thinner in trunk, and young women should not wear skirt too early.

(4) "The deficiency-type pathogen and abnormal weather must be prevented in time"

It refers to that people must know how to recognize the pathogenic factors and keep away from them timely. In spring, it may be pleasant when it is warm with sunlight, sometimes it may be cold when it rains continuously. Changeable weather in spring often cause infectious diseases of respiratory system, like flu and mumps, skin diseases like neurodermitis and urticaria, as well as gastro-intestinal diseases. Therefore, we must pay much attention to the changes in weather, especially the influence on human body, to avoid attack of the deficiency-type pathogen and abnormal weather.

4.1.1.2.2 Daily Life Nursing in Summer

Yang qi is exuberant in summer, the heaven yang qi goes down from above, the earth yin qi goes up from below, leading to the integration of yin and yang qi and prosperity and flourishing of all living things.

(1) The principle of daily life nursing in summer

With extremely exuberant characteristics of yang qi in summer, people should keep consistent with the growing tendency of all living things, comply with the strong yang qi in nature to nourish yang qi rising the body, and nourish heart qi to assist yang qi. People should not only protect themselves from summer-heat pathogen in summer and pathogenic dampness in long-summer, but also need to pay attention to protecting yang qi in the human body. All the aspects of health preservation should follow the general rule of "cultivating yang qi in spring and summer" to lay a foundation for health promotion in autumn.

(2) Maintenance of daily activities

In summer, people should adapt to early sunrise and late sunset. It is good for people to go to bed later and get up earlier in the morning. As the daytime lasts longer, they should have a nap at noon to restore energy. They are likely to be attacked by wind-cold-dampness in summer, because the striae and interstices are loose and the sweating pores are open. People should not prefer coolness too much or have too much cold drink, which will result in deficiency of *center qi*, meanwhile, the summerheat pathogen accompanied by wind-cold pathogen will take the chance to invade the human body. So in summer, people should not dress too few, and should pay more attention to keep the abdomen and the back warm since *du mai* is on the back, which governs yang qi of the whole body. The circulation of yang qi in the body will be blocked if the back gets cold. The point of the bellybutton belongs to the *ren mai*, the major function of which is to adjust qi and blood of yin channel. Catching cold on bellybutton and the back will not only affect the spleen and stomach causing abdominal pain, diarrhea, etc. but also result in dysmenorrhea and menstrual disorder. In the meantime, it is inadvisable for people to sleep outside or sleep in air conditioning rooms with air-conditioner blowing too hard. People should not stay in the passageway or under the eave, and should keep away from the slit of windows and doors in case of the invasion of wind pathogen. People should neither take a cold shower, swim in cold water to relieve heat nor walk in rain in order to avoid the invasion of cold-damp pathogen while the sweating pores are open. When it is too hot, taking a warm bathe or towel off sweating softly by warm and wet towel is strongly advised in order to avoid the striae and interstices shutting down immediately in cold circumstance and consequently preventing smooth-flowing of qi and leave the pathogenic factors in the human body. The sunshine is sufficient in summer for its longer sunlight time. One should get out in the sun as often as possible to promote yang qi in the human body. One should carry on some outdoor exercises as possible as one can and it can promote sweat excretion which regulates the human body fluids and takes away the waste from the body. When doing exercises in summer, it is better to do exercises in the morning or the evening and in a place like a park or garden where there is abundant of fresh air. Moderate physical exercises should be chosen like taking a walk, jogging etc.

(3) Avoiding pathogenic factors to prevent diseases

The excessive summerheat will lead to dizziness, chest oppression, nausea, thirst, even coma. Hence, doing labor work or physical exercise should avoid burning sunshine and necessary protection should be taken. In summer, one should protect himself from pathogenic dampness which prevails in the long summer. If pathogenic dampness and pathogenic heat work together, yang qi of the spleen and stomach is easily get hurt so that fluid in the body cannot normally metabolize. The diseases caused by summerheat pathogen and pathogenic dampness are not easy to be cured. So one should avoid living in wet environment and avoid sleeping in the humid place for a long time. Simultaneously, people should be cautious about common summer illness such as "common cold in summer," heatstroke, bacillary dysentery, acute gastroenteritis, solar dermatitis, food poisoning and so on.

4.1.1.2.3 Daily Life Nursing in Autumn

In autumn, yang qi falls gradually and yin qi rises little by little in nature, formed together with the transition from the abundant yang qi to the profuse yin qi. The rising and falling of yin-yang in body also correspond with waxing and waning of yin-yang in nature. The qi movement transfers from the opening in strong state of yang qi into the accumulation in the abundant state of yin qi. It is also called rising in summer transferred to gathering in autumn.

(1) The principle of daily life nursing in autumn

The principle of daily life nursing in autumn should follow the basic rule of "nourishing yin in autumn and winter" to foster the yin qi, gather the mature, care the lung and prevent the troubles from the autumn dryness. People should follow natural rules that yin qi grows gradually from weak to prosperous and then take cultivating yin qi of body as the most important task to build a good foundation for the winter storage.

(2) Maintenance of daily activities

In autumn, people should adapt to the dry weather and restraining characteristic in nature to work and rest, sleeping early to comply with the collection of the yin essence and getting up early to comply with the extension of yang qi. In the daily activities, people should avoid overtiredness and excessive perspiration to protect yang qi from injuring and yin fluid from consuming. Exercise for health preservation in autumn should be classified into the following three levels, firstly, the static-oriented exercises like *qigong* which involves rhythmic breathing coordinated with slow stylized repetition of fluid movement, a calm mindful state, and visualization of guiding qi through the body; secondly, the moderate exercise aiming at relaxing the bones and muscles without sweating profusely and labor-consuming, such as the *taijiquan*, the *taiji* sword, walking; thirdly, the vigorous exercise with large amount of motion, suitable for the obese people to lose weight.

(3) "Enduring cold in autumn" to defend yang qi

The old saying of "keeping warm in spring and enduring cold in autumn" is a principle for health preservation in four seasons. The "keeping warm in spring" is helpful to raise yang qi, while "enduring cold in autumn" contributes to defend it. "enduring the cold in autumn" is effective for cultivating health in the autumn, which has been paid much attention to in both the ancient and modern times, because the weather in autumn is cool but not yet too cold to endure at this time, people should comply with the principle of storing up yin essence and defending yang qi in the autumn, and do some cold-resistant exercise intentionally to strengthen their physique gradually avoiding over-dressing-induced perspiration which will lead to the consumption of yin fluid and leaks of yang qi. Of course, "enduring cold in autumn" should be carried on according to different people and weather, for instance, the old and the young children whose resistance is weak should pay attention to keeping warm and adding clothing in time in the deep autumn.

(4) Evading the deficiency-type pathogen and abnormal weather to prevent diseases

The weather changes greatly and all the heat pathogen, dryness pathogen and cold pathogen exist in the autumn. So people should be cautious in daily life to prevent the pathogenic factors from invading the body before getting sick. In autumn, people should mainly pay attention to the prevention of the following illnesses: the bronchial asthma which often relapses suddenly when the autumn weather turns from hot to cool; constipation being caused by autumn dryness which could consumes the human body fluid resulting in intestinal dryness; the autumn diarrhea which is a typical seasonal sickness, which is the reason that much attention must be paid to maintaining abdominal warm for the babies and infants, since the weather in autumn becomes cooler and cooler, the children are likely to catch cold in the abdomen.

4.1.1.2.4 Daily Life Nursing in Winter

In winter, yang qi in nature is hidden and the yin qi works as a commander to control the accumulation and storage of everything. Yang qi is also accumulated in body complying with the changing rule of natural yin-yang movement.

(1) The principle of daily life nursing in winter

The principle of health preservation should comply with the hiding and storing characteristic in winter, keep up with the tendency of storing energy in nature to nourish yin essence of the human body, gather the vitality and maintain yang qi and keep warm against cold, furthermore, people should protect the kidney qi to establish the foundation for generating and rising in the next spring.

(2) Maintenance of daily activity

The cold pathogen in winter is very likely to damage yang qi in body. The basic principle of daily activity is to keep away from the cold and protect yang qi. People especially the old should go to sleep early and not get up before sunrise in cold winter, because in winter, the night becomes longer and the coldness is heavier. Going to sleep early may keep yang qi in body to prevent the coldness from invading, and getting up late may ward off the cold of the night. It's the basic measure to keep warm in the cold that the yang qi in body should follow the yang qi in nature. In winter, people, especially the old and the weak, should pay more attention to keep the head, neck, back and feet warm. The wind-cold pathogen tends to invade human body from back which is the yang within yang to cause respiratory and cardiovascular diseases. In addition, "cold invades from the feet", so people should pay attention to keep the feet warm, which can protect people from catching cold in winter. Otherwise, the viscera may be affected by the encroaching cold pathogen resulting in abdominal pain, diarrhea and so on.

(3) Disease prevention and health preservation in winter

The coldness is the strongest predisposing factor of lots of diseases in the severely cold winter. When human body gets over stimulation of coldness hypertension, heart diseases, cranial vascular disease and other diseases related to the circulatory system can be induced. Coldness may cause the coarseness and rahagades of exposed skin, the frostbite on the ear, nose, finger and so on. The facial paralysis can be induced in winter if the head is attacked by the cold air or cold wind suddenly. To keep warm in winter is the key to prevent all above diseases.

4.1.2　Living Regularly, Working and Resting Moderately

4.1.2.1　Living Regularly

"Living regularly" contains the following meanings: working and resting on time, avoiding oversleep, doing exercises moderately to strengthen tendons and bones, eating three meals every day at fixed time and in fixed amount, taking meat with vegetables, combining exertion and rest, keeping still and active alternatively. When this has been achieved, people can live out their lives according to *Su Wen* (*Basic Questions*). "Living regularly" is the important rule of adjusting spirit and qi. People can maintain spirit and qi, possess full of energy and exuberant vitality if they have regular living and reasonable work and rest. Otherwise, people will be lack of energy and their vitality will decline if they live irregularly.

4.1.2.2　Working and Resting Moderately

Overstrain in TCM includes mental overstrain, sexual overstrain and labor overstrain. Excessive desires is one kind of the mental strains, it is caused by over preference which is nerve-racking. For this reason, the measures should be taken to conserve the spirit for health cultivation by cutting the origin of excessive desires and reduce desires. With regard to labor overstrain, "No overwork and over-rest" is the principle according to *Peng Zu She Shen Yang Xing Lun* (*Peng Zu health cultivation theory*), it refers to that people should neither be overtired, but increase activity gradually in their daily life, nor take too much rest, because it will make qi and blood stagnating causing dysfunction of the tendons and bones. If we keep still without enough movement and even no movement, it will induce stagnation of essence, flaccidity of tendons and even decrease of longevity. Longtime lying injuries qi; longtime sitting injuries flesh. Although sexual desire is human nature, it should be under control. As the old saying goes, sexual activities brought both benefits and harm to people, if people can take it reasonably, it will bring health benefits, otherwise it will harm people.

4.1.3　Sleeping Abstemiously

Sleeping abstemiously means that sleeping in proper ways according to the law of nature and changes of yin-yang, so as to keep sleeping quality and get rid of tiredness, and restore energy. The ultimate purpose is to help people to strengthen constitution, prevent diseases and increase longevity. TCM attaches more importance to the rationality of sleep and holds that sleep and diet are important for health preservation. One third of the lifetime is spent on sleeping which is not only the physiological need, but also the essential way to assure health and regain energy.

TCM believes that the movement of celestial bodies and the change of yin and yang contribute to the alternation of day and night which is regard as yang and yin respectively. The body should comply with the law of the alternation of day and night. It is better to go to sleep when yin qi gets much more than yang qi, and it is better to get up in the opposite case.

4.1.3.1　Do and Don't for Sleeping Environment

4.1.3.1.1　Do and Don't before Sleep

(1) Calm down before sleep avoiding excessive reading or consideration.

Exultancy and rage may give rise to spiritual unpeace, excessive reading and consideration induce qi disorder and stop yang transforming into yin. Don't take vigorous activity before sleep in case affecting sleep quality. Slow down the breathing rate before sleep. People can guide themselves into relaxation and meditation by means of sitting still, taking a walk, watching slow rhythmic TV programs, listening to low and slow music, and so on, which is helpful to produce yin, then prosperous yin can bring sleep.

(2) Warm the feet

There are two major points listed as follows: firstly, to wash feet with hot water before sleep to make the blood circulate downward to feet and relieve the brain congestion to promote sleep; secondly, to massage *yong quan* (KI 1) point in the sole, which is an important point of the kidney meridian. Modern medical studies have proved that massaging the feet frequently can regulate the functions of automatic nerves and endocrine system, and promote the blood circulation, ultimately, help to relieve fatigue, improve sleep quality and prevent and treat the cardio-cerebral-vascular diseases.

(3) Eat several small meals, neither too much nor too little

It is stated in the ancient book that "going to bed immediately after eating too much will impair qi". Eating too much before sleep may result in dysfunction of the spleen and stomach. And it is difficult to fall into sleep when people feel hungry before sleep. Drinking tea or coffee can excite the central nerves and make it difficult for people to fall into sleep. In addition, drinking too much water before sleep causes frequent urination at night, especially for the old people which will affect their sleep. People with poor sleep can drink milk or yogurt and eat food with the effect of cultivating heart yin, such as a thick soup cooked with sugar candy, lily and lotus, which has a good effect of improving sleep. Take a rest after eating for about 30 minutes before sleep.

4.1.3.1.2 Do and Don't during Sleep

(1) Avoid wind and fire

The wind pathogen can invade the brain easily leading to face paralysis and hemiplegia if the head faces towards the door and windows or the door and windows are open when people are sleeping. The fire pathogen is easy to attack the upper *jiao* causing dry pharynx, red eyes, nose bleeding and even headache if the head faces towards the fire or heating facilities when people are sleeping.

(2) Avoid speaking and singing at sleep onset

The ancients said that "the lung like the bell is the marquee of the five organs. It should be constringed when people lie down to rest". If people speak and sing before they go to bed, the lung may shake, then the five organs can't be calm, as a result, the quality of sleep will be influenced.

4.1.3.2 Sleeping Time and Posture

4.1.3.2.1 Sleeping Time

Sleeping at noon (11am-1pm) and at midnight (11pm-1am) is one of the traditional sleeping regimens in China. TCM believes that yin and yang in the world connect each other at noon and midnight, when the qi and blood in body are very unbalanced, so people had better go to bed at that time. According to the change of yin and yang in a day, it's the time of the most prosperous yin qi and the weakest yang qi from 11 pm to 1 am, so it is better to go to sleep to foster yin in body, moreover, it's also good time to nourish the liver for the qi and blood in the meridian just arriving in liver and gallbladder at that time. Modern study shows that the function of every organ in the human body is the weakest from 0 to 4 o'clock in the morning and the sympathetic nerve in the human body is the weariest from 11am to 1 pm. So sleeping at noon and midnight is more accordant with physical rules and can achieve double results with half effort. However, a too long nap at noon is not good for the body, half an hour or an hour is enough.

The sleeping time may vary by age, gender, constitution, environment, etc., while the recommend sleeping time is 8 hours, and the younger they are, the longer sleeping time and the more times they need.

4.1.3.2.2 Sleeping Posture

There are three kinds of sleeping position: supine position, prone position and lateral position. The one who sleeps in lateral position resembles a lying dragon, with *ren mai* and *du mai* connected, yin and yang harmonized. TCM health experts believe that lateral position is the most appropriate sleep position. When people lie in prone position with back upward and belly down, though limbs keep forceful and qi circulates smoothly, five viscera is under stress, leading disharmony of yin and yang, causing difficulty in sleeping peacefully. When people sleep with supine position, limbs are stretched and relaxed, while yin and yang conversed, yin channel is upward and yang channel is downward, *du mai* are under stress. As a result, though yin channel gets smooth, yang qi can't be stimulated, when falling asleep, yang qi will be trapped by turbid yin, and qi can't reach distal extremities.

4.1.3.2.3 Sleeping Direction

The sleeping direction is closely interrelated with health. The ancient doctors have already given some opinions on it. Some advocate the sleeping direction should be decided on the yin-yang characters of the four seasons. They argue that people should sleep towards the east in spring and summer since spring and summer pertain to yang and while people should sleep towards the west in autumn and winter because autumn and winter pertain to yin, which are accordant with the principle of "cultivating yang in spring and summer, and nourishing yin in autumn and winter". Some believe that people should sleep towards the east in all the four seasons. They believe that the head, on the top of the body, controls all the yang of the body, towards which qi and blood circulate. The east pertains to spring and helps to raise qi of everything in nature. So people sleep towards the east in order to elevate the clear and lower the turbid to make the head clear. Most of them hold that people should avoid facing the north. They claim that the north which pertains to water is in charge of winter and cold. Cold qi may directly hurt the essential yang and original spirit of the body if people sleep facing the north.

4.1.4 Normal Urination and Defecation

4.1.4.1 Smooth Defecation

Ancient TCM masters attached much importance to smooth defecation. In *Lun Heng* (*Essays of Criticism*) written by Wang Chong (27-97AD), a Han Dynasty (202BC-220AD) thinker, recorded that "if we want to live long, we should keep our intestines clear, if we want to live longer, we should keep our intestines clean." it pointed out the importance of smooth defecation which will be good for longer life span, otherwise piles, anal fissure and bowel cancer may occur.

To develop good bowel habits, we should keep regular schedule, regular meals and defecation, we should also let defecation take its own pace, avoiding holding stools when there is the feeling of bowel movement, and strain during bowel movements.

Paying attention to diet adjustment, we should eat a variety of foods but whole grains -based, take more plant foods and drink plenty of water.

4.1.4.2 Normal Urination

As an old saying goes, "To live long, urine should be clear; to live longer, urine should be clean". Keeping urine clear and clean is the guarantee for health. Normal urination is positively correlative with the level of such viscera function as lung, spleen, kidney and bladder. Water metabolism status can reflects whether viscera function is normal or abnormal, especially for kidney qi, because kidney is the motive power of metabolism, adjusting each link in water metabolism, "kidney governs water" in TCM theory.

　　Small meals, vegetarian diet, waiting a little longer to drink after the meal, no drinking until feeling thirsty are strongly recommended. Holding urine and strain during urination is harmful to health.

(Hao Yufang　Zhou Fen)

4.2　Dietary Nursing

　　Diet is essential for human being to maintain life activities, and it has always been an important factor for promoting health and longevity. Proper diet can help enhance health, prevent ailments and treat diseases. Improper diet, however, may cause diseases, promote ageing and reduce life expectancy. TCM advocates preserving health and even treating diseases with the aid of dietary intervention.

4.2.1　Property and Flavor of Food

　　Based on the TCM theory of "the homogeneousness between medicine and food", food, similar to medicine, has four kinds of properties including coldness, hotness, warmness, and coolness; and five kinds of flavors including pungent, sweet, sour, bitter and salty flavors. Therefore, choosing diet based on different properties and flavors of food can balance cold and heat with five flavors well distributed, which will be beneficial to health protection and treatment while supplying nutrition.

4.2.1.1　Four Properties of Food

　　The food cold in nature has the function of clearing heat, releasing fire-toxin and detoxification, and nourishing yin, and is used to cure heat syndromes. Examples of food with cold property are watermelon, radish, mung bean, lotus seed and so on.

　　The food warm in nature has the effect of warming the center, assisting yang and dissipating cold, and is therefore used to treat cold syndromes, such as lamb, carp, walnut, litchi and so on.

　　Some foods are mild in nature, which are called "food with mild-nourishing function". They tend to have nourishing effect, such as pork, yam, peanut, egg and so on.

4.2.1.2　Five Flavors of Food

　　The food pungent in nature has the effects of dispersing and promoting the circulation of the qi and blood, and is used to treat superficial and mild illnesses caused by external pathogens, qi stagnation, blood stasis, etc. Examples are ginger, garlic, distilled spirit, etc.

　　The food bitter in nature has the effects of clearing heat, relaxing the bowels and eliminating dampness, and is indicated for fire-heat syndrome, constipation due to excessive heat, and damp-heat syndrome. Examples are apricot kernel, balsam pear, etc.

　　The food sour in nature has the effects of inducing astringency, arresting discharge, promoting appetite, promoting the secretion of saliva, and is used to cure sweating due to debility, chronic diarrhea, spontaneous seminal emission, enuresis, etc. Examples are rosa roxburghii, haw, etc.

The food sweet in nature has the effects of nourishing and normalizing the function of the spleen and stomach, relieving spasm and pain, and is usually effective in treating deficiency syndrome, spleen-stomach disharmony, various pains, etc. Examples are as honey, Chinese-date, etc.

The food salty in nature has the effects of softening hardness, relieving constipation by purgation, and is used in treating constipation, scrofula, mass in lower abdomen, etc. Examples are seaweed, kelp, etc.

Some foods such as Chinese watermelon with unobvious flavor are called "bland flavor", which can promote urination and percolate dampness, classified into sweet flavor. Some astringent in nature such as persimmon are classified into sour flavor due to the two flavors often coexist in one food.

Each food has its own nature and flavor. Therefore, they should not be treated separately but should be taken into consideration as an integrated whole.

4.2.2 Basic Principle of Dietary Nursing

4.2.2.1 Balancing Yin and Yang, Reinforcing Healthy Qi and Dispelling Pathogen

A harmonious and balanced state of yin and yang is maintained in normal circumstances. If changes of balance between yin and yang occur, either predominance or subordination of one side over the other, it results in various degrees of diseases.

The occurrence and development of diseases mainly involve two aspects, healthy qi in the body and the invading pathogenic qi. The development of diseases is a process of conflict between healthy qi and pathogenic qi with either predominance or subordination, which can all be summarized and explained by means of imbalance of yin and yang. Therefore, the basic principle of dietary nursing is to regulate yin and yang by reinforcing the deficient and reducing the surplus so as to restore the relative balance between yin and yang. The purpose of dietary nursing is to restore healthy qi and purge pathogenic qi so as to maintain the integrity of the viscera, balance of yin and yang and body recovered.

4.2.2.2 Balancing Flavors of a Variety of Food in Diet

Huang Di Nei Jing (*The Yellow Emperor's Inner Classic*) stated that "The five kinds of grains are basic foods; five kinds of fruits are supplementary foods; five domestic animals are beneficial foods; and five kinds of vegetables are nourishing foods. The favorite taste and smell of food, if matched to the body, could replenish vital essence and qi". The above statement has generalized the structure and compositions of an optimal diet, which includes a variety of sources: grains, meat, vegetables and fruits. Diet arranged like this is rich in diversity, well-balanced in meat and vegetables, which may prevent indulgence in any flavor so as to be well-proportioned in various nutritions.

In addition, the five flavors of food have relative tropism to different organs, the sour flavor enters the liver; the bitter, the heart; the sweet, the spleen; the pungent, the lung; and the salty, the kidney. They play different roles in the body and may have much to do with the function of five *zang* organs. If the five flavors can not meet the needs of the internal organs, the correlated *zang-*

qi would be ups and downs. As a result, normal functions of the five *zang* organs would decline accordingly. For example, having more food with sweet flavor would cause jam and flatulence, which helps catch phlegm, and damage the spleen and stomach. The five flavors properly mixed can nourish the five *zang* organs, replenish qi and strengthen health.

----- Supplementary reading 4-1 ---

You are what you eat

It is a prominent method of dietary prescription for life cultivation in TCM and has aroused much controversy. Nourishing one organ with corresponding animal organ would achieve superior effects than herbal plants. Therefore, the method has widely been used in food therapies. Li Shi-zhen, a famous doctor in Ming-dynasty, said, "the stomach, heart, blood, bone, marrow, skin of animals can be used to tonify the stomach, heart, blood, bone, marrow, skin of people.". Nourishing a part of human body with food having similar function or similar shape like walnut imaged the brain of human being, has the effect of tonifying kidney and supplementing brain. For example, Kidneys cooked with walnut is recommended medical formula to cure kidney deficiency, symptoms include dizziness and tinnitus, soreness in the waist, seminal emission, etc.

4.2.2.3　Choosing Food based on Differentiation of Causes and Syndromes

Diet based on differentiation of causes denotes that food is chosen to benefit health, which is used to solve problems according to the actual conditions instead of taking a single standard.

Generally speaking, health preservation practice should be in accordance with individuality, geographical environment, seasons, syndrome and illness. Good examples are diet in correspondence to seasons, diet on constitution differentiation.

Dietary nursing should be given based on the person's age, sex, constitution, personality, psychological status and occupation, etc. Senile stage in which function of five *zang* organs is declining. As senile people favors food over medicine, diets with tonics are suitable to supplement the lung, the spleen and the kidney to promote the process of metabolism, and to prevent the diseases and prolong life.

People should choose reasonable diet according to different season to restore health because the climatic changes in four seasons could influence people's physiology and pathology. The weather is very cold in winter, so choose Dang Gui Sheng Jiang Yang Rou Tang (Chinese Angelica, Fresh Ginger, and Goat Meat Decoction) to tonify kidney and warm yang.

Human beings living in different geographical locations develop different adaptability to environment, resulting in different constitution and different diseases. In the southeast area of China, the climate is hot and humid, so light food with the effects of excreting dampness is suitable for the people there. In the northwestern region, it's cold and dry, so the warm and hot food which can promote fluid production and moisten dryness is suitable for the people there.

When making food recipes, factors such as yin and yang, exterior and interior, deficiency and excess, cold and heat, must be seriously taken into account. For instance, for yang deficiency pattern, it is better to offer sweet and warm food, such as longan, Chinese yam, Chinese date.

4.2.2.4 Balancing Diet Composition, Choosing Beneficial Foods and Avoiding Contraindicated Foods

Food is for everyday life care, but it should be used in proper proportions in terms of composition so as to obtain complete nutrition to support human life. Reasonable diets should include meat and vegetables, whole-grain food and purified food, moderate cold and heat food, so as to protect spleen and stomach. Unhealthy dietary habits or indulgence in certain foods should be rectified. Contraindicated foods that are unfavourable to health or even aggravate disease should be avoided.

For example, the following foods are diet taboo during illness.

(1) Raw and cold foods: cold drinks and snacks, raw vegetables and fruits, etc. The patients with cold syndrome, deficiency syndrome, deficiency-cold of the spleen and stomach, and the patients susceptible to wind-cold should avoid raw and cold foods.

(2) Sticky food: foodstuff made of sticky rice, barley and wheat, including traditional Chinese rice-pudding, sweet dumplings made of glutinous rice flour (for the Lantern Festival). The patients with spleen deficiency and the beginning of external contraction, are unsuitable to eat sticky food especially in summer wet season.

(3) Greasy food: fatty, fried, and frying oily food, milk product, etc. The patients with spleen deficiency, phlegm-dampness, are better not to eat greasy foods.

(4) Pungent food: The patients with heat syndrome or yin deficiency with internal heat should not have the pungent things like ginger, onion, garlic, hot pepper, wine, etc.

(5) Meat and sea food: The patients with asthma, or skin eruption, macula and papule should not have sea food, mutton, dog meat, etc.

(6) Stimulating food: Food which can make new disease get worse, and old disease relapses, such as fish, shrimp, crab, bean sprout, crown daisy, leek, chicken head, etc. The patients with asthma, skin disease, allergic physique, should not eat meat and sea food, pungent food, and some special food like coriander.

4.2.3 Diet based on Differentiation of Constitution

Constitution refers to effective organic function and relatively stable physical feature affected by inheritance, and postnatal factors in accordance with natural and social environments. Constitution determines the liability and tendency to certain pathogenic factors or diseases. Health preservation in accordance with individuality, for instance, diet based on constitution differentiation should be according to different constitution.

4.2.3.1 Balanced and Peaceful Constitution

Feature: Harmony of qi and blood, yin and yang, is characterized by moderate posture, sanguineness, full of guts, etc.

Dietary nursing: Moderate constitution is the source of heath. For people of moderate constitution, "diet is the priority of health preservation". The principle of dietary recuperation for them is to balance diet, eat and drink moderately, avoid hunger or binge eating; have meals regularly; chew foods thoroughly before swallowing; massage abdomen and take a walk after meals so as to nourish and recuperate qi and blood, yin and yang. "Diet should include coarse and fine food without being too sweet and salty; people should have three, or four or five meals a day with being 70 to 80 percent full".

4.2.3.2 Constitution of Qi deficiency

Feature: Constitution of qi deficiency is characterized by fatigue, dispiritedness, shortness of breath, no desire to speak, spontaneous sweating, etc.

Dietary nursing: To replenish qi to invigorate the spleen, reinforce and tonify original qi. Hence, foods with the effects of replenishing qi can be used for dietary recuperation, such as rice, millet, Chinese yam, potato, hyacinth bean, carrot, mushroom, tofu, chicken, eggs, beef, and cauliflower, etc. Qi-tonifying medicated diet can be also used for gradual recuperation, for example, ginseng lotus soup, astragalus steamed chicken.

4.2.3.3 Constitution of Yang deficiency

Feature: People with this constitution appear pale and puffy, aversion to cold with cold limbs, etc.

Dietary nursing: People with yang deficiency constitution should include in their diet a larger proportion of foods which are sweet and warm in nature, and the principle of warming and supplementing the spleen and kidney should be adopted. The common yang-tonifying foods include mutton, hairtail, shrimps, chestnut, leek, onion, etc. People with yang deficiency constitution should keep away from foods that are cold, raw, bitter even in summer. The prescription for warming and recuperating the spleen and kidney yang is suitable to be used in winter such as Gui Sheng Jiang Yang Rou Tang (当归生姜羊肉汤, Chinese Angelica, Fresh Ginger, and Goat Meat Decoction).

4.2.3.4 Constitution of Yin deficiency

Feature: The physique is marked by emaciation. Main manifestations include dry mouth and throat, feverish sensation in the palm and soles, flushed face, etc.

Dietary nursing: People with yin deficiency constitution should take in more foods with the effects of nourishing liver and kidney yin. These foods include sesame, sticky rice, honey, sea pumpkin, oyster, hard shell clam, white fungus, sugarcane, duck meat, milk, etc. These foods are sweet and cold in taste and cool in nature, which have the actions of nourishing yin. People with vigorous fire due to yin deficiency, should abstain from astringent food, warm-hot foods, and fried foods.

4.2.3.5 Constitution of Phlegm-dampness

Feature: The physique is marked by overweight. Main manifestations include chest oppress and too much sputum, sticky greasiness taste in the mouth, whitish greasy coating, etc.

Dietary nursing: For people of this constitution, spleen should be fortified to resolve damp and resolve phlegm to reduce damp. Appropriate foods include barley, red bean, hyacinth bean, peanut, crucian carp, carp, radish, Chinese yam, bamboo shoot, chufa, and jelly fish etc. Medicated diet is also advisable for improving constitution such as Poria Cake, Apricot Kernel.

Obese people with phlegm-damp constitution should not overeat and choose less fatty, sweet, greasy foods, and foods that are astringent and cold in nature, and also not drink too much alcohol.

4.2.3.6 Constitution of Damp-heat

Feature: People with this constitution present with dirty complexion, susceptibility to acne, reddish tongue with yellow and greasy fur, bitter taste in the mouth and thirst, etc.

Dietary nursing: Principles for recuperation include clearing and resolving damp and heat, elimination of pathogens through purgation and dieresis. Recommended fragrant vegetables include coriander, agastache to remove internal damp qi, or foods like coix seed, lotus seed, poria, white gourd, small red bean, horse bean, duck meat, crucian, carp, kelp, balsam pear, cucumber, watermelon, Chinese cabbage, celery, cabbage, carrot, mung bean sprout and so on.

People should have less sweet and greasy food and not overeat vegetables and fruits that are warm and hot such as pepper, garlic, litchi, mango, and avoid alcohol, cream, pluck and so on.

4.2.3.7 Constitution of Blood Stasis

Feature:People with this constitution are inclined to have dark complexion, dark and purple lips and mouth, dark tongue proper with spots of blood stasis or with ecchymosis, etc.

Dietary nursing: Recommended foods have the effects of promoting qi and blood circulation by resolving blood stasis, including walnut meat, rape, black soybeans, tangerine peel, black fungus, and rose, etc. Appropriate amount of alcohol is advisable as it can promote qi and blood circulation, and help drug potential. Medicated diet is also advisable for improving constitution such as Hawthorn Porridge, Peanut Porridge. Foods which are cold, cool, warm and dry, greasy and astringent are contraindicated, such as persimmon, guava, egg yolk and so on.

4.2.3.8 Constitution of Qi Stagnation

Feature: It is marked by fragility and depression due to long-term emotional upsets and stagnation of qi, low spirits and irritancy, fullness and distention in the chest and hypochondrium, migratory pain, generally accompanied by frequent sighs, or foreign body sensation in the throat, or distending pain of the breast, etc.

Dietary nursing: Foods that have the effects of regulating qi to alleviate mental depression can be used, including orange, radish, onion, chrysanthemum, rose, fennel, sword bean, etc. so as to soothe the liver and rectify qi, recuperate of functional activity and regulate temper to keep good mood. People with qi stagnation constitution should have less food that are astringent including ebony, pumpkin, pickle, strawberry, plum and lemon for fear of stagnant functional activity resulting in coagulation.

4.2.3.9 Idiosyncrasy

Feature: Idiosyncrasy is due to weak basis and inherent factors, including innate or inherent physical defects, allergic reactions, etc.

Dietary nursing: People with idiosyncrasy should plan their individualized diet based on their condition. For those with allergic constitution should be in lest of various kinds of allergic foods, and reduce times of allergic attacks. For example, for asthma due to allergic food and drink, diet should be light. Foods that are cold, astringent, fatty, sweet and greasy and dispersing food should be avoided, including alcohol, fish, shrimp, crab, pepper, fat meat to avoid triggering latent phlegm and inveterate diseases.

Peng Zu

There was a macrobian who devoted himself to health preservation in ancient China. He was good at cooking pheasant soup, proficient in nourishing with drug and the methods of daoyin. He once cooked the soup for Emperor Yao and was awarded with the Peng City, thus known as "Peng Zu". During the reign of Emperor Shun, he followed Yin Shou-zi, and became a hermit in the Wuyi Mountain; The King of Shang once consulted him about the way of longevity. He never pursued fame or fortune, but focused on self-cultivation, Peng Zu became the symbol of health and longevity.

4.2.4 Health Preservation with Diets in accordance with Four Seasons

The time change in a year manifests as the four seasonal alteration in turn and the daytime length in difference; the climate changes perform in alteration of warm spring, heat summer, cool autumn and cold winter; the change of everything in the world shows as the generation in spring, the growth summer, the reaping in fall and the storage in winter. All the changes reflect waning and waxing of yin and yang in four seasons. Therefore, health preservation in four seasons is to adjust yin-yang in the human body according to rise and fall of yin-yang in nature, thereafter the vital activities within the human body can correspond to changes of nature. Health preservation, like eating with seasonal changes, people should choose reasonable diet according to different season to promote health.

4.2.4.1 Spring

Spring refers to the three months crossing over six solar terms including Spring Beginning, Rain Water, Insects Awaken, Vernal Equinox, Pure Brightness, Grain Rain.

In spring, it's warm and sunny; yang qi is generated and emanative, therefore raw and cold, viscous and greasy food should be avoided. Eating light food like wheat, chicken liver, duck blood, spinach, banana, etc. is suitable for people. Therapeutic recipe is recommended as Scrambled Egg with Leek, Vinegar Soak Soybeans, Celery Porridge, etc.

TCM points out that east in five directions, sour in five flavors and blue in five colors are related to spring in four seasons and have a connection with the liver in the human body. Therefore, health preservation with diets should raise yang qi, regulate liver function, and food with blue color and sour taste could be selected to help generate in spring. In this case, the vigorous liver easily subjugates and restricts the spleen, thus, "taking less sour-taste foods and more sweet foods" could replenish the spleen.

4.2.4.2 Summer

Summer refers to the three months crossing over six solar terms including Summer Beginning, Grain Full, Grain in Ear, Summer Solstice, Slight Heat and Great Heat.

In summer, it's sweltering; the light food, which can quench thirst, promote the production of body fluid and remove summer-heat, such as watermelon, white gourd, mung bean soup, dark plum and adzuki bean soup, lotus leaf porridge and so on are suitable. Cold, cool, and greasy food should be avoided. It is appropriate to choose food warm in nature, and pay attention to hygiene in order to avoid illnesses coming through the mouth.

The principle of dietary nursing is that south in five directions, bitter in five flavors and red in five colors in correspondence with summer in four seasons. All have a connection with the heart in the human body and weather dominating is burning hot. Therefore, health preservation with diets should promote growth and raise yang qi, regulate heart function, and food with red color and bitter taste, such as bitter gourd, lotus seed, tomato, should be the first choice to help grow in summer.

TCM points out that latter summer, a period between summer and autumn, is another season concept besides the four seasons. Dampness is the main climate in it and easily injure spleen yang, food like coix seed, hyacinth bean, Chinese yam and so on, can tonify the spleen and clear dampness.

4.2.4.3　Autumn

Autumn is a period of three months crossing over six solar terms including Autumn Beginning, Heat' End, White Dew, Autumn Equinox, Cold Dew and First Frost.

In autumn, it's dry with the summer-heat gradually reducing; the food nourishing yin and moistening the lung like sesame seed, honey, pineapple, dairy product, sugar cane, lotus root, glutinous rice, etc. are appropriate for people. Pungent foods such as onion, ginger, and hot pepper should be avoided. Replenishing recipe may include food that can promote the production of body fluid based on the food of normal-nourishing nature, such as Autumnal Pear Paste, Tremella and Saccharum Soup.

Corresponding to the autumn climate, the taste of acrid and the color of white goes with the lungs. Food of acrid-nature and white-color can nourish yin, moisten dryness and raise the lung, which means to focus on the astringent tendency in the autumn season. The predominant lung qi can easily hurt the liver, thus, "taking less pungent foods and more sour foods" is advised to protect the liver.

4.2.4.4　Winter

Winter is a period of three months including six solar terms such as Winter Beginning, Slight Snow, Great Snow, Winter Solstice, Slight Cold and Great Cold.

In winter, it's bitterly cold with everything withering; food with the effects of nourishing yin and replenishing yang such as cereal, mutton, egg, black fungus, beef, black sesame, Anguille are appropriate.

Moreover at this time it is proper to nourish and store the essence, warm and tonic food is beneficial. For this season, replenishing means supporting healthy energy to generate internal yang qi and strengthen the resistance for the coming spring plague. Recommended herbal recipes are Stewed Chicken with Chestnuts, Eight Treasures Congee, and Saute Sea Cucumber with Scallions, etc.

The diet also should support "concealment" and nourishing of the kidney which is related to winter. Since the kidney correspond to black in five colors and salty taste in five flavors, black and salty food are advised. Yin-nourishing and yang-concealing food should be selected, which aligns with the hiding tendency of the winter season. Because water restricts fire, "less salty and more bitter foods" should be selected to nourish the heart.

All in all, health preservation with diets in four seasons must follow the rule of yin and yang all the time, and the basic principle of "cultivating yang in spring and summer, nourishing yin in autumn and winter". TCM points out that a day can also divided into four seasons like spring to the morning, summer to midday, autumn to sunset, and winter to midnight, so people had better pay attention to health preservation by day and preserve *zang-fu* organs by hour so as to synchronize with the rhythm of nature and maintain health.

(Chen Yan)

4.3 Emotional Nursing

The so-called seven emotions refer to joy, anger, anxiety, thinking, sorrow, fear and fright. The seven emotions are mental activities of people which are closely related to physiological activities and function of human viscera. The seven emotions are not pathogenic when they are kept properly and normally. Only when the emotional stimuli are too abrupt, strong and continual to go beyond the normal range of human physiological activities can they disturb the movement of qi, disharmonize the viscera, yin and yang, qi and blood, and consequently causing diseases. The seven emotions may not only cause various diseases, but also deeply affect the development of diseases which may be either aggravated or relieved. Therefore, nurses should try their best to help patients to eliminate their adverse emotional stimuli such as tension, fear, anger, worry and help the patients to regulate emotions, maintain good spirit and promote health.

4.3.1 The Theory of Spiritual Cultivation

The theory of spiritual cultivation results from the long-term exploration and practice. It involves cultivation of mind with quietness, virtue cultivation, moderate sentiment and desire, internal concentration of spirit, conformance with the four seasons, regulation of the heart spirit, etc. It reflects the connotation of "harmony" in health preservation. When one can keep their mind tranquil and empty, true qi will come along naturally, how can any illness occur?

4.3.1.1 Cultivating the Mind with Quietness

The thought of cultivating the mind with quietness advocated by *Lao Zi* (571BC-471BC) and *Zhuang Zi* reflects the standpoint of accumulation of essence to preserve mind in Taoism, which refers to complying with the natural laws, clearing the mind, eliminating all distractions, and having few desires. So qi will gather together with mind concentrating, and scatter with mind dispersing. Accumulation of essence without preservation of spirit is like a tree without root. It is better to keep a sound mind with quiet spirit. Excessive distracting thoughts would dissipate mind.

4.3.1.2 Temperament and Virtue Cultivation

Many scholars in ancient China had noticed the close relationship between virtue, man's psychological state and life span. Good cultivation of virtue and temperament can maintain the balance of yin and yang of the *zang-fu* organs. Self-cultivation and accumulation of virtue, harmony between yin and yang make for a longer life with flexible and swift actions. Good moral cultivation helps one to keep broad-minded and optimistic mental state.

4.3.1.3 Mind Cultivation

In the regimen in TCM, "keeping the mind in the interior" is the base of disease prevention and treatment as well as the core of mind cultivation. It mainly refers to self-control and regulation of man's consciousness, thoughts and mental state in order to keep the harmony between human body and environment. Quiet mind is of great importance to health, so it is asserted that man's desire should be controlled to a proper extent by rationality and willpower.

4.3.1.4 Seasonal Regulation of Mental Activity

"Unity of man and nature" and "correspondence between man and nature", which reflects the interaction between man and nature, are about man and natural laws in the field of ancient philosophy in China. From a perspective of health cultivation, our emotion activities should change depending on seasonal climate to comply with natural discipline. Spring and liver belong to wood, wood is active in spring, so man should be delighted in spring. Summer and heart belong to fire, people may get angry in hot, so they should calm down to release yang qi in body. When autumn begins, yin qi increasingly becomes predominant while yang qi declines. People should adapt their emotion to the characteristics of autumn preserving stabilized emotion and peaceful mind at this time, in order to avoid the aberration of yang qi and the damage caused by the brumal pathogenic factor in autumn. In winter, yang qi is incubated while yin qi is exuberant. At this time, it is better to keep mental power and spirit peaceful.

4.3.2 Regulation of Unhealthy Emotions

Emotional changes can directly affect physiological function of the human body. It is stated in the *Su Wen* (*Basic Questions*) that "diseases cannot be cured if people are lack of spirit and volition." Famous experts in ancient times advocate again and again that "a good doctor surely cures physical disease on the premise of curing mental troubles." So strengthening emotional nursing is of great importance to improve disease rehabilitation and maintain health. There are following methods of emotional nursing which can be chosen from based on individual actual condition in order to achieve the best effect.

4.3.2.1 Nursing of Inter-Restriction Among Emotions

The nursing of inter-restriction among emotions here also known as mutual restriction between seven emotions, is to use one emotion to restrict another emotion in order to relieve or eliminate bad mood and to keep good mental state. It is stated in *Su Wen* (*Basic Questions*) that "excessive anger impairs the liver, grief restricts anger; excessive joy impairs the heart, fear restricts joy; excessive thinking impairs the spleen, anger restricts thinking; grief impairs the lung, joy restricts grief; excessive fear impairs the kidney, thinking restricts fear." This nursing method is formed on the basis of inter-restriction and inter-promotion relationship among the seven emotions, yin-yang and the five organs. One emotion which can restrict the other one can be used to transfer and disturb the other emotion if it becomes excessive enough to damage people's health, in order to harmonize the emotions. It is a special method of psychological nursing and rehabilitation in TCM.

The nursing of inter-restriction among emotions should be applied after the patient has known it. Don't abruptly use the method without any preparation. In addition, the nurses should master the patients' sensitivity to emotional stimuli in order to choose a proper stimulation, neither too strong nor too weak.

4.3.2.1.1　Using Joy to Restrict Grief

Using joy to restrict grief in accordance with fire restricting metal, means cheering the patient up by using humorous and amusing words or exciting words in order to restrict his excessive sad emotion and cure the related diseases. The nursing method can be applied in the diseases manifesting depression caused by excessive sadness.

----- Supplementary reading 4-3 --

Here is a case recorded in the ancient book Yi Yuan Dian Gu Qu Shi (The Fun Allusion of Medicion, In the Qing Dynasty (1616~1911AD), a milord always felt depressed and wore a long face with knitted eyebrows, so his family specially invited a famous doctor to make a diagnosis and give treatment for him. After asking about his disease history and feeling his pulse, the doctor determined that the man had menstrual irregularities. After hearing this diagnosis, the man laughed and said: "I am a man, it is impossible for me to have menstrual irregularities and it is so ludicrous." Hence, he would laugh when recalling the case.

Zhu Dan-xi (1281-1358AD), a famous doctor, once met a young man who cried and felt sad all the time for his wife's unexpected death shortly after their marriage, and he finally fell ill. Though he had seen many famous doctors and used all valuable medicines, but all his efforts were in vain. After feeling his pulse, Zhu Dan-xi (1281-1358AD) said: "The pulse shows you are pregnant, and you have been pregnant for several months." The young man laughed and said: "Confounding man with women, you are such an empiricist." Hence, he would laugh and tell the jape to others. Then he got good appetite and good mood, and his disease was cured. The above two stories are typical cases of applying the nursing of joy restricting grief.

There are two common ways to practice: firstly, to make the patient happy and eliminate the diseases caused by excessive sadness and worry by joking with the patient or using unserious words; secondly, if the patient feels unhappy for his unfulfilled demand, his demand should be satisfied to relieve his bad mood for his rehabilitation.

4.3.2.1.2　Using Grief to Restrict Anger

Using grief to restrict anger according to the method of metal restricting wood, means making the patient sad by words or other methods in order to restrict his excessive anger and eliminate related diseases. In clinical practice, nurses can set different situation or make the patient sad with grievous and touching words to arouse his sorrow emotion. Threatening words can also be used to make the patient fearful and then grieved. Grief makes qi consumed so that the depressed qi in the chest can be dispersed.

4.3.2.1.3　Using Anger to Restrict Thinking

Using anger to restrict thinking according to wood restricting earth, means making the patient angry with different methods in order to restrict his excessive thinking and eliminate related diseases.

----- Supplementary reading 4-4 --

It is recorded in the ancient book that "a rich woman had bad sleep for two years because of over thinking. Zhang Zi-he (1156-1228AD) said: 'Your pulse is slow because the spleen which is associated with thinking in emotion is affected.' So he took her money and drunk for several days with her husband in order to make her angry. Then the woman got angry, perspired, then felt sleepy that night. After she had slept for nine days, she ate food and her pulse went back to normal".

Another case is also recorded. "A young man who lived in the green-dragon bridge area caught a strange disease that he liked staying in a dark room alone and was afraid of the light. His disease would get aggravated when he was exposed to the light once in a while. One day Li Jian-ang, a famous doctor passed by his house, and was invited to examine the young man. The doctor didn't give prescription after examining, but he took the young man's writing and read it incorrectly. The young man asked angrily: 'Who read it?' Then Li Jian-ang read more loudly. The young man was very angry so he ran out and took the writing from the doctor and sat down beside the light, condemning him: 'You don't understand the sentences, how could you read it so loudly?' He recovered after his anger which gave full vent to her pensiveness emotion."

The two cases have shown that over thinking could affect the adjustment of human behavior and activity, then qi can't move but stagnates instead, or yin and yang disharmonize. Because excessive yang can't harmonize with yin, people have bad sleep. When people get angry, the upward flowing qi may break the qi blockage, the excited yang may be released with perspiration, then yin and yang become balanced and disease is cured.

4.3.2.1.4　Using Thinking to Restrict Fear

Using thinking to restrict fear according to the method of earth restricting water, means restricting the patient's excessive fear and eliminating those related diseases by making him think.

----- Supplementary reading 4-5 --

It is recorded that "a familiar customer had not come for a long time. Yue Guang asked him why, the man said: 'Last time I came here, you gave me alcohol, when I just wanted to drink, I saw a snake in the glass, and I felt nausea and suffered from disease after drinking.' Guang heard that there was a bow on the wall, the reflection of which in water looked like a snake, so he took the drink and put it on the same place and said to the man: 'What do you see in the drink?' The man said: 'The same.' Guang told him the reason. He understood."

The case of "self-created suspicion" shows that the diseases suffered from fear can be treated by thinking to release fear and tension, then to eliminate disease and recover health.

4.3.2.1.5　Using Fear to Restrict Joy

Using fear to restrict joy according to water restricting fire, means restricting the patient's excessive joy and eliminating related diseases by using different methods to terrify him. The nursing method can be used to treat the diseases manifesting excitation and manic.

----- Supplementary reading 4-6 ---

One story is recorded in the Ru Men Shi Qin (Confucians' Duties to Their Parents), Doctor Zhuang examined a patient who suffered from disease due to over-joy. After feeling his pulse, Zhuang said to the man: "I will go to take drug and I won't come here again in several days." And then the patient felt unsettled, fearful and sad. He thought the doctor wouldn't come to see him because he had caught serious disease. He cried sadly and told his relatives: "I will die." But doctor Zhang knew that is the sign of his recovery, so he came to console him.

Another story is recorded in the Hui Xi Yi Shu. A man who newly became the Number One Scholar fell ill suddenly on his way back home to announce this good news. A doctor was invited. After examining, he told the man: "Your disease cannot be cured, you will die in seven days, you should hurry on with your journey and go home as soon as possible." The man lost his spirits and hurried on with his journey day and night. Seven days had passed, but he was still alive. His servant said to him: "Here's a letter the doctor asked me to give you when you arrived home." The letter said: "After you have become the Number One Scholar, you were over-joy, which injures your heart, no drugs is suitable for you, so I frightened you by saying that you were dying to treat the disease. You are safe now."

4.3.2.2　Empathic Therapy

Empathic Therapy means a series of methods to transfer or change one's emotion and attention with certain measures to dispel bad emotion, it applies to patients who worry so much about his condition and the unknown consequences arising from the disease that set him in depression, worry and even fear. To those people, we can divert their attention from their disease to other things, or change the surrounding environment to protect them from harmful stimulation. However, the specific methods about empathic therapy should be employed flexibly based on the different psychological states and characteristics of different people.

4.3.2.2.1　Empathic Therapy with Music, Chess, Book, Painting and Calligraphy

It is said in the ancient book *Bei Shi* that "listening to the music and reading books can cultivate spirit." It is also stated in another book *Li Lun Pian Wen* (*Rhymed Discourse on External Remedies*) that "reading books and listening to the music are more effective on curing diseases caused by the seven emotions than taking medicine." So one could do such activities according to one's interests as calligraphy, painting, music, etc. to get rid of gloomy mood, smooth the flow of qi and foster the mind. *Ou Yang-xiu* (1007-1072AD) recorded in his book *Song Yang Zhi Xu* that he once suffered from the disease caused by anxiety and his focusing on music gradually helped him to dissipate his disease as if it had never occurred.

4.3.2.2.2 Empathic Therapy with Physical Exercise

When a person is hysterical or quarrelling with others, it is better to divert his attention to physical exercises like playing ball game, walking, *taijiquan* and so on, because mental tension can be eased by physical tension. Traveling can help to dissipate worry and improve rehabilitation of the patient. When people are under excessive anxiety and unhappiness, they should take a walk in the suburban area and enjoy natural scenery which can help to regulate his passive emotion and ease his tension by enchanting blue sky with interspersed cloud and intoxicating fragrance of flower mingled with bird chirping.

4.3.2.3 Method of Persuasion

The method of persuasion means persuading patients by using correct and wise words to correct his viewpoint, realize the harm brought by his behavior, relieve his unnecessary worry, boost his confidence in fighting against the disease, follow doctors and nurses' advice to achieve early recovery.

If the method is used properly and skillfully, enlightening patients with reason, examples or emotionally moving, being targeted, people's mental burden will be relieved, confidence will be boosted, mental and physical condition will be improved.

----- Supplementary reading 4-7 --

It has been pointed out in Huang Di Nei Jing (The Yellow Emperor's Inner Classic) that doctor should inform the patient of the harm of a disease, impart the curability to the patient, guide the patient with the principles of treatment and relieve mental burden of the patient. This is the origin of the persuasion method. That means a few aspects, firstly, "informing the patient of the harm of a disease" refers to tell the patient the character, causes, harm, severity of the disease in order to arise his attention, to make him treat his disease correctly, neither neglecting nor fearing. Secondly, "imparting the curability to the patient" refers to telling the patient that he will recover as long as he cooperates with the doctors and nurses and follow their advices, which can enhance his confidence in conquering the disease. Thirdly, "guiding the patient with the principles of treatment" refers to telling the patient the concrete measures about taking care and treatment. Fourthly, relieving mental burden of the patient refers to help him to relieve negative mental state and overcome bad mood.

In the history of TCM, many famous doctors recorded their experience of curing diseases with the method of persuasion. It has been recorded in *Si You Zhai Cong Shuo* (an ancient book) that Kuang Zi-yuan felt depressed and caught a disease because he failed to be an official in the government. An old monk diagnosed him and pointed out that he had too much desire; and he had to give up his excessive desire if he wanted to recover from the disease. He took the monk's advice and recovered after sitting quietly for months.

4.3.2.4 Method of Restraining

Restraining is a method to prevent drastic emotions through regulating feelings and controlling sentiments to achieve psychological balance.

TCM regimen believes that internal injury caused by excess of seven emotions is the main reason for attack of diseases. Extreme emotion is harmful to the body, so people should lay stress on spiritual cultivation and emotional regulation to maintain psychological balance. *Huang Di Nei Jing* (*The Yellow Emperor's Inner Classic*) points out that intelligent people should keep moderate joy and anger to preserve health. *Yi Xue Xin Wu* (*Medical Revelations*) concludes four important points of regimen, one of which is to avoid anger.

Delighted mood is helpful to the human body. But sudden over-joy makes qi sluggish, that is, heart qi dispels. The heart governs the blood and vessels. Heart qi deficiency will cause failure of qi to circulate the blood. Disability of blood circulation results in blood stagnation in vessels of the heart and then induces palpitations, angina, stroke and even death.

----- Supplementary reading 4-8 --

It is recorded in Yu Yi Cao written by Yu Chang (1585-1664AD), a famous doctor in Qing Dynasty, that a man got a new position and was jaunty, he died because of over joy before he went home. It is recorded in Yue Shu Zhuan that Niu Gao (1087-1147AD) was too excited because he had beaten Wan Yan (?-1148AD), he laughed three times and then died. It is recorded in Ru Lin Wai Shi that Fan Jin took part in the test several times when he was young, he failed every time. When he was more than fifty years old, he finally succeeded. He turned manic suddenly because of over joy. Those are the cases to show that over joy injures the heart.

Moderate anger helps regulate qi and calm the emotions. But over anger injures the liver and then the liver qi cannot flow smoothly. If liver qi invades the head, people will feel headache marked by redness in the face and eyes, pain in liver region; or people are quiet, don't say anything, in most serious case, people's limbs may be twitch and asphyxia and even resulted in death. When people meet annoying things, it is normal that they feel moderately worried. But if they are over worried, depressed, low-spirited, strained with bad sleep, the function of *zang-fu* organs will be maladjusted, people will have palpitations, stomachache, poor appetite, insomnia and so on.

When people get problems, they will think about it but over-thinking would result in many diseases. TCM holds that pensiveness leads to qi stagnation, the spleen is associated with thinking of seven emotions. So pensiveness is most likely to impair spleen qi which will lead to dysfunction of the spleen and stomach, manifesting poor appetite, distention in stomach, abdominal pain and so on.

It can be known from the above that extreme emotions do great harm to body, so people should consciously pay attention to controlling their own emotions. Don't be over-excited when encountering with good things and don't be too sad when encountering with bad ones. Immunity of the human body can be improved greatly by avoiding the unpleasant negative mood such as anger, depression and sadness, and keeping in an optimistic state. If the function of the brain and the entire nervous system can be improved and the function of all the organs are consistently harmonized, the mild psychological disorders or diseases such as anxiety, insomnia, headache, neurasthenic, can be avoided, even the chance of catching severe psychological diseases such as schizophrenia can be also prevented.

(Hao Yufang　Zhou Fen)

4.4　Physical Exercise Care

Regular physical exercises could help maintain health, enhance physique and delay aging. Traditional Chinese exercises include a variety of forms, such as *Taijiquan*, *Taiji* sword, *Wu Qin Xi* (five-animal exercises), *Ba Duan Jin* (Eight-section exercise), *Yi Jin Jing* (Channel-changing Scriptures), etc. Each of these has its own characteristics with different styles and requirements. This section focuses briefly on introducing effects and key points of *Taijiquan*, *Wu Qin Xi* (five mimic-animal exercise), and *Ba Duan Jin* (Eight-section exercise), as well as regular requirements and key points for physical exercises care.

4.4.1　Traditional Chinese Exercises

4.4.1.1　*Taijiquan*

Taijiquan is a treasured cultural legacy of the Chinese people. It is characterized by graceful gestures, soft actions, therefore is suitable for both men and women, the old and the young. It is also not limited by season or time. *Taijiquan* has been widely practiced in China for its benefits on improving physical fitness, preventing and treating diseases.

4.4.1.1.1　Functions

Firstly, it can improve respiratory function and increase lung capacity. When practicing *Taijiquan*, one should breathe deeply down to the pubic region (*dan tian*) with even, fine, deep, long, slow breath while enlarging chest and abdomen, which is good for maintaining flexibility of the lung tissues, increasing chest movement, vital capacity and improving respiratory ventilation and air exchange function.

Secondly, it can improve cardiovascular function and enhance vessel flexibility. *Taijiquan* involves movement of every muscle and joint in the body, all of which need to be harmonized with conscious breathing. Thus, it can ensure venous blood's return to heart, improve blood and lymph circulation and enhance vessel flexibility.

Thirdly, it can improve the function of nervous system. People are required to focus the mind solely on the movements of the form to bring about a calm and clear mental state. The brain concentrates on directing all organs to coordinate body action. Therefore, the self-control ability of the nervous system is increased, and the function is improved consequently which is good for resting the brain and eliminating fatigue.

Finally, it can help dredge the meridian and nourish qi. As long as one keeps practicing *Taijiquan*, it can help people dredge the *ren mai*, *du mai*, *dai mai*, and *chong mai*. Subsequently, it has effects on increasing the qi in pubic region (*dan tian*) which keeps people energetic, vigorous and healthy.

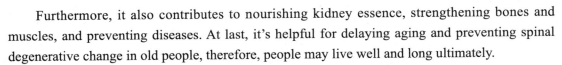

Furthermore, it also contributes to nourishing kidney essence, strengthening bones and muscles, and preventing diseases. At last, it's helpful for delaying aging and preventing spinal degenerative change in old people, therefore, people may live well and long ultimately.

4.4.1.1.2 Key Points

Keep head up with neck straight: The head and neck should be lifted up, kept straight, and relaxed. It is good for keeping balance of the body weight.

Keep chest held in with back straight, shoulder and elbow relaxed: It refers to the gesture of the chest, back, shoulder and elbow. The chest should be held inward; the back should be straight; the shoulder and elbow should be relaxed in a natural way. Keep two sides of the shoulder on the same lower level, and keep the elbow little curved and flexible and be held when the arm stretches or shrinks.

Keep eyes and hands coordinated with the waist as pivot. Move your footsteps quietly like a cat. Differentiate empty steps and full ones. When practicing Taijiquan, one must keep upper and lower part coordinated with each other as a whole, which requires that the movements are initiated from the waist, the eyes move with hands, and that bow steps alternate with empty steps until the legs have force and can move steps slowly and softly.

Lead movement with mind rather than force only: Induce the movements with the mind first, then put forth one's force guided by one's mind, to the extent that the force can't be shown externally yet there is intense force internally, namely exerting force without being shown.

Combine mind and qi and breathe down to the pubic region: It refers to cooperative breathing with mind. One should adopt abdominal respiration and the inspiration and expiration should match with the opening and closing of the action.

Seek peaceful mind from the movement, and combine movement and peace: It means that the body is moving but the mind is calm, namely the physique is moving but the heart is static. One should concentrate all the thoughts on practicing Taijiquan.

Keep every movement even and continuous: It means that the speed of each action should be even without stop.

4.4.1.2 *Ba Duan Jin* (Eight-Section Exercise)

Ba Duan Jin (Eight-section exercise), namely eight individual movements, which is also named as Eight-Section Brocade, because of the eight individual forms of the movements are characterized by a silken quality energy and also like a piece of brocade. It's a kind of aerobics originating from the Song Dynasty (960-1279) with more than 800 years' history. Ba Duan Jin (Eight-section exercise) is suitable for all the people especially for the old people and people with chronic diseases due to its simple actions and moderate motions.

Traditionally, Ba Duan Jin (Eight-section exercise) contains both a standing and a seated set of eight postures. Generally speaking, there are two major schools of standing style: the Southern and Northern Schools. The former prefers gentler actions and the latter prefers firmer actions. However, by analyzing the literature review and their movements, we can tell that they share the same origin. In the modern era, the Southern School of standing version is more widely practiced.

4.4.1.2.1   Functions

Ba Duan Jin (Eight-section exercise), often viewed as an excellent practice which has been purported to enhance health and well-being with many benefits, including improving the function of neurohumoral regulation, strengthening blood circulation, soft massaging effect on abdominal portion, regulating effects on nervous system, cardiovascular system, digestive system, respiratory system, immune system and motor organs, improving mental and physical health, delaying the aging and increasing longevity. Besides, *Ba Duan Jin* (Eight-section exercise) also has preventive and curative effects on headache, dizziness, scapulohumeral periarthritis, lumbocrural pain, indigestion, neurasthenia, etc.

4.4.1.2.2   Key Points

When practicing *Ba Duan Jin* (Eight-section exercise), one should calm down and concentrate on the pubic region (*dan tian*) point, with the head up, mouth closed, tongue tip touching upper palate, eyes looking at the front horizontally, body relaxed and breathing naturally.

Breathe evenly and naturally: The fluid movement should be coordinated with rhythmic breathing, which should be deep, long, even and calm. Every movement should coordinate with breath and mind. Use the mind to induce practicing.

Concentrate on pubic region (*dan tian*): The exercise requires "using the mind to induce actions". Body movements should be guided by the mind while actions shouldn't be stiff with a good mood and peaceful mind. Mind coordinates movements as a whole smoothly. It lays stress on "omphaloskepsis", so mind training is more important than body training.

Combine relaxing and contracting: When one practices this exercise, he should fully relax muscles and nerves, stabilize the body gravity first and then do the movements according to the key points. Pay attention to releasing and holding of force. When releasing the force it should be natural and when exerting force it should be well distributed and stable.

The eight-sectional exercise is a healthy exercise including eight consecutive sections. Specific procedures are listed as follows:

(1) Pressing Up to the Heavens with Two Hands (*Shuang Shou Tuo Tian*)

This move is said to stimulate the "Triple Warmer" meridian (*Sanjiao*). It consists of an upward movement of the hands, which are loosely joined and travel up to the center of the body.

(2) Drawing the Bow and Letting the Arrow Fly

While squating in a lower horse stance, the practitioner imitates the action of drawing a bow to either side. It is said to exercise the waist area, focusing on the kidneys and spleen.

(3) Separating Heaven and Earth

This resembles a version of the first piece with the hands pressing in opposite directions with one up and one down. A smooth motion in which the hands switch positions is the main action, and it is said to especially stimulate the spleen and stomach.

(4) Wise Owl Gazes Backwards or Look Back

This is a stretch of the neck to the left and the right in an alternating fashion.

(5) Sway the Head and Shake the Tail

This is said to regulate the function of the heart and lungs. Its primary aim is to remove excess heat (or fire) from the heart. In performing this section, the practitioner squats in a low horse stance, places the hands on thighs with the elbows facing out and twists to glance backwards on each side.

(6) Two Hands Holding the Feet to Strengthen the Kidneys and Waist

This involves a stretch upwards followed by a forward bend and a holding of the toes.

(7) Clenching the Fists and Glare Fiercely (or Angrily)

This repeats the second piece, and is largely a punching movement either to the sides or forward while in horse stance. It is aimed at increasing general vitality and muscular strength.

(8) Bouncing on the Toes

This is a push upward from the toes with a small rocking motion on landing. The gentle shaking vibrations of this piece is said to "smooth out" the qi after practice of the preceding seven pieces.

4.4.1.3　*Wu Qin Xi* (Five-Animal exercises)

Wu Qin Xi (Five-animal exercises) is a group of exercises for health care by imagery of the Five Animals-Tiger, Crane, Deer, Monkey, and Bear. It was developed on the basis of the experiences of Hua Tuo (145-208), a predecessor who was a famous ancient Chinese physician two thousand years ago. It's popular for its effects of preventing and treating diseases, strengthening joints and bones, delaying the aging process and prolonging the life span.

4.4.1.3.1　Functions

Mental health: When doing five animals exercise, the exercisers should adjust their mind before and during every unit. Therefore it can relieve mental nervousness and enhance mood stability so as to keep mental health.

Physical health: Each of the five animals exercise has its own advantage. However, they form a systematic whole. If one keeps practicing it, it may achieve the effects of regulating qi and blood, reinforcing viscera, inducing meridians, stretching muscles, and lubricating joint.

Respiration adjustment: Practicing five animals exercise can dredge channels and meridians and promote the circulation of qi and blood, strengthen the function of the lung in controlling respiration and the function of the kidney in governing reception of qi. Only if qi can flow smoothly, blood can flow smoothly, and sufficient qi makes people energetic, and then improve health.

4.4.1.3.2　Key Points

Relaxing the whole body: Completely relax, keep in a good mood and in high spirit so as to make blood and qi flow freely. Relax the whole body in case it is over stiff or tense.

Rhythmic breathing: Breathe slowly, quietly and naturally with abdominal respiration. When one breathes in, the mouth should be closed with the tongue tip touching the upper palate. "Breathing in with the nose and out with the mouth."

Empty mind, focus meditative state: Focus the attention on the parts according to mind concentration, so as to coordinate mind and qi.

Acting naturally: The five animals exercise has its different characteristics in actions, such as slowness of a bear, lightness of a monkey, robustness of a tiger, softness of a deer, and activeness of a crane. When one practices, the actions should be stretched naturally and conducted according to their own characteristics.

4.4.2 Regular Requirement and Key Points of Physical Exercise Care

4.4.2.1 Combination of Static and Dynamic Exercises

When using exercise care, one should combine static exercises with dynamic exercises. Naturally regulate the respiration and mentality, balance, both physique and spirit should be given attention to when doing exercise internally and externally. Move the body with a state of inner peace, the moving body is for the physical health and the inner peace is for the mental health. Therefore, doing exercises can get both physique and spirit trained so as to ultimately benefit internal and external harmony. It embodies the idea of "dynamic to static", "dynamic in static", "the static against the dynamic" and "dynamic and static combination".

4.4.2.2 Persistence

Doing such exercises is not a one-time thing. One should persist in doing it for a long time with certain intensity regularly in order to keep healthy.

4.4.2.3 Doing Moderate Exercise, Step by Step

The amount of exercise should vary with different individuals, and build up gradually. Generally speaking, if one does not feel overtired after exercise, it indicates the intensity of the exercise is appropriate.

Heart or pulse rate is also used as a measure of exercise intensity. For a healthy adult, it is proper to increase the heart rate to 140 times per minute, while for the old people, it is better to increase to 120 times per minute. If one loses appetite, gets headache, feels exhausted and sweats excessively after doing exercise, it means that one may take too much exercise which exceeds the body range and may cause damage to the body.

4.4.2.4 Taking Exercise at the Right Time

Generally speaking, it is better to do exercise in the morning, as the air is fresher. Doing exercise outsides helps to exhale more carbon dioxide and inhale more oxygen to improve metabolism. However, strenuous exercise is not allowed before/after naps or before sleep at night in case of exciting the nervous system and affecting sleep. Furthermore, do not take strenuous exercise before/after meals, for it can lead to hypoglycemia. While taking strenuous exercise after meals, it may not only affect digestion, but also result in gastroptosis or chronic gastroenteritis.

4.4.2.5 Doing Exercise Suited to Each Individual

Physical exercise should be chosen according to one's interest as well as one's own condition. Old people had better choose slow and gentle exercises which can relax muscles and enable all the parts of the body to take part in, such as walking, *Taijiquan*, jogging, because their muscle strength is decreasing, their nervous system is of poorer response and their coordination ability is also poorer.

For people who are young and strong, they can choose vigorous intensity activities such as long-distance running, and basketball. Exercises should also be chosen according to various occupations. For example, teachers, shop assistants, et al. may easily develop varicose veins of lower limbs due to longtime standing. Thus, when doing exercise they should choose leg lifting. Sedentary office staff should choose such excises as chest expanding, straightening up, and heading up etc.

(Su Chunxiang)

5

Practical Self-Nursing of Traditional Chinese Medicine

Human body is an organic whole. Any local pathological change is closely related to the pathological changes in the corresponding internal organs. Malfunction of any part is sure to affect the whole function. Protection and care targeted at a particular part according to the actual conditions of each individual will have direct influence on the physiological functions of the whole body.

5.1 Proper Care of the Oral Cavity

It is well known that disease may enter through the mouth which is one of the "open doors" of the human body. Good oral health care and prevention against oral diseases may not only protect us from oral and dental diseases but also help to prevent and cure many diseases of the whole body.

5.1.1 Oral Cavity Care by Strengthening the Tooth

Experts on health preservation in ancient China point out "health preservation of any living things starts from care of the tooth". Forming good hygienic habits and paying attention to health care by strengthening the tooth is an important task of health preservation.

5.1.1.1 Rinsing the Mouth Frequently

It is recorded in *Li Ji* (*The Book of Rites*) that "as soon as the roosters sing, people will wash their faces and rinse their mouths". It is said in the *Qian Jin Yao Fang* that "gargling several times after eating prevents the tooth from decaying and keeps the mouth fragrant." Gargling helps to clear away odorous qi and food residua in the mouth, and clean the mouth and the tooth. After each meal or eating sweet food, it is necessary to rinse the mouth immediately. A variety of liquids can be used to rinse the mouth, e.g. water, tea water, saliva, saline, vinegar, solutions of Chinese medicinal substances.

5.1.1.2 Brushing the Tooth in the Morning and Evening

Tooth brushing aims to clean the oral cavity, massage the gum, promote blood circulation and enhance the ability of preventing diseases. The times of tooth brushing should be adjusted according to the needs and the actual possibility. It is suggested that one should "brush the tooth in the morning and in the evening, and gargle after meal", and that brush tooth before going to the bed is more important than in the morning. In addition, more attention should be paid on the right method of tooth brushing, which is to brush the tooth upright along crevice between the teeth, from interior to exterior with moderate strength. If brushing the tooth across or with excessive strength, one cannot clean the feculence between the teeth and may hurt the tissues around the tooth, resulting in gum atrophy.

5.1.1.3 Clicking the Teeth Frequently

It is pointed out in *Bao Pu Zi* (*Analects of Bao Pu-zi*) by Ge Hong of the Jin dynasty that "those who click their teeth over three hundred times every early morning have strong teeth that will never become loose." Since ancient times, many of those who live a long life have paid special attention to tooth-clicking, especially in early morning. They have benefited a lot from this. The specific way to practice the tooth-clicking exercise is to get rid of distracting thoughts, relax the mind, close the mouth and tooth lightly, and then click the upper teeth with the lower teeth gently. Click first the molars 50 times, then the incisors 50 times, and finally stagger a little bit to click the canine 50 times, once every morning and evening.

5.1.1.4 Massaging the Lip

This means to close the mouth, keep the four fingers of the right hand together to massage and rub the outer side of lips in a clockwise direction and then counterclockwise direction until they become warm and red. Lip massage accelerates blood circulation of the oral cavity and the gum, keeps the tooth healthy and firm, prevents dental diseases, and keeps the face lustrous and beautiful.

5.1.1.5 Correct Way of Chewing

It is advisable to chew on both sides or alternatively, while chewing only on one side should be avoid. The disadvantages of chewing only on one side are listed as follows: first, it may cause dental hypersensitiveness or pulpitis to the frequently used side; second, it may cause gingival atrophy to the disused side, which in turn causes dental diseases; third, it may cause the face to become distorted.

5.1.1.6 Proper Diet

Oral and dental diseases are related to malnutrition in some way. Therefore, proper intake of nutrition is essential. Vitamin A, D and C, calcium, phosphorus, protein and so on are indispensable nutritional elements for dental development. One should eat moderate sum of fresh vegetable and fruit containing vitamin C and food rich in vitamin A, D, C, calcium, phosphorus, protein such as animal's liver, kidney, yolk and milk. Women in gestation and lactation periods, infants and little children in particular should take these foods more to guarantee the development of dental enamel.

5.1.1.7 Correcting Habit Disturbance

Bad habits are another cause of dental diseases. Children should form the hygienic habit of not sucking the fingers and biting pencils. It is improper to use toothpicks or match sticks to pick the tooth after meal because it may easily damage gingival tissues and even lead to infection and ulceration.

Those who smoke a lot for a long time often have dark brown stains on the surface of their teeth. Those stains may cause calculus deposition, and bacterial stains in certain parts may aggravate periodontal disease. Tobacco contains a variety of harmful elements. The chemical elements in cigarette smoke can irritate the periodontal tissue directly or go immediately into blood circulation, and cause chronic damage to the periodontal tissue.

5.1.1.8   Preventing Medicine-induced Tooth Damages

Dental diseases should be treated in time. However, medicines harmful to the tooth should be avoided. It is especially unsuitable for women in gestation and lactation periods, infants and little children to take medicines containing tetracycline and oxytetracycline. Otherwise, the use of the above-mentioned medicines is likely to make the teeth turn yellow and lead to permanent yellow teeth, or cause hypoplasia of dental enamel and dental caries.

5.1.2   Health Care by the Saliva in the Oral Cavity

Saliva is a special kind of body fluid. TCM holds that saliva is a natural tonic closely related to vitality. Therefore, it was awarded as "golden liquid and jade-like fluid", "manna", "water from the Hua Chi Pond" by ancient people. Rinsing the mouth with the saliva and swallowing it, also named as "fetal food" in ancient China, is a strongly recommended way to enhance our health.

5.1.2.1   Functions of the Saliva

It is stated in *Su Wen* that "the spleen produces saliva while kidney produces spit." The saliva is dominated by the spleen and kidney which are the prenatal and the postnatal bases of the human body and are closely related to health and longevity. Therefore, saliva has a special value in health care.

5.1.2.1.1   Moisturizing Food and Facilitate Digestion

The amylase in the saliva decomposes the amylum into maltose, which is further decomposed into dextrose so that the food has undergone a preliminary digestion.

5.1.2.1.2   Cleaning the Oral Cavity and Protecting Alimentary Tract

The saliva has an effect of cleaning the oral cavity, protecting the tooth, counteracting stomach acid and restoring gastric velum etc.

5.1.2.1.3   Detoxifying

After the saliva and food are fully mixed together, chemical change happens in the oral cavity to make the carcinogen malfunctioned. So the saliva is regarded as a natural agent of preventing cancer. The saying in TCM health preservation studies goes that "to chew food well before swallowing can promote longevity."

5.1.2.1.4   Postponing Senescence

It is pointed out in *Yang Xing Yan Ming Lu* (*Recordings of the Art of Health and Life Preservation*) that "drinking the jade-like spring (saliva) can extend one's lifespan and get rid of various diseases". All these functions have been proved true by long-term practice of experts on health preservation and qigong masters. Furthermore, the saliva also has the function of preventing and curing diseases, healing the wounds. The saliva contains a variety of components of blood plasma, many kinds of enzymes, vitamins, minerals, organic acids and hormones.

Regular secretion of a large amount of saliva participates directly in the metabolism of human body, improves the functions of hair, bones, muscles, blood and *zangfu* organs, strengthens immunity, prevents diseases, and live a long and healthy life.

5.1.2.2   Health Care by Swallowing the Saliva

There are many ways to rinse the mouth with saliva and swallow saliva. The following two methods are frequently used.

(1) Normal Method of Swallowing the Saliva

One may take a sitting, standing or lying position, keep calm and patient, lick the palate, or extend the tongue outward to the outer side of the teeth on the upper jaw and stir up and down, and then extend the tongue inward to the inner side of the teeth on the upper jaw and stir up and down, right and left. This method is called "the red dragon stirring the heavenly pool" by ancient Chinese people. Wait until the saliva fills the whole mouth, and then swallow it in 3 times downward to *Dan Tian* (丹田, pubic region), or click the teeth for 36 times and rinse the mouth with the saliva and then swallow it. Repeat the whole process for 3 times and swallow the saliva for 9 times altogether in each practice. The best timing for this exercise is in the morning and in the evening. If time is permitted, one can also repeat for more times.

(2) Practicing Qigong and Swallowing the Saliva

Static qigong is the most suitable one. Specific practice form can be chosen according to their preference. The specific way is to get rid of thoughts, concentrate the mind on *Dan Tian*, place the tongue against the palate, close eyes slightly, relax, adjust the breath, sit in meditation and achieve absolute mental tranquility. When breathing in, place the tongue against the outer side of the upper teeth, and lick them continuously to accelerate saliva secretion; when breathing out, put the tip of the tongue down, lead qi upward from *Dan Tian*, open the mouth slightly, breathe gently and slowly, and swallow the saliva slowly in 3 times after it fills the mouth. One can practice this exercise for half an hour every morning and evening. The two methods mentioned above are easy to follow. As long as one keep practicing for a long time, one will attain abundant qi and energy, young looks, intelligent ears and eyes, good health and longevity.

5.2   Facial nursing

Facial nursing is also known as beauty care. Face is the place to which the qi and blood of the *zangfu* organs flow upward and with abundant blood circulation. TCM believes that different parts of the face relate to different *zang* organs, e.g. the left cheek relates to the liver, the right cheek relates to the lung, the forehead relates to the heart, the chin relates to the kidney, and the nose relates to the spleen. The face has a very close relationship with the channels and collaterals of the *zangfu* organs in general and the heart in particular. Similarly, changes in the face reflect the prosperity and decline and pathological changes of the channels and collaterals. As it is exposed on the top of the body, the face is usually the first victim when the six pathogenic factors attack our body. Face is the reflection of health condition of the body. So much importance should be attached to face care for health preservation.

5.2.1　Facial Care by Washing Scientifically

Face is the place to which the essential qi of the *zangfu* organs flow upward. Washing face frequently can promote the flow of qi and blood, promote the energy and qi of the *zangfu* organs to flow upward. But the quality, the temperature of water used to wash face and the times of washing face should be corresponding with the physical characters of the human body.

The soft water is suitable for washing face because it contains little minerals and has the effect of intenerating the skin.

The temperature of water used to wash face is different based on the skin style. Non-oily skin and mixed skin had better use the water with the temperature higher than 30℃ but lower than body temperature. The suitable water may not only help easily wash dust on the face, but also make pores open in order to clean deep-seated derma. If the temperature of the water used to wash face is higher than the normal body temperature, the vigor of blood vessel in the face becomes weak and the skin is easy to be laid-back, dry and appear wrinkles. For the oily skin person, it is unsuitable to use cold water to wash face because cold water makes the pores contract so that it can't clear a great deal of sebum, dust, cosmetic residua and so on accumulated on the face, which has no effect of face care and may easily induce or aggravate the acne. In addition, washing face with cold water and warm water by turns is suggested. This not only helps clean face, but also makes superficial blood in the face dilate and contract, strengthens blood circulation to make the skin beautiful.

It is advised to wash face with soap and latex at least twice a day (in the morning and evening). The right way to wash the face is that middle finger and ring finger are gently used to move from the center to peripheral and from bottom to the upward drawing a circle. Soap or latex together with warm water is used to knead bubble and then place it on the face, massage gently for 1 minute. Then wash with cold water because cold water reinforces blood circulation and improves the skin elasticity.

5.2.2　Facial Care by Massage

Experts of health preservation in different generations emphasized that "face should be scraped frequently". Ancient people pay more attention to facial beauty by massage.

Facial massage falls into two categories. One is performed directly on face, that is direct facial massage, and the other is performed by massaging the channels and collaterals away from the face to achieve the purpose of beautifying the face, that is indirect facial massage. There are many methods of massage and here only introduce a traditional method.

Peng Zu Facial Massage (*Qian Jin Yi Fang, Supplement to 'Important Formulas Worth a Thousand Gold Pieces'*): After getting up in early morning, rub and pull the ears gently with both hands; then rub the scalp and comb the hair with the fingers; and lastly rub the two hands together until they are warm, and wipe the face with the warm hands from up to down for 14 times. This massage exercise may help stimulate the circulation of qi and blood in the face, brighten the face, keep the hair from growing gray, and prevent head diseases.

5.2.3 Face Care by Diet

In order to prevent premature aging of facial skin, one should pay attention to the nutritional balance of diet and increase food taking that is good for the skin. From the perspective of TCM, to practice beauty diet, one should follow the principles of health preservation in daily diet. It is recorded in ancient books of TCM that many kinds of food preserve beauty such as sesame, honey, fragrant mushroom, cow's milk, goat milk, sea cucumber, pumpkin seed, lotus root, wax gourd, cherry, and wheat. Modern scientific experiments also prove that the food mentioned above is rich in nutrition, containing many vitamins, enzymes, minerals and amino acid. The above food makes the facial skin delicate, bright and rosy, and extends lifespan. In addition, preservation of beauty and health care can also be done through medicated diet. Beauty congee: Use an appropriate amount of *nuo mi* (glutinous rice) and *yan wo* (dried cubilose) to make congee, which is called *yan wo zhou* (cubilose congee). It serves to moisturize the lung, nourish the spleen, and preserve beautiful facial appearance. Use a suitable amount of carrot and *jing mi* (Oryza Sativa L.) to make congee that strengthens the stomach, nourishes the spleen, smoothes the skin and preserves beauty. Use a certain amount of *yi yi ren* (Semen Coicis) and *bai he* (Bulbus Lilii) to make congee that relieves internal heat, moisturizes dryness syndrome, and cure flat wart, acne and flecks on the face.

5.2.4 Face Care by Medicinal Substances

Face care by Chinese medicinal substances refers to the use of beauty preservation formulas to make the skin delicate and fair, nourish the skin, prevent and get rid of wrinkles, and eradicate facial skin diseases. There are many formulas, which fall into two categories, those for oral administration and those for external use.

5.2.4.1 Formulas for Oral Administration

Formulas for oral administration can be further divided into two subcategories. One is oral administration of Chinese medicinal substances to regulate the functions of *zangfu* organs, qi and blood, channels and collaterals in order to achieve the purpose of moisturizing and whitening the skin, preventing and getting rid of wrinkles, and preserving beautiful look. The other is to use formulas aiming at promoting blood flow and removing blood stasis, expelling wind and removing cold, clearing heat and detoxification, detumescence and eliminating stagnation in order to cure various diseases that affect facial beauty.

For example, *Sui Yang Di Hou Gong Mian Bai San* (Whitening Powder for the Concubines of the Emperor Yangdi of the Sui Dynasty) from *Yi Xin Fang* (*Prescriptions at the Heart of Medicine*): Take *ju pi* (Citri Reticulatae Pericarpium) 30g, *dong gua pi* (Benincasae Exocarpium) 50g, and *tao hua* (peach flower) 40g, pound them into fine powder. Take 2g of the powder each time and three times a day. This remedy performs the function of drying dampness and dissipating phlegm, promoting blood circulation and nourishing the face.

Drinking medicated wine may also be helpful. For example, *gou qi zi* (Fructus Lycii) vinum from *Yan Nian Fang* (*Recipes to Extend Years of Life*) may nourish the liver and the kidney and preserve facial beauty. *tao hua* (peach flower) beauty wine from *Tu Jing Ben Cao* (*Illustrated Classics of Materia Medica*) can moisturize the face and bring the color of peach flower to the face. Generations of research and practice have proven that the following medicinal substances can moisturize the skin and increase the elasticity of the skin. They are *bai zhi* (Radix Angelicae), *gou qi zi* (Fructus Lycii), *xing ren* (Semen Armeniacae), *tao ren* (Semen Persicae), *hei zhi ma* (Semen Sesami), *tao hua* (peach flower).

5.2.4.2   Beauty Powder for External Use

Beauty powder for external use is either spread over the face or used to wash the face. The powder can be absorbed by the skin and can get rid of wrinkles, and guard the body against climatic evils. According to modern researches, beauty powder for external use can nourish the skin, increase immunity of the skin, protect cells on the skin surface and enhance the elasticity of the skin. *Yu Rong Xi Shi San* (from *Dong Yi Bao Jian, Precious Mirror of Oriental Medicine*): Take *lv dou fen* (green gram starch) 60g, *bai zhi* (Radix Angelicae), *bai ji* (Rhizoma Bletillae), *bai lian* (Radix Ampelopsis), *bai jiang can* (Bombyx Batryticatus), *bai fu zi* (Rhizome Typhonium), and *tian hua fen* (Radix Trichosanthis) 30g each, *gan song* (Radix Nardostachydis seu Rhizoma), *shan nai* (Rhizome Kaempferiae), and *mao xiang* (Herba Aristolochiae Mollissimae) 15g each, and *ling ling xiang* (strong-fragrant loosestrife herb with root), *fang feng* (Radix Saposhnikoviae), and *gao ben* (Rhizoma Ligustici) 6g each, and two troches of *fei zao jia* (Chinese coffee tree fruit) and grind them into fine powder. Use the powder every time when washing the face. It performs the function of expelling wind, moisturizing the skin, dredging the channels and collaterals, making the skin fragrant, and giving a jade-like color to the face.

5.2.5   Face Care by Psychology

TCM holds that "Facial appearance is determined by the heart." Rosy cheeks and pretty face, full energy, and graceful bearing come from healthy psychological state. Lao Zi (517-471BC) pointed out in his *Dao De Jing* (*The Classic of the Virtye of the Tao*) that the intangible was more important than the tangible in the world. One's mood not only affects the physiological functions of the human body, but also exerts a direct influence on the skin color. Be good at relieving psychological pressure. In daily life, try to be optimistic and open-minded, avoiding emotional stress.

5.3   Proper Care of the Hair

The standards for beautiful hair of Chinese people are as follows: Hair is black and lustrous, thick and dense. Therefore, early gray hair, withering and dry hair, less hair and hair loss are all regarded as pathological conditions. Besides being the sign of health, the hair itself performs the function of protecting the head and brain. At the same time, healthy and graceful hair plays a specific role in enhancing physical beauty, making people look full of energy and glow with health.

TCM believes that "the kidney dominates the bones and their essence manifests in the hair", and that "the hair is the surplus of blood." With abundant kidney essence, qi and blood, one may have healthy and graceful hair. The hair is closely related with the five *zang* organs and the flourishing and withering of the hair can directly reflect the vicissitudes of the qi and blood of the five *zang* organs. The change of the hair reflects the change of mood, the physiological and pathological changes as well. When the seven modes of emotion go to extremes, it can also cause changes in the hair. Generally, the process in which the hair turns from black to gray and to white is the process the essential qi in the human body turns from strong to weak. Therefore, experts on health preservation take much count of hair care and regarding it as one of the important measures for a healthy and long life.

5.3.1   Hair Care by Combing and Massage

Health preservation experts in ancient times advocated that "hair should be combed frequently". It is said in *Zhu Bing Yuan Hou Lun* that "if one combs the hair over one thousand times, the hair will not turn white". Combing hair can promote the flow of qi and blood, dispel wind and improve eyesight, nourish and strengthen the hair, improve the quality of sleep, and be very significant for health care and preservation. TCM considers that head is the place to which yang qi flow upward and the place where many acupoints, blood vessels and nerves are located. Massage the scalp by comb stimulates nerve twigs and acupoints which conduct through the nerves and channels and act on pallium to adjust the function of channel system and nervous system, improve tense state of cephalo-nerves, and promote local blood circulation. The suitable time for combing is usually in early morning, before taking a nap and before going to bed at night. Other spare time is also possible for this exercise. Combing in early morning is the best because morning is the time when yang qi rises. Combing in the morning helps to raise yang qi of the human body. The correct way is to comb hair from the front to the back, and then from the back to the front; from the left to the right; and then from the right to the left. Repeat the same procedure for dozens or hundreds of times. Lastly, arrange the hair and comb it until it becomes smooth and lustrous.

One can combine combing with finger massage, stretch and separate the ten fingers and thumbs, use the finger pulps or finger tips to massage the hair from the front hairline to the back hairline along a circle, and then massage from the right and left sides to the top of the head. Apply strength evenly and repeat for 36 times until the scalp becomes slightly warm. Combing and massage can be done either in combination or separately.

5.3.2   Hair Care by Proper Way of Washing

It is recorded in *Lao Lao Heng Yan* (*Common Saying for Senile Health Preservation*) that "health preservation experts say that hair should be combed frequently but should not be washed frequently. Washing hair against the wind is likely to cause wind syndrome of the head." Washing the hair too frequently will remove the protective sebum from hair, shorten the lifespan of hair, and more seriously induce hair ringworm fungus inflection. Generally speaking, dry hair should reduce washing times, while oily hair should be washed more frequently. The water used to wash hair should neither be too cold nor too hot and the best temperature range is from 37 to 38℃. If the water temperature is too low, it will be difficult to wash away filth from hair. If the temperature is too high, the hair will be damaged and become slack, crisp and easy to break. As for the choice of hair lotion, neutral soap or shampoo should be used for dry and neutral hair, and ordinary soap, sulfur soup or alkaline shampoo should be chosen for oily hair. As the shin of infants is very delicate and skin of the old is very dry, they may use soap or shampoo made from fat. Don't twist hair by towel after washing. Dry the hair naturally. Don't use the hair drier to blow hair. If it is necessary, the temperature should be lower and the time should be shorter. The intensity of wet hair decreased obviously and easy to be broken. Don't go to bed until the hair is dry, otherwise it is easy to catch dampness and heat pathogen and damage hair.

5.3.3 Hair Care by Diet

Daily diet should be diversified and with a reasonable mix to reach a balance of the acid and the alkali in the body, which plays an important role in preventing presenility of the hair. It is advised to have an appropriate amount of natural food that is rich in protein, iodine, calcium, and vitamin A, B and E, such as fresh milk, fish, eggs, beans, green vegetables, melons and fruits, and coarse food grain. Black sesame, Chinese date, peach seed, almond, semen pini koraiensis, mushroom, Chinese yam, soybean, lily bulb, arillus longan, strawberry, and peanuts are all nutritious agents for hair care and beauty. One can choose some of them according to one's own condition. One of the congees for hair beauty preservation is Xian Ren Zhou (Congee for the Immortal) from *Zun Sheng Ba Jian* (*Eight Discourses on the Art of Living*): Use an appropriate amount of *he shou wu* (Radix Polygoni Multiflori Preparata) and *jing mi* (Oryza Sativa L.) to make congee. Taking the congee regularly can nourish the liver and the kidney, replenish qi and blood, blacken the hair and preserve a beautiful and young look.

5.3.4 Hair Care by Medicinal Substances

Hair care by medicinal substances is the method of using Chinese medicinal substances for hair care under the guidance of TCM theories. Hair care by medicinal substances can not only preserve hair health and beauty but also strengthen hair and cure hair disease. Medicinal substances for hair care can be divided into two types: medicinal substances for internal administration and those for external use.

5.3.4.1 Medicinal Substances for External Use

Choose different Chinese medicinal substances to wash the hair according to different situations. The medicinal substances can perform their functions directly on the skin tissue and the hair to achieve the purpose of keeping hair healthy. External medicinal substances perform such functions as nourishing, cleaning, making hair fragrant, thick and black, and preventing and curing hair loss. Experts on medicine and health preservation in ancient times have many records on it. Two of them are introduced as follows.

(1) *Xiang Fa San* (Hair Fragrance Powder) from *Ci Xi Tai Hou Yi Fang Xuan Yi*, (*Selected Medical Prescriptions for Empress Dowager Cixi with Comments*): *ling ling xiang* (strong-

fragrant loosestrife herb with root) 30g, *xin yi* (Flos Magnoliae) 15g, *mei gui hua* (Flos Rosae Rugosae) 15g, *tan xiang* (Lignum Santali Albi) 18g, *chuan da huang* (Rhubarb) 12g, *gan cao* (Radix et Rhizoma Glycyrrhizae) 12g, *dan pi* (Cortex Moutan) 12g, *shan nai* (Rhizome Galanga Resurrectionlily) 9g, *ding xiang* (Flos Caryophylli) 9g, *xi xin* (Radix et Rhizoma Asari) 9g, *su he xiang you* (Styrax oil) 9g and *bai zhi* (Radix Angelicae Dahuricae) 9g. Grind the medicinal substances into fine powder, pour *su he xiang you* (Styrax oil) into the powder, homogenize the powder and the oil, and dry it in the open air. Spread the medicinal substances paste on the hair, and use fine-toothed comb to comb the hair. This recipe makes the hair clean and fragrant. Long-term use helps the hair to grow again from where the hair lost and prevents the hair from graying even at an old age.

(2) *Ling Fa Bu Luo Fang* (Hair Loss Prevention Recipe) from *Ci Xi Guang Xu Yi Fang Xuan Yi* (*Selected Medical Prescriptions for Cixi and Guang Xu with Comments*): Take three *fei zi* (Semen Torreyae), two *hu tao* (walnut), and *ce bai ye* (Cacumen Platycladi) 30g, pound them and immerge them in snow water. Use the liquid to wash hair. This formula prevents hair from falling and makes hair black and lustrous, and it is especially effective for hair loss caused by the heat in blood.

5.3.4.2 Medicinal Substances for Oral Administration

The medicinal substances for oral administration keep the hair healthy by regulating the functions of the whole body and promoting the flow of qi and blood. There are many Chinese medicinal substances that perform such functions, e.g. *hu ma* (Semen), *you cai zi* (Chinese colza), *he tao* (Semen Juglandis), *hei da dou* (black soybean). There are various forms of Chinese medicinal substances for oral administration such as medicinal broth, slurry, vinum, pellet and pilula.

Gua Zi San (Sunflower Seeds Powder) from *Qian Jin Yi Fang, Supplement to the Invaluable Prescriptions*: Take *gua zi* (sunflower seeds), *bai zhi* (Radix Angelicae Dahuricae), *dang gui* (Radix Angelicae Sinensis), *chuan xiong* (Rhizoma Chuanxiong), and *zhi gan cao* (Radix et Rhizoma Glycyrrhizae Praeparata cum Melle) 60g each, and grinding them into powder. Take about 1g after each meal, 3 times a day. Drink it with wine or soup. Regular use of this powder activates blood circulation, replenishes blood, makes hair beautiful, nourishes the skin, anti-aging and prevents the hair from early graying.

5.4 Proper Care of the Eyes

The eyes are closely related to *zangfu* organs and channels, which is the general reflection of essential qi and spirit of the human body. *Ling Shu* points out that "the essential qi of the five *zang* organs and the six *fu* organs all flow upward to the eyes". Therefore, eye care should stress both the care of the eyes themselves and the care of the relation between the part (eyes) and the whole human body. Health preservation experts all view eye care as an important task of health preservation and accumulate many effective methods and measures, which are summarized below.

5.4.1   Eye Care by Eyeball Movement

Eyeball movement refers to a variety of exercises of rolling eyes in order to strengthen the functions of eyes.

5.4.1.1   Eyeball Movement

This exercise adds luster to the eyeballs, makes them more sensitive, gets rid of cligo lentis and nephelium, and remedies nearsightedness and farsightedness. The specific practice is to close eyes after waking up in the morning, move eyeballs from right to left and from left to right 10 times respectively; then sit with open eyes, look at the upper left corner, upper right corner, lower left corner and lower right corner one by one, and repeat the procedure 4-5 times. Before going to bed in the night, roll the eyeballs with eyes shut for about 10 times.

5.4.1.2   Looking into the Distance

Looking at views in the distance helps regulate the functions of the eyeballs and avoid decrease of eyesight due to eyeball distortion. For example, look at mountains, trees, prairie, blue sky, white clouds, bright moon or starry sky in early morning or at night.

5.4.2   Eye Care by Massage

5.4.2.1   Pressing the Eyes

It is recorded in *Sheng Ji Zong Lu* (*Comprehensive Recording of Divine Assistance*) that one is advised to rub the hands and press them on the eyes. The process is rubbing the palms together until they are warm, open the eyes and press the two palms on the two eyes to warm the two eyeballs with the warmth. When the palms become cool, rub them again and press them on the eyes. Repeat this 3 to 5 times. Doing this exercise several times every day gives warmth to the eye and facilitates the flow of the yang qi, refreshes oneself and improves eyesight.

5.4.2.2   Pinching Canthus of the Eyes

Hold breath and pinch the four canthus till one feels slightly short of breath, then take a breath and end the exercise. Repeat the procedure 3 to 5 times. Keep doing this exercise several times every day.

5.4.2.3   Pressing Acupoints

Use the first finger pulp or the first joint of the thumb to press *si zhu kong* (SJ 23), *yu yao* (EX-HN4), *cuan zhu* (BL 2), *si bai* (ST 2), *tai yang* (EX-HN5). The strength should be from gentle to heavy and one have the sensation of sourness and distention, and then massage gently for several times. The method has the effect of strengthening and improving eyes and treating ocular diseases.

5.4.3   Eye Care by Closing the Eyes and Taking a Rest

Experts on health preservation in ancient times advocated that "do not look at one thing for long" which indicated that eye care is closely related to vitality preservation. In daily life, study and work, one should try not to read, write, watch TV for a long time, when asthenopia occurs, try to get rid of distracting thoughts, relax the mind, close the eyes and sit quietly for 5 to 10 minutes or do this exercise several times every day. This method helps to cure asthenopia and regulate mood and temperament and cures ocular diseases.

5.4.4 Eye Care by Diet

Generally speaking, taking more vegetables, fruit, carrot, animal's liver, or oil of fish liver helps to protect the eyesight. Avoid food rich in fat, hot and pungent. Meanwhile, medicated diet and food therapy may be used complementarily to nourish the liver and brighten the eyes.

5.4.5 Eye Care by Medicinal Substances

TCM holds that asthenopia is closely related to the spleen, liver, kidney, qi and blood. Therefore, eye care by Chinese medicinal substances starts primarily from invigorating the spleen, nourishing the liver, tonifying the kidney and reinforcing qi and blood. Medicinal substances for eye care fall into two categories: those for oral administration and those for external use, which are chosen according to different conditions.

For example, Pillow for Eyesight Improvement: pillows made *of qiao mai pi* (buckwheat seed spermoderm), *lv dou pi* (green gram spermoderm), *hei dou pi* (Glycinis Testa), *jue ming zi* (Semen Cassiae), *ju hua* (Flos Chrysanthemi) can expel wind, dissipate heat, clear the liver-heat and improve eyesight.

It is advised to take Chinese medicines according to different conditions. For example, asthenopia and dryness of the eyes are due to yin deficiency of the liver and kidney. Those who want to tonify and nourish the liver and kidney may choose *Liu Wei Di Huang Wan* (Six-Ingredient Rehmannia Pill), *Qi Ju Di Huang Wan* (Lycium Berry, Chrysanthemum and Rehmannia Pill) and *Shi Hu Ye Guang Wan* (Vision Improving Bolus of Noble Dendrobium). People who are easily to get visual fatigued and being physically weak in daily life is insufficiency of qi and blood. *Ba Zhen Wan* (Eight-Gem Bolus) can be used to nourish both qi and blood. Those who suffer from asthenopia, weak physique and lack of appetite due to insufficiency of spleen qi may choose *Bu Zhong Yi Qi Wan* (Center-Supplementing and Qi-Boosting Bolus).

5.5 Proper Care of the Ears

The ears are considered as the orifices of the kidney in TCM. The functions of the ears are related to all of the five *zang* organs in general and to the kidney in particular. The hearing ability of the ears reflects the functions of the *zangfu* organs such as the heart, the kidney and the brain.

5.5.1 Ear Care by Avoiding Intensive Use of Hearing

Intensive listening consumes the essential qi and damage the audition.. *Huai Nan Zi* (*The Masters of Huainan*) points out that "five voices clamor the ear and make the ear not sharp". Working or studying in a noisy environment, one must take necessary protective measures such as controlling the noise source. In noisy surrounding, one should open the mouth consciously in order to diffuse the sound waves entering the auditory canal, to relieve excessively pressure on the ear drum and tympanic membrane of the inner ear, and to achieve good self-protection.

5.5.2　Ear Care by Massage

Ear massage consists of the following steps:

(1) Massage the sulcus auriculae posterior: Massage the front and the back of the two sulcus auriculae posteriors with the index fingers for 15 times respectively.

(2) Press the auricle: Press down the auricles with both hands for 15 times.

(3) Shake and pull the ears: Shake and pull the two auricles with the thumbs and the index fingers for 15 times, but do not pull too hard.

(4) Flick the ears: Flick the ears with the middle fingers for 15 times.

(5) Knock the occipitals: Cover the two ear holes with the two palms, place the thumbs and fingers on the back of the head, and knock slightly the hind brain for 24 times with the index, middle and ring fingers of both hands, and then uncover and cover the palms on the ears for 10 times continually. This exercise inflates the auditory canals and vibrates the eardrums so it is known as the "occipitals-knocking therapy".

Ear massage accelerates qi and blood circulation in the ears, mobilizes the healthy qi in the body to enhance body resistance against diseases and strike a relative physiological balance. Besides, this exercise adds luster to the skin of the outer ears, slows the aging of eardrum, prevents chilblain on the ears, and prevents and cures ear diseases. In addition, it invigorates the original qi of the kidney, strengthens constitution, prevents aging, helps to keep fit and facilitates longevity.

5.5.3　Ear Combing

It is suggested to use soft thin brush to comb the ears.

5.5.3.1　Brushing the Back Auricles

Fold the auricle and brush the back auricles 20 to 30 times until the local skin turns slightly red with heat sensation; or use the thenar of hands to rub if the thin brush is not available.

5.5.3.2　Kneading the Cochlea

Press and knead bilateral cymba conchae (the depressions on the superior part of the helix crus) with ventral aspect of the index fingers of both hands 10 to 20 times; and then press and knead cavity of concha (the depressions on the inferior part of the helix crus) 10 to 20 times; then brush the above two areas with thin brush until the heat sensation.

5.5.3.3　Brushing the Helix

Brush the bilateral auricular lobes 20 to 30 times from upward to downward; then hold the two ears tightly and lift and pull the bilateral helixes 3 to 5 times upward or downward respectively. Or use ventral aspect of finger in case the thin brush is not available.

One of the clinical applications is preventing and curing auricle chilblain. Wash the ears with decocted eggplant pieces or the root part of eggplant and then apply the ear combing method until the obvious heat sensation of the local area.

5.5.4 Ear Care by Medicated Pillow

Chinese people in ancient times used medicated pillows for the ear care. Two kinds of medicated pillows are introduced as follows.

Ju hua Pillow: Put dried *ju hua* (Flos Chrysanthemi) 1, 000g, *chuan xiong* 400g, *dan pi* (Cortex Moutan) and *bai zhi* (Radix Angelicae Dahuricae) 200g each into the pillowcase and let the fragrance of the medicinal substances volatilize slowly. Each medicated pillow can be used continuously for about half a year. Modern medical studies have proven that this medicated pillow contains many kinds of essential oil and fulfils the functions of clearing the liver, improving the eyesight, lowering blood pressure, preventing viruses and bacteria, removing heat to cool blood, promoting blood flow and removing blood stasis. Those who use chrysanthemum pillow for a long time will feel refreshed and energetic.

Ci shi Pillow: Taoist health preservation in ancient times advocates the use of *ci shi* (Magnetitum) pillow and *bai mu* (Cypress) pillow. The magnetite pillow is made by inlaying magnetite into the wooden pillow. Using the pillow for a long time helps to improve hearing and eyesight. The cypress pillow is made of cypress board with 120 small holes on the four sides of the pillow. Put *dang gui* (Radix Angelicae Sinensis), *chuan xiong* (Rhizoma Chuanxiong), *fang feng* (Radix Saposhnikoviae), *bai zhi* (Radix Angelicae Dahuricae), *dan pi* (Cortex Moutan), and *ju hua* (Flos Chrysanthemi) into the pillow, cover the pillow with a cloth bag and let the fragrance of the medicinal substances volatilize gradually. The health preservation principle of the medicated pillow is to cure diseases by smelling the special fragrance given out by the medicinal substances in the pillow and being influenced by the magnetic field of the magnetite.

5.6 Proper Care of the Nose

Huang Di Nei Jing points out that "the air from the lungs passes through the nose." Nose is the gateway of the respiratory passage and the first defense against pathogenic microorganism, dust. With the hairs and nasal mucus in the nasal cavity, there are often many bacteria and dirt in the nose and sometimes it may become the disease source that disseminates bacteria. Therefore, it is of vital importance to maintain good nose care in order to efficiently prevent respiratory disease.

5.6.1 Nose Care by the "Nose Bath" Exercise

"Bathing the nose" means bathing the nose with cold air or cold water. It is suggested to bathe the nose with cold water in the four seasons of the year. Cleaning the nasal cavity with cold water when washing face in the morning can improve blood circulation of the nasal mucous membrane, strengthen the ability of the nose to adapt to weather changes, and prevent cold and other diseases of the respiratory passage.

People working in the seriously polluted environment, with dry nasal cavity or after nasal operation can go to hospital for nasal medicated rinsing. Nasal rinsing can relieve the nasal discomfort effectively. It can also be done with rinsing or light brine at home: immerse nostril in salt water and inspire the liquid into the nasal cavity. Make the liquid thoroughly contact the nasal mucous membrane for a while, then expire the water. Repeat this for 1 to 3 minutes and care to prevent choke due to the water irritating the windpipes. Drip several drops of vegetable oil into the nasal cavity to keep the cavity moist.

5.6.2 Nose Care by Massage

Nose massage consists of the following manipulations: pulling the nose, rubbing the nose, scraping the nose, rubbing the nasal tip, and massaging *yin tang* (EX-HN 3), all of which may help to improve blood circulation in the nose, add luster to the outer skin of the nose, nourish the lungs, prevent cold and cure many kinds of rhinitis.

Pulling the nose: Use the thumb and index finger to clamp the two sides of nasal root, and pull them downward hard for 16 consecutive times.

Rubbing the nose: Rub the thenar eminences of the two palms together until they become warm, press them on the two sides of the nose, rub up and down between the nasal root and the *ying xiang* (L120) point for 24 times.

Scraping the nose: Scrape the bridge of the nose downward with fingers for 36 times.

Rubbing the nasal tip: Rub the nasal tip for 36 times with fingers of each hand respectively.

Massaging *yin tang*: Press *yin tang* (located between the two brows) with the finger pulp of the middle, the index and the ring finger for 16 times, or use the middle fingers to press *ying tang* from the right and the left alternatively. This massage enhances the hyperplasia ability of epithelia of the nasal mucous membrane, stimulates the olfactory cells and sharpens the olfactory sensation.

5.6.3 Nose Care by Medicinal Substances

It is advised to keep the appropriate moisture of the nasal cavity. Excessive dryness in the nose may cause the nasal mucous membrane to chap and bleed. In dry weather, one can take some medicinal substances to take proper care of the nose, e.g. drip some compound recipe mint oil into the nostril or take some Vitamin A and D to protect the nasal mucous membrane. One can also take some Chinese medicinal substances. Please consult the following two formulas for reference.

Run Bi Tang (Decoction Moistening the Nose): *tian dong* (Radix Asparagi) 9g, *hei zhi ma* (Semen Sesami Nigrum) 15g, *sha shen* (Radix Adenophorae) 9g, *mai dong* (Radix Ophiopogonis) 9g, *huang jing* (Rhizoma Polygonati) 9g, *yu zhu* (Rhizoma Polygonati Odorati) 9g, *sheng di* (Radix Rehmanniae) 9g and *chuan bei mu* (Bulbus Fritillariae Cirrhosae) 9g. This formula moistens the lung and nourishes the spleen. Taking the medicated decoction with ingredients of more or less the above mentioned amount moistens and nourishes the nose.

Jian Bi Tang (Decoction for Nose Care): *cang er zi* (Fructus Xanthii) 27g, *chan yi* (periostracum cicadae) 6g, *fang feng* (Radix Saposhnikoviae) 9g, *zhi gan cao* (Radix et Rhizoma Glycyrrhizae Praeparata cum Melle) 4.5g, *yi ren* (Semen Coicis) 12g, and *bai he* (Lilli Bulbus) 9g. This formula aims at resisting wind and keeping the nose fit, moistening the lung and strengthening the spleen, and harmonizing the lung qi and nourishing the spleen qi. It has good health-care and prevention effects for those who are liable to catch cold and running nose.

5.6.4   Correcting Poor Habits

While caring the nose, one should pay attention to the following several aspects:

First, the most frequent action of the patients with coryza is blowing the nose. Incorrect action can make nasal antrum full of nasal grume and become the hotbed of growing of pathogen. So the correct way of blowing nose should be developed. Press the right and left wings of the nose to the nasal septum alternatively to get rid of the nasal discharge. Do not pinch the two nostrils tightly or blow the nose to remove the nasal discharge in case of increasing the pressure in the nose and the pharyngeal portion, which may cause the nasal discharge to flow back into the ears.

Second, don't pick the nose and don't pluck or cut the vibrissa. Because the board of nose is the medically named "dangerous triangle part", the inflammation is possible to invade into cranial cavity if not controlled. So it is better to abstain from the bad habit of picking the nose.

The third improper habit is swallowing nasal mucus. This action may easily irritate the throat, the intestine and the stomach. Nasal mucus contains tiny injurant and allergen like dust and bacteria, which would irritate the mucous membrane of throat and arouse cough, and lead to chronic faucitis after a long period. The bacteria and virus swallowed into the intestine and stomach would irritate the mucous membrane and cause illness.

5.7   Proper Care of the Cervical Vertebra

Researches have shown that over recent years the morbidity of cervical syndrome is rising and seems to occur at an earlier age. Improper care of the cervical part keeps it in an unhealthy position for a long time, causes chronic strain of the tissues around the cervical vertebra, and leads to fibrositis and gradual cataplasia.

5.7.1   Cervical Vertebra Care by Correct Sitting Posture

Morbidity of cervical syndrome is high among those who have to bend over their desk working for a long time. While incorrect posture is one of the important causes of cervical syndrome. Therefore, a correct sitting posture is of vital importance for prevention against the syndrome.

The correct sitting posture is sitting straight up in a natural and comfortable way, straighten the upper body, tighten the abdomen, draw in the lower mandible slightly, keep the two legs close to each other, lean the head forward slightly, and keep the head, neck, shoulder and chest in natural and normal physiological curve. At the same time, pay attention to the appropriate distance of the desk and the chair.

In addition, try to get rid of some unhealthy habits in daily life. For example, do not lean against sofa or lie halfway down on the bed when watching TV. Do not play *mah-jong* for too long and remember to change body postures from time to time.

5.7.2   Functional Exercises on Cervical Vertebra

Looking at close quarters for a long period, especially keeping the state of nutation easily affects cervical vertebra and leads to eyes fatigue. Therefore, those who have to work over their desks for a long time, try to do some exercises every 0.5 to 1 hour. It is better to raise the head and look into distant for about half minute. It is suggested to do some cervical exercise according to its motor function characteristics, including bending forward and backward, bending right and left, rotating right and left, and turning clockwise and anticlockwise in circles. One may also do part exercise such as shrugging shoulders and pulling arms in circles.

One may practice the "Phoenix" (*Feng Huang*, Chinese characters) exercise for cervical care regularly. The specific practice: Close the eyes, imagine that the chin is a pen, keep the body still and write the two unsimplified Chinese characters "鳳凰" in the air, write 10 times successively and repeat the exercise 3 times a day. This exercise can be done at any time, during breaks or while waiting for the bus and it will have great effects. This exercise moves various joints and links the cervical part with gentle and systematic movements and without too big movement range and it is helpful for the prevention and cure of cervical syndrome.

5.7.3   Cervical Vertebra Care by Proper Use of the Pillow

The early symptoms of cervical syndrome are the abnormal change of the physiological curve of the spine in the cervical part such as lessening, straightening and backward protruding of the curve. Therefore, prevention against abnormal change in the physiological curve of the cervical spine is the key to the prevention of cervical syndrome. One may achieve the goal by proper use of the pillow. Choose pillows that match the physiological curve of the cervical vertebra, particularly those are soft and with good air permeability. The best shape of pillow is cylindrical and with a diameter of about 20cm. When lying on bed, one should place the pillow under the neck so that the muscles at the back of the neck may relax and the cervical vertebra may remain in a normal physiological curve. The middle of pillow should be concave and two ends of the pillow should be slightly higher than the middle part, and make the cervix contact the pillow completely but not hang in the air, so that the head can rest in a relative fixed place and the neck will not make any abnormal movement during the sleep. The pillow also keeps the neck warm. The pillow should not be too high or too low, too soft or too hard. In addition, notice the sleeping posture and don't pronate. The pillow people use for lying sideways should be as high as their shoulder.

It has been proved that cervical vertebra care by medicated pillow has some curative effects for chronic insomnia, cervical syndrome, high blood pressure, nerve headache, tension headache, migraine headache, dizziness, anxiety disorders and depression. There are 12 ingredients for the pillow listed as follows: *chuan xiong* (Rhizoma Chuanxiong), *wu zhu yu* (Fructus Evodiae), *chuan wu* (Radix Aconiti Preparata), *cao wu* (Radix Aconiti Kusnezoffi), *dang gui* (Radix Angelicae Sinensis), *mo yao* (Myrrha), *xi xin* (Herba Asari), *wei ling xian* (Radix Clematidis), *gan cao* (Radix

Glycyrrhizae), *bing pian* (Borneolum Syntheticum), *zhang nao* (Camphora) and *bo he* (Herba Menthae Haplocalycis). Grind the first 9 ingredients into fine grain, put in some vinegar and stir fry the grain on small fire until there is scotched flavor, add *bing pian*, *zhang nao* and *bo he* into it and mix all the ingredients together. Then wrap the medicament with dry silk cloth to make the pillow. Use it in the night and seal it in a plastic bag in day time.

5.7.4 Cervical Vertebra Care by Self-Massage

Self-massage: Massage such points as *wan gu* (SI 4), *wai guan* (TE 5), *jian zhong* (SI 15) and *feng chi* (GB 20), and turn the neck slowly at the same time for 10 to 15 minutes each time, twice a day.

Kneading the neck: Hold the hind neck with the palm, pinch the nape with strength of the four fingers and the root of the palm for 6 to 9 times each time and three times a day. Doing this exercise is very helpful for health care of the cervical vertebra.

5.8 Proper Care of the Hands and Feet

The hands and feet are the cross-connecting place of the yin channel and the yang channel of the upper limbs and the lower limbs. The rise and fall of qi and blood, yin and yang of the body have close relation with the functional status of the hands and feet. Experts on health preservation in ancient China pay much attention to the health care of the hands and feet.

5.8.1 Proper Care of the Hands

In daily life, the hands are the most easily contaminated part of the body. Improper care of the hands will result in many diseases. The following are methods of hand care.

5.8.1.1 Swinging the Hands

Clench the both fists gently and swing the upper limbs from the front to the back, first to the left side, then to the right side. Afterwards, drop the upper limbs at the two sides of the body and swing the hands. Repeat the above movement for 24 times respectively. The exercise has the actions of limbering up the muscles and joints, promoting qi flow and blood circulation of channels and collaterals, making the upper limbs healthy. It may prevent the joint diseases of the shoulder, elbow and wrist, regulate qi and blood, prevent and cure hypertension.

5.8.1.2 Hand Care by Massage

Massage of the hands can be carried out in combination of massage of the upper arm. The exercise goes as follows: put the hands together and rub them until they are warm. Put one palm on the back of the other, rub the upper hand back and forth from the finger tips to the wrist of the lower hand until the area is warm. Exchange hands and repeat the exercise. The massage can be carried out at bedtime in the evening or after waking up in the morning. This exercise can improve blood circulation of the skin, enhance metabolism and absorption of nutrition, make the muscle strong, remove wrinkles, increase the glossiness of the skin, make it smooth and prevent chilblain.

5.8.1.3　Hand Care by Medicinal Substances

Hand care by medicinal substances can make the skin smooth and tender, clean and rosy. The following are two formulas:

Qian Jin Shou Gao Fang (*Invaluable Hand Mastic Recipe*), from *Qian Jin Yi Fang*: *tao ren* (Semen Persicae) 20g, *xing ren* (Semen Armeniacae) 10g, *ju he* (Semen Citri Reticularae) 20g, *chi shao* (Radix Paeoniae Rubra) 20g, *xin yi ren* (biond magnolia flower kernel), *chuan xiong* (Rhizoma Chuanxiong) and *dang gui* (Radix Angelicae Sinensis) 30g each, and *da zao* (Fructus Jujubae), *niu nao* (ox brain), *yang nao* (goat brain), *gou nao* (dog brain) 60g, each, make all of these ingredients into mastic. After washing the hands, apply the mastic to the hands and avoid being burned by fire. This mastic can smooth the skin, protect the hands and prevent wrinkles.

Tai Ping Shou Gao Fang (Tai Ping Hand Mastic Formula), from *Tai Ping Sheng Hui Fang* (*Tai Ping Sacred Remedies*): Gualourang (melon flesh) 60g, *xing ren* (Semen Armeniacae) 30g, and an appropriate amount of *feng mi* (honey). Make all the ingredients into mastic. Apply the mastic to the hands at bedtime every evening. It can prevent chapping, and make the skin white, tender and elastic.

5.8.2　Proper Care of the Feet

As the old saying that "trees' withering starts from the root, and people's aging begins with the feet" and that "it is good to protect the root when planting trees, and protect feet when preserving people's health." The feet are very important to the health of the body. Discomfort of the feet is a sign for presenility of the body and pathological changes. Health care therapy of the reflex zones of the feet has been regarded as one of the supplementary medical therapies and widely applied in clinic.

5.8.2.1　Foot Care by Keeping Warm

The normal temperature of the tiptoes of healthy people is about 22℃, and the sole is about 28℃. The most comfortable temperature is 28 to 33℃ of the feet. If the temperature falls below 22℃, people are susceptible to catch cold and other diseases. According to TCM, "every disease starts from coldness and the coldness comes from the feet." So it is important to keep the feet warm in cold days. Shoes and socks are supposed to be able to keep the feet warm, and they should be slightly loose, soft and comfortable. Shoes should be waterproof with good air permeability, and be changed in time. Keeping the feet warm is an important way to prevent diseases, which is effective in preventing cold, rhinitis, asthma, and angina.

5.8.2.2　Foot Care by Bath and Wash

Experts on health preservation believe that "the feet are the bottom of the body and they should be washed every night." A folk song about the curative effects of washing the feet everyday saying that: "Wash the feet in spring to strengthen yang, wash the feet in summer to remove summer humidity, wash the feet in autumn to nourish the lung and bowels, wash the feet in winter to warm *Dan Tian*. Wash the feet at bedtime to have a good sleep, and wash the feet after long walk to remove the tiredness." Wash the feet with warm water can stimulate the acupoints of the feet, enhance the blood circulation, regulate *zangfu* organs, dredge channels and collaterals, and calm the nerves, so as to keep fit and prevent diseases.

Apart from washing the feet with warm water, one can also wash the feet with medicated water.

(1) Take *xia ku cao* (Prunellae Spica) 30g, *gou teng* (Uncariae Ramulus cum Uncis) and *ju hua* (Flos Chrysanthemi) 20g each, and *sang ye* (Folium Mori) 15g, decoct them with water and bathe the feet in the medicated water once or twice a day and 10 to 15 minutes each time. It is especially suitable for patients suffering from high blood pressure.

(2) Take *tou gu cao* (Tuberculate Speranskia Herb), *xun gu feng* (Herba Aristolochiae Mollissimae), *lao guan cao* (Herba Erodii) 30g each, *huang hao* (Herba Artemisiae Annuae) 20g, and *ru xiang* (Olibanum), *mo yao* (myrrha), *tao ren* (Semen Persicae) 10g each, decoct them with water and bathe the feet when the water is hot. Do the bathe twice a day. It is applicable for patients suffering from arthritis in lower limbs.

(3) Take *su mu* (Sappan Lignum) 30g, *tao ren* (Semen Persicae), *hong hua* (Flos Carthami), *tu yuan* (eupolyphaga), *xue jie* (Daemonoropis Resina) and *ru xiang* (Olibanum) 10g each, and *zi ran tong* (pyritum) 20g, pour hot water into the medicinal substances and bathe the feet immediately. It is applicable for foot injuries.

(4) Take *ding xiang* (Flos Caryophylli) 15g, *ku shen* (Radix Sophorae Flavescentis), *da huang* (Radix Rhei et Rhizoma), *ming fan* (alumen) and *di fu zi* (Fructus Kochiae) 30g each, and *huang bai* (Cortex Phellodendri) and *di yu* (Radix Sanguisorbae) 20g each, and decoct them with water and obtain the solution. When the solution is no longer hot, bathe the feet in the solution for 10 to 15 minutes, 5 to 6 times every day. Take one bathe a day and it can cure dermatomycosis pedis.

5.8.2.3 Foot Care by Massage

Foot massage is simple and easy to follow and it is one of the simplest methods of self-care and disease prevention. Foot massage is to massage the acupoints of the feet, stimulate the reflex zones, relax the muscle, improve blood circulation, regulate the functions of the *zangfu* organs, balance yin and yang, relieve tiredness, and prevent local diseases of the foot and overall diseases of the whole body. The following are methods of food massage.

(1) Massage of *yong quan*: yong quan (KI 1) is an important acupoint in the Channel of Foot-Shaoyin, the reflex zone of the kidney. At bedtime after washing the feet, grasp the tiptoes with one hand, and massage *yong quan* with the other hand for 30 to 60 times until the foot is warm. Then massage the other foot. This exercise can regulate the function of the liver, strengthen the spleen, make sleep peaceful and strengthen the body.

(2) Foot massage: One may use fingers, finger joints, and tools such as massage sticks and massage balls to carry out foot massage. Rub or press the feet according to the body conditions. As for daily health care, massage every reflex zone for 2 to 3 minutes, first the left foot and then the right one. Massage the feet for about 30 minutes each time. The strength applied should be in the order of "light, heavy and light" with one's endurance as the upper limit. If abnormal sore, distension, prick, paralysis, pain, or prints in the shape of nodus, trabs or psammosum appear during the massage, which shows that the corresponding parts of the body may suffer from some functional diseases, so these parts should be massaged in particular.

5.8.2.4 Foot Care by Medicinal Substances for External Use

In autumn or winter, because of the block of channels, the feet will have dry skin and may even chap. Apply traditional Chinese medicinal substances with the functions of removing cold, promoting blood circulation, and moistening the skin of the feet can prevent diseases effectively. One formula is introduced as follows.

Dong Yue Run Zu Fang Lie Fang (*Recipe for Moistening the Feet and Preventing Chap in Winter*): Prepare mastic with *zhu zhi you* (pig fat) 12g, *huang la* (yellow wax) 60g, *bai zhi* (Radix Angelicae Dahuricae), *sheng ma* (Rhizoma Cimicifugae), and *zao jia* (Fructus Gleditsiae) 3g each, *ding xiang* (Flos Caryophylli) 1.5g, and *She xiang* (Moschus) 0.6g. Wash the feet and apply the mastic to them. This formula can remove coldness, prevent chap and relieve swelling.

5.9 Proper Care of the Chest, Back, Waist and Abdomen

The chest, back, waist and abdomen is the place where the *zangfu* organs locate. The functional vicissitudes of the four parts above are directly related to the activities of the *zangfu* organs. Experts on health preservation all put great emphasis on proper care of these parts. Proper care of these parts can improve the circulation of qi and blood, coordinate and enhance the relationship among parts of the body, improve metabolism, strengthen the body and prevent diseases.

5.9.1 Proper Care of the Chest

Chest is the position of the heart and lung, the circulation of qi and blood and cold or warm in the chest directly affects the function of *zangfu* organs, the basic methods of chest care include attention to keep warm and self-massage.

5.9.1.1 Chest Care by Clothes

Experts on health preservation in TCM believe that "the breast should be protected all the time". It is recorded in *Lao Lao Heng Yan* (*Common Saying for Senile Health Preservation*) that "although the summer is hot, one should wear clothes with short sleeves made of hemp cloth in order to protect the chest." It means that the protection of the chest emphasizes on keeping warm and avoiding cold to protect the yang of the chest. This is more important for the old and the weak. In daily life, people wear waistcoats and jackets to protect the yang qi of the chest and back.

5.9.1.2 Chest Care by Massage

Massage the breast: sit or lie on the back. Use the palm of left hand to massage the breast from upper left to lower right, and the palm of right hand to massage from upper right to lower left. Do the massage by two hands alternately for 30 minutes. Then rub the two breasts with the two hands in clockwise and anticlockwise directions, each for 30minutes, and from right to left and up to down, each for 30 times. Women can do the breast grasping exercises: Cross the two forearms, hold the left breast with the right hand and the right breast with the left hand, and then use fingers and thumbs to grasp the breast. Grasping and loosing the breasts once accounts for one time, repeat the procedure for 30 times. Massage of the breast can stimulate yang qi, improve qi and blood circulation and enhance the functions of the heart and lung, so as to prevent diseases such as chest distress, asthma, cough and palpitation.

Grasp the muscle of the chest: cross the two hands on the chest. Use the thumbs to press the front of the armpit, apply the index and middle fingers to press the inferior armpit and grasp the muscles. This method can promote qi and blood circulation and enhance the function of the respiratory system.

Clap the chest: clap the chest gently with the soft palm or void fist. This can enhance the function of the heart and lung and help to discharge phlegm, which can be used to prevent and treat the illness of respiration system and circulation system.

Push the chest and flank: Put one palm on the upside of the same bosom, push downwards and slantingly by the middle of two nipples until the flank of the opposite side. This method has the effect of comforting the chest and regulating qi, relieving cough and disperse phlegm, antiasthma and appeasing retch, comforting the liver and smoothing the gallbladder, helping to digest food and eliminating stasis.

5.9.2   Proper Care of the Back

The back is the place where the foot *taiyang* bladder channel and *du mai* pass by. All the back-*shu* acupoints of five *zang* organs concentrate at the back. Since the warm or cold of the back has direct connection with functions of *zangfu* organs. The exercises and massage of the back can improve the immunity of the body, regulate blood pressure, enhance the functions of the heart and improve the digestive functions.

5.9.2.1   Back Care by Keeping It Warm

There are three ways of keeping the back warm:

Protect the back with clothes: try to keep the back warm by wearing clothes in daily life. Put on or take off clothes timely to protect the back.

Expose the back to the sun to warm it: expose the back to the sun while avoiding wind to warm the back, activate yang and improve health.

Avoid wind and cold: since the back is the place where the back-*shu* acupoints concentrate, it can be easily invaded by wind and cold and thus suffer from diseases, especially when perspiring, do not turn the back to fans in case the body is invaded by wind-cold evil.

5.9.2.2   Back Care by Frequent Pounding and Massaging

Doctors and experts on health preservation in ancient China all emphasized on the importance of back protection, and propose such exercises as pounding the back, rubbing the back, pinching the spine to protect the back.

(1) Pounding by oneself: this exercise can harmonize the five zang organs and six fu organs, improve the circulation of qi and blood, stretch muscles, stimulate yang qi, strengthen the heart and benefit the kidney, so as to increase the vigor of human body. Process: stand with two legs separated. Relax the whole body and half clinch the two fists, and let them droop down naturally. When pounding, first turn round the waist, let the two fists swing with the waist and knock back

and forth on the back and the lower abdomen alternatively. If turning the waist right and left once accounts for one time, repeat the process for 30 to 50 times. Pound the body from down to up, and then up to down.

(2) Rubbing the back by oneself: this exercise can prevent common cold and relieve soreness in the waist and back, chest distress and abdominal distension. It can be carried out during bath with a wet towel at the back, grasp the two ends of the towel tightly and rub it against the back until the back is warm. Please notice not to overexert and to avoid injuries of the skin.

5.9.3 Proper Care of the Waist

Waist is the middle point of the body. It is the hinge of human activities with many movements and weight loading. Traditional Chinese martial arts emphasize much on "waist as the axle" and "waist as the dominant part", regarding the movements of the waist as the foundation of vital movement. Since daily life and work are especially likely to cause waist strain, it is very important to take proper care of the waist.

5.9.3.1 Waist Care by Using It Properly

Before moving or lifting heavy objects, one should keep the two legs at the same distance as the width of the shoulder, bend the knees, and energize abdominal muscles. At the moment, the simultaneous effort of muscles of the thighs and shanks disperses the pressure on the waist. If one lifts heavy objects from the ground with the knee joint straightened, the pressure on the waist will increase by 40% over the previous position. In that case, ligaments, muscles and intervertebral discs of the waist will be easily injured. Therefore, when moving objects, one should not bend the waist, but bend the knees, keeping the waist at its normal curvature of the upstanding posture and avoiding the concentration of pressure on the waist. If the objects are too heavy, it is not recommendable to move them forcefully.

Standing upright is the best posture for the joint of the lumbar vertebra. When one bends the waist, the burden on the tissues of the waist will increase in certain degree. Bending the waist for a long time will cause lumbar muscle strain, which, in turn, may develop into strain and cataplasia of the backbone (column vertebral). But if the angle of bending is less than 20 degrees, the burden on the waist is comparatively small. Therefore, it is necessary to keep the back straight and upright in daily life, and avoid bending the waist to work for a long time, to ease the burden on the waist.

5.9.3.2 Waist Care by Doing Traditional Exercises

There are many traditional Chinese exercises for waist care. Many of them stress on waist movements, such as *Wu Qin Xi* (Five-animal Mimic Exercise), *Yi Jin Jing* (Sinew-transforming Exercise), *Ba Duan Jin* (Eight-section Brocade), and *Taiji Quan*. These exercises intend to strengthen the waist and keep healthy through movements such as loosening the hip, turning the waist, and bending and lifting the head.

5.9.3.3 Waist Care by Regular Massage

"Waist is the mansion for the kidneys." Massage of the waist fulfils the functions of warming and nourishing the kidney yang, strengthening the waist and kidney, and lubricating the bowels to relieve constipation. It also stretches muscles, improves the circulation of qi and blood, removes fatigue of waist muscles, and relieves spasm and pain of the waist and makes the waist nimble, strong and healthy.

(1) Massage of the waist: Rub the hands and make them warm. Put the palms closely to the sides of the spine at the part of the waist. Rub the two sides of the waist up and down along straight lines. Repeat the procedure for 108 times until the waist becomes warm. Keep rubbing the waist every day. It will promote qi to activate blood circulation, warm the body, dispel the cold, strengthen the waist and tonify the kidney.

(2) Rubbing and pressing the acupoint of *ming men* (GV 4): Clench the right or left hand into a fist and put the protuberant part (edge of the fist) formed by the articulation manus of the index finger at the acupoint of *ming men*. Press and rub the acupoint clockwise for 9 times and counter-clockwise for 9 times. Repeat this process for 36 times. Keep the mind on *ming men*. Massage of the acupoint every day will warm the kidney yang and strengthen the waist and the spine.

(3) Massage of the acupoint of *yao yan* (EX-B 7): Clench the two hands into fists, and put the protuberant parts of articulations digitorum manus of the index fingers on the two acupoints of *yao yan* on both sides. Press and rub the acupoints clockwise for 9 times, and then anticlockwise for 9 times. Repeat this process for 36 times. Focus the mind on the acupoints of *yao yan*. Massage of the acupoints every day will promote blood circulation to remove meridian obstruction, and strengthen the waist and the kidney.

(4) Knock the lumbosacra: Clench fists with the four fingers holding the thumb. Knock the two sides of spine at the waist and pars sacralis rhythmically with the back of fists. Knock both the left and the right parts for 36 times. Focus the mind on the lumbosacra, and keep thinking loosening the lumbosacra. Knocking the lumbosacra every day will activate the blood, stretch muscles, and strengthen the body.

5.9.4　Proper Care of the Abdomen

Since the abdomen is the place where the six *fu*-organs locate, proper care of the abdomen can enhance the functions of digestive system and urogenital system, prevent and cure diseases such as obesity, hypertension and gynecological diseases.

5.9.4.1　Abdominal Care by Keeping It Warm

Experts on health preservation in ancient China paid great attention to keeping the abdomen warm. It is said in *Lao Lao Heng Yan* (*Common Saying for Senile Health Preservation*) that "the abdomen is the energy source of five *zang*-organs. So it needs to be warm. Since elder people are weak in original qi, it is better for them to keep the abdomen warm." The book advocates the old and the weak to use the bib or girdle.

(1) Bib: Pound *ai ye* (Folium Artemisiae Argyi), make it soft, spread it evenly, and cover it with silk wadding or cotton. Put the mixture into a double-layered bib. Attach the bib to the abdomen.

(2) Girdle: It is also known as the "waist ornamental", i.e. a piece of cloth with the width of about 7 or 8 *cun* (1 *cun*=1/3 decimeter) tied to the waist and abdomen. Cao Ci-shan, an expert

on health preservation, notes that girdles may "protect the abdomen at the front, the waist at the side, and *ming men* (GV 4) at the back and they are very beneficial." The two methods mentioned above can be supplemented by adding other medicaments with warming effect to enhance the function of warming the abdomen.

5.9.4.2   Abdominal Care by Massage

Massage of the abdomen can not only cure local diseases at the abdomen, but also promote and regulate the functions of all the organs and tissues of the whole body. According to clinic practices, massage of the abdomen has the therapeutic effects and adjunctive therapeutic effects on diseases such as coronary heart disease, high blood pressure, diabetes, gastrointestinal dysfunction, baby dyspepsia, irregular menstruation, climacteric period syndrome, dysmenorrheal. It can also improve human body resistance against diseases, and prevent the invasion of wind, cold, summer heat, moist, dryness and excessive internal heat.

The health regimen of the abdomen massage has a history of thousands of years, which is a good self-care method for the middle-aged people and the old. TCM points out that "the spleen and stomach are the root of life acquirement", "six-*fu* organs takes dredging as nourishment". These views indicate that the functions of digestion, assimilation and excretion have the affinity with human health. Abdomen massage can enrich *five-zang* organs, dredge and reconcile six-*fu* organs, dispel the external pathogenic factors and dismiss the internal evil symptoms.

Abdomen massage can be done without time or posture limitation. While the best time of doing abdomen massage is at night while lying on the back before sleeping. It is noticeable to discharge the bladder before doing abdomen massage. Don't do it just after overeating. It is inadvisable to do abdomen massage for the patients with local skin infection, acute abdominal inflammation or abdominal tumors.

Massage by oneself: The specific practice is rub two hands to make them warm first, and overlap them on the surface of the abdomen. Rub the abdomen with the palms in a clockwise direction around the navel from small cycle to larger cycle for 36 times. Then massage the abdomen anticlockwise for 36 times in the same manner. It can be done either standing up or lying down, after meals or at bedtime. The massage will invigorate the spleen and the stomach, assist digestion, help to sleep peacefully, and prevent stomach intestine diseases. The massage should be done gently and slowly but not carelessly or rudely. The whole process lasts for 10 to 15 minutes. It is not appropriate to do the massage either to patients within 1 hour after meal or to drunken people.

(Qiao Xue)

6 TCM Nursing for Common Diseases

TCM nursing for common diseases, which is a part of clinical nursing of TCM, involves basic concepts, basic patterns and nursing interventions of common diseases. Nursing interventions include daily life nursing, administration, diet and symptoms. Nursing based on pattern differentiation is emphasized in TCM nursing. This chapter covers nursing interventions for common cold, insomnia, stomachache, dyspepsia, constipation, and dysmenorrheal, etc.

6.1 Common Cold

Cold is an externally contracted disease, mainly characterized by nasal obstruction, nasal discharge, sneezing, headache, aversion to cold, fever, and discomfort in body. Cold occurs in every season, especially in spring and winter. Cold which is widely popular with similar symptoms in a period time is called as influenza. Influenza is often caused by epidemic toxin.

6.1.1 Basic Patterns

6.1.1.1 Wind-Cold Fettering the Exterior

Serious aversion to cold, slight fever, absence of sweating, headache and body aches, nasal congestion, watery nasal discharge, sneezing, a thin and white coating, a floating and tight or floating and moderate pulse.

6.1.1.2 Wind-Heat Invading the Exterior

Fever, slight aversion to wind and cold, headache, nasal congestion, yellow nasal discharge, red and sore throat, cough, a red tongue border with a white or tiny yellow coating, a floating and rapid pulse.

6.1.1.3 Summerheat-Damp Attacking the Exterior

Distending pain and heaviness in the head, nasal congestion, runny nose, fever, slight aversion to wind and cold, absence of sweating or scanty sweating, chest oppression, vomit, a yellow and greasy coating, a soggy and rapid pulse.

6.1.1.4 Qi-Deficiency

Fever, aversion to cold, headache and body aches, cough, nasal congestion, spontaneous sweating, lassitude and lack of strength, qi deficiency and laziness to speak, a pale tongue with white coating, a floating and weak pulse.

321

6.1.1.5   Yin-Deficiency

Fever, slight aversion to wind and cold, headache, absence of sweating, dizziness, vexation, thirsty and dry throat, feverish feeling in palms and soles, cough with little sputum, a red tongue, a thready and rapid pulse.

6.1.2   Nursing Interventions

6.1.2.1   Environment and Daily Life Nursing

6.1.2.1.1   Keep the ward room quiet and clean with fresh air. Regularly ventilate and sterilize the room. Avoid wind pathogen re-attacking the patient when the room is being ventilated. For patient with wind-cold or qi-deficiency, keep the room warm. For patient with wind-heat or yin-deficiency, the temperature should be lower and the humidity should be moderate. For patient with summer-dampness, drop the temperature and humidity.

6.1.2.1.2   Advise the patient to have enough rest and sleep to recover energy. Strong physical labor or intense sports exercises should be avoided in mild cases. For severe cases, patient should be advised to lie and rest on bed to avoid too much energy consumption and immunity compromised.

6.1.2.1.3   People with influenza should be quarantined. Sterilize the air once to twice a day; avoid throwing away objects in contact with the patient's oral and nasal secretion, and sterilize the utensils every day.

6.1.2.1.4   Ask the patient to adjust clothes according to the changes of weather to avoid exogenous pathogen re-attacking the body.

6.1.2.2   Administrative Nursing

6.1.2.2.1   It is unsuitable to decoct diaphoretic drug for a long time as they often contain volatile active ingredients.

6.1.2.2.2   After taking warm-pungent diaphoretic drug while it is hot, it is better for the patient to cover up and sweat. Patient with excess constitution can take hot soup to promote sweating. Patient with weak constitution can take hot thin porridge to nourish stomach qi and fluids in order to promote sweating. Cool-pungent diaphoretic drug should be taken while it is warm. Slight sweating all over the body is preferred after administration. Wind exposure and heavy sweating should be avoided.

6.1.2.3   Dietary Nursing

6.1.2.3.1   Insipid and digestible diet and semi-fluid or fluid diet such as porridge and noodle are advised as the digestive function of spleen and stomach is lowered. Patient should drink plenty water, eat fresh vegetable and fruit. Pungent, hot, greasy, and fried food should be avoided. Stop smoking and drinking.

6.1.2.3.2   Wind-cold pattern: eat food of pungent and dispelling nature such as ginger to dispel cold pathogen.

6.1.2.3.3   Wind-warm pattern: use mint leaf and chrysanthemum tea to clear heat.

6.1.2.3.4   Summerheat-damp pattern: avoid eating raw, cold and sweet food; drink agastache, eupatorium tea.

6.1.2.3.5   Qi-deficiency pattern: eat food of warm nature such as chicken soup;

6.1.2.3.6   Yin-deficiency pattern: eat food of cool nature such as white fungus.

6.1.2.4 Symptomatic Nursing

6.1.2.4.1   If the patient has a fever and aversion to cold, avoid applying cool or cold compress with ice bag for fear that the striae of the skin (pores) and muscles get obstructed. Otherwise, evils may be kept within the body when perspiration is obstructed. If the patients has a high fever and slight aversion to cold, apply warm compress or acupuncture point to let blood out to subside fever. If the patient is invaded by wind-cold pathogen, apply tuina (Chinese medical massage) on points of *da zhui* (DU 14), *qu chi* (LI 11), *feng chi* (GB 20), *he gu* (LI 4), etc. or combined with moxibustion. If the patient is contracted by wind-warm pathogen, needling points of *da zhui* (DU 14), *qu chi* (LI11), *chi ze* (LU 5), *he gu* (LI 4), etc., or do blood-letting on points of *shi xuan* (EX-UE 11). If the patients feel tired and heavy in the head and body, pinch points of *yin tang* (EX-HN 3), *tai yang* (EX-HN 5), and neck, and/or scrape the patient's neck and back along both sides of the spine, or chest, elbow fossa, popliteal fossa.

6.1.2.4.2   If the patient has nasal obstruction, push and press along the two sides of nose to the root of nose, or press with finger or apply acupuncture on *ying xiang* (LI 20).

6.1.2.4.3   If the patient feels pain in the head and body, apply massage from the point of *yin tang* (EX-HN 3) to *tou wei* (ST8), *tai yang* (EX-HN 5) and press *yin tang* (EX-HN 3), *yu yao* (EX-HN 4), *tai yang* (EX-HN5), and *bai hui* (DU 20) as well; and apply grasping manipulation from the top of head to *feng chi* (GB 20), *da zhui* (DU 14) along bladder meridian; and then press and rub *da zhui* (DU 14), *qu chi* (LI 11), and grasp *jian jin* (GB 21) and *he gu* (LI 4); pat bladder channel on the back until the skin becomes slightly red.

6.1.2.4.4   Cupping: it's indicated for pain in the head and body. Apply moving cupping along the bladder channel or retained cupping on the points of *da zhui* (DU 14), *fei shu* (BL 13), etc.

6.2 Insomnia

Insomnia is a condition in which one frequently fails to get normal sleep. Mild insomnia refers to difficulty in falling asleep, frequently waking up during sleep or being unable to fall back asleep, while severe insomnia refers to inability to fall sleep through the whole night.

6.2.1 Basic Patterns

6.2.1.1 Deficiency of Both the Heart and Spleen

Profuse dreaming, susceptibility to wake up, palpitation, poor memory, dizziness, dizzy vision, weakness of the limbs, mental fatigue, a lusterless complexion, a pale tongue with a thin coating, a thready and weak pulse.

6.2.1.2 Vigorous Fire due to Yin Deficiency

Vexation, sleeplessness, palpitation, poor memory, vexing heat in the five centers (chest, palms and soles), soreness and weakness in the lumbar region and knee joints, dizziness, tinnitus, a dry mouth, a red tongue with a scanty coating, a thready and rapid pulse.

6.2.1.3　Heart Deficiency with Timidity

Profuse dreaming, waking up with a start, timidity, palpitation, shortness of breath, lassitude, a pale tongue with a thin coating, a wiry and thready pulse.

6.2.1.4　Phlegm-Heat Harassing the Interior

Sleeplessness, heaviness of the head, vexation, a bitter taste in the mouth, chest oppression, profuse sputum, dizzy vision, a red tongue with a yellow and greasy coating, a slippery and rapid pulse.

6.2.1.5　Liver Constraint Transforming into Fire

Sleeplessness, profuse dreaming, vexation and agitation, irascibility, red eyes, a bitter taste in the mouth, constipation, bloody urine, a red tongue with a yellow coating, a wiry and rapid pulse.

6.2.2　Nursing Interventions

6.2.2.1　Daily Life Nursing

6.2.2.1.1　Provide good environment to help sleep: Keep the bedroom quiet, and avoid noise; use smooth and comfortable mattress; maintain appropriate temperature and humidity in the room.

6.2.2.1.2　Instruct patients to have a regular life cycle and develop a good sleep habit.

6.2.2.1.3　Advise patients to go out for a walk after dinner to relax.

6.2.2.2　Administrative Nursing

Generally, take sedative drug half an hour before sleep. Don't take them at the same time if other drugs need to be taken such as anti-hypertension drug. To observe adverse effects such as dizziness, headache, etc. if other sedative drugs are taken.

6.2.2.3　Emotional Nursing

Relieve emotional stress and different stimulating factors of the mind, avoid excessive thinking. Advise people with liver constraint transforming into fire to keep good mood. For people with heart deficiency with timidity who are timid and frightened and afraid to sleep alone, advise their family to provide private and safe living environment or give more help and care.

6.2.2.4　Dietary Nursing

Take moderate amount of food for dinner, and avoid taking too much or too little. Avoid taking too greasy food and too late. Don't drink strong tea, liquor or coffee at dinner or after dinner. Drinking a moderate amount of warm milk before sleep is better.

6.2.2.5　Symptomatic Nursing

6.2.2.5.1　The commonly used points for acupuncture and tuina (Chinese medical massage) are *bai hui* (DU 20), *nei guan* (PC 6), *shen men* (HT 7), *san yin jiao* (SP 6), *yong quan* (KI 1). It's more effective to do massage before sleeping and gentle massage is also appropriate.

6.2.2.5.2　Soak feet or bath in warm water or herbal medicine water half an hour before going to bed.

6.2.2.5.3　Advise patients to apply relaxation techniques such as deep and slow breathing training, or listen to relaxing music to calm the mind and promote sleep.

6.2.2.5.4　Aromatic agents such as lavender essential oil or incense are applied to make people happy and help them to sleep.

6.3   Stomachache

Stomachache, also called epigastric pain, is a symptom characterized by frequent pain in the upper abdominal area. Gastric pain is usually caused by cold, irregular emotions, or improper diet.

6.3.1   Basic Patterns

6.3.1.1   Pathogenic Cold Attacking the Stomach

Sudden onset of stomachache, aversion to cold and preference for warmth, the pain that can be alleviated by warmth but is aggravated by cold, absence of thirst, or preference for warm drinks, a thin and white coating, a wiry and tight pulse.

6.3.1.2   Food Retention

Stomachache, epigastric fullness and abdominal distension, belching with acid reflux, or vomiting with undigested food, pain that can be alleviated by vomiting or flatus, incomplete defecation, a thick and greasy coating, and a slippery and excess pulse.

6.3.1.3   Qi Stagnation in the Liver and Stomach

Distending pain in the stomach cavity, frequent belching, incomplete defecation, stomachache that is always triggered by emotional factors and radiates to the costal regions, a thin and white coating, and a deep and wiry pulse.

6.3.1.4   Spleen and Stomach Damp-heat

Stomachache, severe pain with sudden onset, or fullness and distending pain, epigastric upset, acid regurgitation, vexation, a bitter or sticky taste in the mouth, a red tongue with a yellow or greasy coating, and a rapid pulse.

6.3.1.5   Stasis Obstruction in the Stomach Collateral

Severe stomachache, stinging or stabbing pain with a fixed location, discomfort upon pressure, or hematemesis or melena, a purple tongue and a choppy pulse.

6.3.1.6   Stomach-Yin Deficiency

Dull stomachache, burning sensation with discomfort, epigastric upset that likes as hunger, poor appetite, a dry mouth, dry stool, a red and dry tongue, a thready and rapid pulse.

6.3.1.7   Deficiency and Cold of the Spleen and Stomach

Dull stomachache, pain that can be exacerbated by an empty stomach and relieved by eating food, a preference for warmth and pressure, vomiting watery fluid, lassitude, or even cold hands and feet, loose stool, a pale tongue, a deep and thready pulse.

6.3.2   Nursing Interventions

6.3.2.1   Daily Life Nursing

6.3.2.1.1   Regulate dressing according to the change of weather. When doing outdoor activities in winter or staying in air conditioned room in summer, pay attention to preventing stomach from being attacked by external cold. People suffering from stomachache should pay more attention to keeping abdomen warm when the weather changes in spring and autumn.

6.3.2.1.2 Keep in good mood, avoid excessive anxiety and relieve stress actively.

6.3.2.1.3 For people suffering from gastric disease, keep regular life, especially take three meals in a fixed time and a fixed quality, and avoid overeating or being hunger.

6.3.2.1.4 People with deficiency pattern should have a good rest and avoid tiredness. People with excess deficiency take a rest when they feel stomachache, and take proper activity after pain is relieved.

6.3.2.2 Administrative Nursing

For patients suffering from being invaded in stomach by cold pathogen or deficiency cold of spleen and stomach, Chinese herbal decoction should be taken while it is hot to dispel cold and relieve pain. People with deficiency pattern should take decoction in small doses multiple times after meal.

6.3.2.3 Dietary Nursing

6.3.2.3.1 Take insipid, warm and easily digestible food. Keep away from alcohol, greasy and spicy food. It's better for people with deficiency of stomachache to take fine, soft food in small amount in multiple meals.

6.3.2.3.2 Pathogenic cold attacking the stomach: take ginger soup and brown sugar but avoid raw and cold food.

6.3.2.3.3 Food retention: restrict food intake and eat only after symptoms relieve.

6.3.2.3.4 Qi stagnation of liver and stomach: take food that can regulate the flow of qi, harmonize the stomach and relieve qi stagnancy in the liver, such as radish, orange.

6.3.2.3.5 Stagnant heat in the stomach: take more vegetables and fruits such as watermelon and apple.

6.3.2.3.6 Stomach-yin deficiency: take fine, soft, juicy food with less eating and more meals.

6.3.2.3.7 Deficiency-cold of the spleen and stomach: take fine, soft, warm, digestible, nutritious semi-fluid food or soft food with less eating and more meals, such as porridge and noodles.

6.3.2.4 Symptomatic Nursing

6.3.2.4.1 Stomachache attacked by external cold can be treated with heat therapy, such as hot compress, cupping, moxibustion. *Wei shu* (BL 21), *pi shu* (BL 20) for cupping;*zhong wan* (RN 12), *zu san li* (ST 36) for moxibustion.

6.3.2.4.2 The excess of stomachache can be treated with *zhong wan* (RN 12), *nei guan* (PC 6), *zu san li* (ST 36) using a reducing manipulation. The deficiency of stomachache can be treated with *zhong wan* (RN12), *pi shu* (BL 20), *wei shu* (BL 21), *zu san li* (ST 36) using a reinforcing manipulation. Stomach caused by qi stagnation of liver and stomach can be treated with *gan shu* (BL 18), *qi men* (LV 14), *tai chong* (LV 3), etc.

6.4 Constipation

Constipation refers to a condition mainly characterized by difficult bowel movement with longer duration or intervals, or difficult and unsmooth bowel movements. It is usually caused by exogenous cold and heat, improper diet, irregular emotion, and deficiency of qi, blood, yin and yang. The main pathogenesis is dysfunction of the large intestine in transportation.

6.4.1 Basic Patterns

6.4.1.1 Excess Constipation

6.4.1.1.1   Excess Heat in the Intestine: Dry and hard stool, abdominal distension and fullness, pain that is execrated by pressure pain, a dry mouth and bad breath, a yellow and dry coating, a slippery and rapid pulse.

6.4.1.1.2   Qi Stagnation in the Intestine: Incomplete defecation, difficult and unsmooth bowel movement, or even distension in the lesser abdomen, frequent belching, a thin coating, a thin and wiry pulse.

6.4.1.2 Deficiency Constipation

6.4.1.2.1   Spleen Deficiency and Qi Weakness: Neither dry nor hard stools, difficult bowel movement, shortness of breath and sweating after exertion, a pale complexion, mental fatigue, a pale tongue with a thin and white coating, and a weak pulse.

6.4.1.2.2   Yin Deficiency and Intestinal Dryness: Dry and hard stool like granules, mental fatigue, restlessness, poor appetite and digestion, soreness and weakness in the lumbar region and knee joints, a dry mouth with little fluid, a red tongue with a scanty coating, a thready and rapid pulse.

6.4.1.2.3   Yang Deficiency of the Spleen and Kidney: Dry and hard stool, or even abdominal pain with a cold sensation, dizziness, palpitation, profuse and clear urine, aversion to cold, cold limbs, a pale tongue with a white and moist coating, a deep and slow pulse.

6.4.2 Nursing Interventions

6.4.2.1 Daily Life Nursing

6.4.2.1.1   Have a good life style; keep regular life and moderate work and rest. Do moderate exercise everyday.

6.4.2.1.2   Keep good habits of defecation on time. It's necessary to have enough time, keep relaxed, and provide private environment for defecation.

6.4.2.1.3   The old, weak people who are difficult to defecate should do exercises to strengthen abdominal muscles.

6.4.2.2 Administrative Nursing

6.4.2.2.1   People with excess pattern take Chinese herb medicine or purgatives in external use following doctor's advice. Avoid using laxative for long time, and don't apply drastic purgative when there is no definite diagnosis.

6.4.2.2.2   People with qi deficiency of spleen frequently take white atractylodes rhizome or Chinese yam to tonify qi. People with yin deficiency and intestinal dryness should take drug on a regular basis.

6.4.2.3 Dietary Nursing

6.4.2.3.1   Take food regularly and moderately. Drink more water, honey water or juice.

6.4.2.3.2   Keep a balanced diet. Take more food rich in fiber such as vegetables, fruits and whole-wheat bread.

6.4.2.4   Symptomatic Nursing

6.4.2.4.1   People with excess constipation can be treated by needling *tian shu* (ST 25), *qu chi* (LI 11), *tai chong* (LV 3) to relax the bowels.

6.4.2.4.2   People with deficiency constipation can be treated by needling *tian shu* (ST 25), *shang ju xu* (ST 37), *da chang shu* (BL 25), *zu san li* (ST 36), *ba liao* to relax the bowels. Apply abdominal massage clockwise to regulate qi activity and strengthen the spleen.

6.5   Food Accumulation/Infantile Dyspepsia

The typical symptoms of infantile dyspepsia are anorexia, indigestion, abdominal distension and disordered defecation. It is often caused by internal damage due to improper feeding and qi stagnation.

6.5.1   Basic Patterns

6.5.1.1   Infantile Food Accumulation

Poor appetite, or vomiting rancid infantile food, vexation and agitation with frequent crying, uneasy sleeping at night, oliguria with yellow-colored urine, loose watery stool, red tongue with greasy coating, a slippery and rapid pulse, purple and red finger venules.

6.5.1.2   Food Accumulation due to Spleen Deficiency

Sallow complexion, sleepiness and fatigue, uneasy sleeping at night, no desire to eat, abdominal distension and willingness to be pressed, vomiting with rancid infantile food, watery stool, a pale tongue with a white coating, a thin pulse

6.5.2   Nursing Interventions

6.5.2.1   Daily Life Nursing

The living environment should be comfortable and clean, sunny with fresh air and in appropriate temperature. Keep regular life and keep the infantile with enough sleep and moderate outside activities. Provide good, quiet environment for eating.

6.5.2.2   Dietary Nursing

6.5.2.2.1   Feed the infantile regularly in a fixed quantity and at a fixed time. The food should be rich in nutrition and easy to digest. Avoid taking fat, sweet and fried food, or raw and cold fruits.

6.5.2.2.2   Regulate food and gradually add supplement food according to the growth and development of the infantile. Don't be picky. Keep a balanced diet.

6.5.2.3   Symptomatic Nursing

Clear away heat in the stomach meridian. Knead *ban men*, internal Eight Diagrams, *si heng wen*, *zhong wan* (RN 12), *zu san li* (ST 36) and lower *qi jie* bones. It is indicated for the pattern of infantile dyspepsia. Tonify the spleen meridian. Knead internal Eight Diagrams, *zhong wan* (RN 12) and *zu san li* (ST 36). It is indicated for the syndrome of dampness retention due to spleen deficiency. Chiropractic therapy can be applied to both patterns listed above. People with abdominal distension can be treated with massage.

6.6   *Bi* Syndrome

The typical symptoms of *bi* syndrome are pain (arthralgia), soreness, numbness, heaviness or with difficulty in bending and stretching of the muscle, tendons and bones, limbs and joints, or even swollen and burning joints in severe cases. It is mainly caused by qi and blood failing to flow smoothly and obstructing the meridians which results from pathogenic wind, cold, dampness and heat due to deficiency of healthy qi and weakness of defensive qi.

6.6.1   Basic Patterns

6.6.1.1   *Bi* Syndrome due to Wind-Cold-Dampness

6.6.1.1.1   Migratory *Bi* (Wind *Bi*): Aching wandering pain in the limbs, joints and muscles without fixed locations, mostly in the upper limbs and shoulders, incapacitation of flex and extendedness, or aversion to wind and cold, a thin and white coating, and a floating pulse.

6.6.1.1.2   Painful *Bi* (Cold *Bi*): Sharp fixed pain which can be relieved by warmth and execrated by cold, incapacitation of flexing and extending, neither red nor warm in local skin, a thin and white coating, a wiry and tight pulse.

6.6.1.1.3   Fixed *Bi* (Dampness *Bi*): Heavy, swollen and aching body and joints, pain in fixed locations, inconvenience to move, a white and greasy coating, soggy and moderate pulse.

6.6.1.2   Heat *Bi* due to Wind-Heat-Dampness

Red, swollen, hot and painful joints which are relieved by cold and execrated by heat and can't be touched, difficulty in moving the joints, fever, aversion to wind, sweating, thirst, vexation and oppression, a red tongue with yellow and dry coating, a slippery and rapid pulse.

6.6.1.3   *Bi* Syndrome due to Phlegm Stasis

Swollen and large joints due to chronic *bi* syndrome, even rigidity and deformity, incapacitation of flex and extendedness, a purple and dark tongue with a white and greasy coating, a thin and choppy pulse.

6.6.1.4   Deficiency of Healthy Qi due to Chronic *Bi* Syndrome

Painful joints, pain that sometimes is relieved but sometime is worsened, weakness and pain in the lumbar region and knee joints, emaciation and lassitude, a pale tongue, a deep, thready and weak pulse.

6.6.2   Nursing Interventions

6.6.2.1   Daily Life Nursing

6.6.2.1.1   The bedroom should be dry and avoid dampness. Don't get wet in the rain, or catch wind after sweating. Take care of clean, ventilation, prevention of dampness and cold. Keep the balance of dry and damp, cold and warm.

6.6.2.1.2   Strengthen the physique, avoid external evils. Avoid catching the evils of wind, cold, dampness and heat.

6.6.2.1.3　People with severe pain in joints are suggested to reduce vigorous exercise and taking a rest properly.

6.6.2.2　Emotional Nursing

At the early stage of disease, patients tend to be low in spirits due to joint pain, general malaise, repeated attack and long duration of the disease. Patients should be encouraged to have confidence in overcoming disease and actively cooperate with various treatments. At the later stage of disease, patients feel depressed and losing confidence in life because of sequelae such as joint deformity and muscle contraction. They should be encouraged to do activities and strengthen independent living ability.

6.6.2.3　Symptomatic Nursing

6.6.2.3.1　Massage, acupuncture or analgesic drug following doctor's advice can be applied to local severe pain to relieve pain. *Jian yu* (LI 15), *qu chi* (LI 11), *chi ze* (LU 5), *he ge* (LI 4), *wai guan* (SJ 5) in the arms can be selected; *huan tiao* (GB 30), *zu san li* (ST 36), *yang ling quan* (GB 34) in the legs can be chosen. Massage for 5 to10 minutes for local pain.

6.6.2.3.2　Moxibustion or moxibustion on ginger is indicated for painful *bì* (cold *bì*) to warm meridian. Massage and plum-blossom needle and so on are indicated for fixed *bì* (damp *bì*) to prevent muscle contraction, joint deformity and relieve symptoms.

6.6.2.3.3　Hot herb compress, fumigating and steaming therapy are recommended in the nursing of *bì* syndrome especially for those due to wind-cold-dampness. These therapies can warm meridian, promote blood circulation and relieve swelling and pain. Pay more attention to the temperature of herbal liquid when it is used externally.

6.7　Dysmenorrhea

The typical symptoms of dysmenorrhea are that the patients have cyclical lower abdominal pain which may spread to lumbosacral region during or before and after menstrual period. When the severe pain can't be endured, it may affect patients' lives and work. It can also be called abdominal pain during menstruation.

6.7.1　Basic Patterns

6.7.1.1　Qi Stagnation and Blood Stasis

Distending pain or intermittent pain in lower abdomen at one or two days before menses or during the menstrual period, pain that refuses pressure, distending pain of the chest and rib-side and breasts, scanty and inhibited menstruation, purple and dark menses with clot, pain that is relieved after clot going out and disappears when the menstrual period has completely finished, purple and dark tongue or tongue with stasis spots, a wiry pulse or wiry and choppy pulse.

6.7.1.2　Stagnation of Cold-Dampness

Cold pain or colicky pain in lower abdomen at several days before menses or during the menstrual period, pain that is relieved by warmth and is exacerbated by pressure, scanty menstruation, purple and dark menses with clot, aversion to cold, cold limbs, blue and white complexion, a dusky tongue with white and greasy coating, a wiry and tight pulse.

6.7.1.3 Qi and Blood Deficiency

Dull pain in lower abdomen and private part with preference for rub and pressure, at one or two days after menses or during the menstrual period, scanty and pale and thin menstruation, soreness and weakness of the lumbar region and knee joints, mental fatigue, lassitude, a lusterless complexion, poor appetite, thin and unformed stool, dizziness, palpitation, pale and teeth-marked tongue, a thin coating, a thready and weak pulse.

6.7.1.4 Damp-Heat Pouring Downward

During or after menstruation, pain in the lower abdomen that refuses pressure with burning sensation, or pain in lumbosacral region, pain in lower abdomen that occurs sometimes at ordinary times and is exacerbated during menstruation, low fever which changes up and down, dusky red and thick menses with clot, yellow and thick leukorrhea, oliguria with yellow urine, a red tongue with yellow and greasy coating, a wiry and rapid pulse or soggy and rapid pulse.

6.7.1.5 Liver-Kidney Depletion

During or after menstruation, dull pain in the lower abdomen that is relieved by pressure, scanty and pale and thin menstruation, dizziness, tinnitus, soreness and weakness of the lumbar region and knee joints, a pale tongue with a thin coating, a deep and thready pulse.

6.7.2 Nursing Interventions

6.7.2.1 Daily Life Nursing

6.7.2.1.1 Keep the environment clean, comfortable and quiet and avoid unfavorable stimulation. Take a rest on the bed when bellyache is serious. Pay attention to keeping abdomen warm and hot compress can be applied to the abdomen.

6.7.2.1.2 Pay attention to keeping clean during the menstrual period. Before and after and during the menstrual period, don't go swimming, contact cold water, do vigorous sports or heavy physical work.

6.7.2.2 Dietary Nursing

6.7.2.2.1 During or before the menstrual period, avoid taking raw and cold, cold-cool, or acid food. People with stagnation of cold-dampness can take brown sugar and Chinese date during the menstrual period.

6.7.2.2.2 Take light, balanced and nutritious food. Avoid taking too cold or too hot food. People with qi stagnation and blood stasis can take moderate amount of safflower every day. People with stagnation of cold-dampness are inhibited to take raw or cold food; People with damp-heat are inhibited to take more spicy and pungent food or strong drinks or drink too much. People with qi and blood deficiency should supplement and take egg, meat, milk product, fresh vegetables, and take ginger mutton soup frequently. People with deficiency of liver and kidney take more black sesame and walnut.

6.7.2.3 Symptomatic Nursing of Symptoms

6.7.2.3.1 Acupuncture to relieve pain: *zhong ji* (RN 3), *san yin jiao* (SP 6), *qi hai* (RN 6), *nei guan* (PC 6) and so on are selected to relieve pain. Acupuncture and moxibustion can be applied together. Patients with stagnation of cold-dampness can be treated with moxibustion on *qi hai* (RN 6), *guan yuan* (RN 4), etc. to warm yang and dispel cold, promote blood circulation, relieve pain. Auricular acupuncture is indicated for pain. Auricular points such as *zi gong* (TF2), *shen men* (TF4), *nei fen mi* (CO18), Liver (CO12), Kidney (CO10) can be selected to prevent pain 3 to 5 days before menstrual period.

6.7.2.3.2   Point application or hot compress to relieve pain: The paste made from for dysmenorrhea is used to relieve pain before dysmenorrheal occurs, which it is renewed each time per 1 to 3 days until patients feel no pain. Abdomen can be applied by hot compress. Put herbs which are 250-500g salt, 250g scallion, 200g chopped ginger into the bag after baking hot, and then put them on abdomen. Be careful not to burn.

6.7.2.3.3   Massage lower abdomen to relieve pain: 3 days before menstrual period, every night overlap with both hands, press on the center of lower abdomen with palms, massage for 10 minutes with counterclockwise rotation from the belly to navel for 30 to 50 times.

6.8   Hypogalactia

It's also called "inhibited lactation". The typical symptoms of hypogalactia are inadequate production of breast milk or even no breast milk for baby feeding after delivery. It often occurs within 2 or 3 months to half a year after delivery.

6.8.1   Basic Patterns

6.8.1.1   Qi and Blood Deficiency

Scanty lactation or absent lactation, thin and clear lactation, soft breast without distension and fullness, mental fatigue, poor appetite, a lusterless complexion, a pale tongue with little coating, a thready and weak pulse.

6.8.1.2   Liver Constraint and Qi Stagnation

Postpartum depressed emotion, scanty and sticky lactation, or inhibited lactation, distending pain of the breasts, fullness and oppression in the chest and rib-side, distension in the stomach cavity, poor appetite, mild fever, a normal tongue with a thin and yellow coating, a wiry and thready pulse or wiry and rapid pulse.

6.8.2   Nursing Interventions

6.8.2.1   Daily Life Nursing

6.8.2.1.1   Create warm, comfortable and harmonious environment. Avoid wind and cold such as air condition in summer after delivery. For the mother, choose a comfortable posture for breast feeding and avoid fatigue due to uncomfortable posture.

6.8.2.1.2   Take sufficient rest and sleep more than 10 hours per day. Avoid over fatigue to affect the secretion of the breast milk. Keep a good posture when sleeping. Don't press breasts when they are distending and pain.

6.8.2.1.3　Do proper exercises, such as postpartum gymnastics, which are helpful to promote qi and blood transformation and transportation, regulate emotion and prompt recovery.

6.8.2.2　Dietary Nursing

Take nutritious, light, digestible food and drink adequate water. Encourage the mother to take nutritional soup. Avoid sour, astringent, greasy and pungent food.

6.8.2.3　Emotional Nursing

Regulate mood, avoid stimulation of bad feelings such as depression or anger. Encourage the mother to actively breast feed. Keep good mood when breast feeding is conducted.

6.8.2.4　Symptomatic Nursing

6.8.2.4.1　Advice the mother to breastfeed her baby as early as possible. Even though hypogalactia occurs, breastfeed is supposed to be done at a fixed time. If the baby is unable to suck, breast pump is used or others suck.

6.8.2.4.2　Wipe the nipples and breast with warm towel before breastfeeding. Teach the mother how to massage breast by herself. For example, massage breast from the edge to the nipple or apply hot compress with hot towel to promote milk secretion.

6.8.2.4.3　For patients with difficulty in milk discharge, do massage or squeeze local breast: massage on the points such as *ru gen* (ST 18), *dan zhong* (RN 17), *qi men* (LV 14), *gan shu* (BL 18), *shao ze* (SI 1), etc. for several minutes with single palm and fingers and help patients to choose supine posture. Comb along the lactiferous ducts to nipples softly for 20 minutes each time, 2~3 times a day, and empty milk in a fixed time to prevent acute mastitis caused by milk accumulation transforming into fire. Apply acupuncture on the points such as *dan zhong* (RN 17), *ru gen* (ST 18), in combination with *shao ze* (SI 1), *tian zong* (SI 11), *he gu* (LI 4), etc.

(Wang Qi　Su Chunxiang)